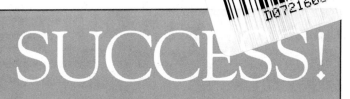

SUCCESS!

for the EMT-Intermediate 1999 Curriculum

Complete Review

Joseph J. Mistovich, M.Ed, NREMT-P
Chairperson and Professor
Department of Health Professions
Youngstown State University
Youngstown, Ohio

Richard A. Cherry, M.S., NREMT-P
Clinical Assistant Professor of Emergency Medicine
Assistant Residency Director
Upstate Medical University
Syracuse, New York

PEARSON
Prentice
Hall

Upper Saddle River, New Jersey 07458

Library of Congress Cataloging-in-Publication Data

Mistovich, Joseph J.
   Success! for the EMT-Intermediate : 1999 curriculum / Joseph
Mistovich, Richard A. Cherry.
      p. ; cm.
   Includes index.
   ISBN 0-13-118427-X
   1. Medical emergencies—Examinations, questions, etc.
   2. Emergency medical technicians—Examinations, questions, etc.
      [DNLM: 1. Emergency Medicine—Examination Questions. WB
18.2 C522r 2006] I. Cherry, Richard A. II. Title.
   RC86.9.M55 2006
   616.02'5'076—dc22   2005007013

Notice: The author and the publisher of this book have taken care to make certain that the information given is correct and compatible with the standards generally accepted at the time of publication. Nevertheless, as new information becomes available, changes in treatment and in the use of equipment and procedures become necessary. The reader is advised to carefully consult the instruction and information material included in each piece of equipment or device before administration. Students are warned that the use of any techniques must be authorized by their medical adviser, where appropriate, in accord with local laws and regulations. The publisher disclaims any liability, loss, injury, or damage incurred as a consequence, directly or indirectly, of the use and application of any of the contents of this book.

Publisher: Julie Levin Alexander
Publisher's Assistant: Regina Bruno
Executive Editor: Marlene McHugh Pratt
Senior Managing Editor for Development: Lois Berlowitz
Project Manager: Sandy Breuer
Editorial Assistant: Matthew Sirinides
Director of Marketing: Karen Allman
Executive Marketing Manager: Katrin Beacom
Senior Channel Marketing Manager: Rachele Strober
Marketing Coordinator: Michael Sirinides
Director of Production and Manufacturing: Bruce Johnson
Managing Editor for Production: Patrick Walsh

Production Liaison: Faye Gemmellaro
Production Editor: Heather Willison,
Carlisle Publishers Services
Manufacturing Manager: Ilene Sanford
Manufacturing Buyer: Pat Brown
Senior Design Coordinator: Christopher Weigand
Cover Designer: Solid State Graphics
Interior Designer: Janice Bielawa
Composition: Carlisle Publishers Services
Printing and Binding: Courier/Westford
Cover Printer: Coral Graphics

Studentaid.ed.gov, the U.S. Department of Education's website on college planning assistance, is a valuable tool for anyone intending to pursue higher education. Designed to help students at all stages of schooling, including international students, returning students, and parents, it is a guide to the financial aid process. The website presents information on applying to and attending college as well as on funding your education and repaying loans. It also provides links to useful resources, such as state education agency contact information, assistance in filling out financial aid forms, and an introduction to various forms of student aid.

Pearson Education Ltd.
Pearson Education Singapore, Pte. Ltd.
Pearson Education Canada, Ltd.
Pearson Education–Japan
Pearson Education Australia Pty. Limited

Pearson Education North Asia Ltd.
Pearson Educación de Mexico, S.A. de C.V.
Pearson Education Malaysia, Pte. Ltd.
Pearson Education, Upper Saddle River, New Jersey

10 9 8 7 6 5 4 3 2 1
ISBN 0-13-118427-X

This book is dedicated to the memory of my father, who provided me with the love and encouragement that allowed me to pursue my dreams. He will always be my inspiration to continue living life to its fullest, no matter what obstacles I encounter. To my beautiful wife Andrea, who continues to be my greatest supporter and best friend. To my wonderful children, Katie, Kristyn, Chelsea, Morgan, and Kara, for helping me get through another project. Your energy, hugs, kisses, and smiles make every day so much brighter! I love you all dearly!

—Joseph J. Mistovich

To all the great folks at Brady who have made my writing career extremely satisfying and enjoyable. I can't thank you enough!

—Richard A. Cherry

Contents

Preface

The purpose of this review manual is to help prepare you for examinations in your EMT-Intermediate course and your certification examination. The manual consists of a series of self-assessment sections that can identify your strengths and weaknesses in relation to the information you are studying. If you are a currently certified EMT-Intermediate, this manual can serve as a refresher tool or as a method to determine where your knowledge has deteriorated and which areas need specific review.

SUCCESS! for the EMT-Intermediate consists of multiple-choice items that are organized according to the U.S. Department of Transportation's (DOT's) National Standard EMT-Intermediate 1999 Curriculum. Enhancement questions are included that are supplemental to the DOT curriculum. Every item has a corresponding answer and rationale. In addition, all items, with the exception of those that are considered "enhancement items," are referenced to specific DOT objectives. This information can be found after the module questions in the "Answers and Rationales" section. Answers and rationales marked with an asterisk are supplemental to the DOT curriculum.

You will also find that many of the answers and rationales are followed by page references that correspond to Brady's *Intermediate Emergency Care* textbook, which will allow you to find more specific information on a topic or concept.

The authors and manuscript reviewers all have extensive knowledge and experience as EMS educators. The items were developed in a "teacher-made test format" to allow you to test your knowledge and understanding of the material. When compiled into a series of sections, the items serve as a self-assessment tool to identify particular strengths and weaknesses in your knowledge and understanding of the information. This allows you to concentrate on specific sections that have been identified as a weakness.

This manual should be used as a tool to better prepare you for your examinations. However, there is no better preparation than studying and understanding the information that has been presented to you in your course. To best ensure your success on the examination, we encourage you to study first until you feel confident that you know the information and then use this manual as a self-assessment to determine how well you know the information. When you have identified areas of weakness, do not simply study the manual or review items. Go back and study the information presented to you, study the textbook, and use other sources to better understand the information. Once you again feel confident you know the material, retest yourself using the review manual to determine if you are better prepared for that section.

We hope this manual assists you in preparing for your examination. However, when it comes time to manage a patient in the prehospital environment, there is no time for preparation. You must draw on your existing knowledge and skills to successfully and efficiently treat the patient. Thus, it is imperative to good patient care that you are truly prepared not only to pass that examination but to take care of each and every patient you encounter to the best of your ability. Good luck in your EMS endeavors!

Joseph J. Mistovich
Richard A. Cherry

Contributors

In preparation for development of *SUCCESS! for the EMT-Intermediate,* well-established educators were sought with years of both clinical and classroom experience. These individuals were responsible for contributing teacher-made test items based on objectives from the U.S. Department of Transportation's National Standard EMT-Intermediate Curriculum for inclusion in this manual. The following individuals contributed a significant number of items to this review manual.

Beth Lothrop Adams, MA, RN, NREMT-P
EMS Quality Manager
Inova Health System
Fairfax County Fire Department
Fairfax, Virginia

Randall W. Benner, MEd, NREMT-P
Director, Emergency Medical Technology
Instructor, Department of Health Professions
Youngstown State University
Youngstown, Ohio

Elizabeth Criss, RN, CEN, MEd
Clinical Educator, Emergency Services
Research Associate, Emergency Medicine
Arizona Health Sciences Center
Tucson, Arizona

Heather M. Drake, BS, RN, EMT-P
New Castle, Pennsylvania

James W. Drake, MS, NREMT-P
EMS Coordinator
Jameson Health System
New Castle, Pennsylvania

Linda K. Honeycutt, EMT-P, I/C
St. Louis, Missouri

Blaine Griffiths, MS, CRNA
Hamilton Anesthesia Associates
Hamilton, Ohio

Edward B. Kuvlesky, AAS, NREMT-P
Battalion Chief, Indian River County EMS
Indian River County, Florida

Reviewers

We would like to thank the following reviewers for their comments and suggestions, which have been helpful in ensuring the accuracy and clarity of questions.

Bill Locke, EMS I/C
Moraine Park Technical College
Fond du Lac, Wisconsin

Bruce L. Gadol, NREMT-B, CCT, EMS I/C
Director of EMS Education
President, Emergency Medical Training Institute
Miami, Florida

Brian J. Wilson, BA, NREMT-P
EMS Education Director
Texas Tech School of Medicine
El Paso, Texas

Christina Blaney, NREMT-P, EMS I
Horry-Georgetown Technical College
Myrtle Beach, South Carolina

Introduction

ABOUT THE SUCCESS! SERIES

SUCCESS! is a complete review system that combines relevant exam-style questions with a self-assessment format to provide you with the best preparation for your exam.

- Build your experience and exam confidence!
- Practice with realistic exam-style questions.

The SUCCESS! program is a complete method for increasing pass rates in many health professions from EMS to Nursing Assisting. We invite you to use our exam preparation system and HAVE SUCCESS!

Prentice Hall's complete SUCCESS! system includes review for the following areas:

Clinical Laboratory Science/ Medical Technology	Massage Therapy
Dental Assisting	Medical Assisting
Dental Hygiene	Nursing Assisting
Emergency Medical Services	Pharmacy Technician
Health Information Management	Phlebotomy
	Surgical Technology

ABOUT SUCCESS! FOR THE EMT-INTERMEDIATE

Prentice Hall is pleased to present ***SUCCESS! for the EMT-Intermediate: 1999 Curriculum*** as part of a review series on the various EMS education levels. The authoritative text gives you expert help in preparing for certifying examinations.

ABOUT THE BOOK

SUCCESS! for the EMT-Intermediate, by *Joseph J. Mistovich and Richard A. Cherry,* has been designed to help students prepare for the written course and certification exams. It can also be used as a review for currently certified EMT-Intermediates. More than 1,000 multiple-choice items are organized by the sections covered in the 1999 U.S. Department of Transportation's (DOT's) National Standard EMT-Intermediate Curriculum. The multiple-choice items are similar to those found on teacher-made exams and certifying exams. Working through these items will help you assess your strengths and weaknesses in each section.

- **Answers and Rationales:** Correct answers and comprehensive rationales are provided to assist you in better understanding each item. Rationales are presented so that you may also learn why answers that you incorrectly gave are wrong. Many of the answers and rationales are followed by page references to Brady's *Intermediate Emergency Care* textbook, where supporting information can be found.
- **DOT Objectives:** DOT objective reference numbers located in the "Answers and Rationales" section allow you to refer to the specific DOT curriculum objective that each item was written from. For the enhancement material that is beyond the DOT objectives, answers and rationales are marked with an asterisk instead of an objective reference number. The DOT objectives are presented in full in the Appendix.

BRADY WEBSITE FOR ADDITIONAL RESOURCES

Visit our website at www.brady-books.com for links to related educational resources. You will want to bookmark this site and return frequently for the most current information about Brady texts and online offerings as you continue on your path to success.

Study Tips

So, you're getting ready for an exam. Congratulations for making it to this point. Now let's help you make the next step—doing your best on this exam. Some people find test taking unsettling, unnerving, and even scary! Use this book as an opportunity to practice physical preparation, information review, and exam techniques.

PHYSICAL PREPARATION

The key to maximizing your potential on a test is to be at your personal best. Along with mental preparation, physical preparation should be included in a good study strategy. Physical preparation includes getting adequate rest and exercising. It also includes eating a balanced meal the night before and the morning of the exam. Your brain works best when it has access to a supply of glucose. So fruits, grains, vegetables, and pasta are important foods. Try to avoid caffeine and foods with high sugar content on the morning of the exam. These foods provide a short burst of energy, but when they are used up, the slump will significantly reduce your ability to function.

Try some physical exercise the days before the exam, although not to the point of exhaustion. Increasing cardiovascular perfusion will also increase perfusion to the brain. More oxygen circulating in the brain can only be good, right? Exercise is also an outlet for stress, making it easier to get a good night's sleep.

INFORMATION REVIEW

Contrary to popular belief, preparing for an exam should not include extensive last-minute studying. You've been studying for months, you know the material, and cramming now will probably cause an intellectual shutdown. Review the material for short periods of time and take frequent breaks. Try study groups of three to five people for review; the active discussion will be an excellent way to reinforce the material and retain the information.

While knowing the material is essential, physical preparation is equally important. Remember, review only in brief intervals, use a study group, and don't cram.

TAKING THE EXAMINATION

An exam is not written by happenstance; it's an art and a science. Each time you take an exam, it's a chance to evaluate your knowledge as well as master the test-taking process. Exams are generally built to measure *minimum* competency. Certification or recertification exams are usually not designed to test total knowledge, ability to expertly function in the field, or even your level of professionalism. They are an attempt to evaluate your reading comprehension and judgment.

There are two basic kinds of questions found on most certification exams—multiple choice and true/false. Each question is built in a specific way to test your ability and your knowledge. Knowing how the questions are constructed may help you during the exam.

Multiple-choice questions consist of two parts: stems and answers. A stem is the actual question part, and the list of answers that follows contains one correct answer and several distracters. Distracters are designed to (what else?) distract you from the correct response. Multiple-choice questions require you to use knowledge, judgment, and expertise to answer the question. Use the process of elimination.

When answering a multiple-choice question, read the question and all the answers first. Then begin the process of elimination, starting with the most obvious incorrect answer and sorting your way through until you're left with one or two possible answers. Got a problem picking from those? Then reread the stem. If it would make it easier, re-phrase the question looking for key words that give you a hint about the answer. Don't forget to look at the grammar—is the stem in plural form or singular? Whatever process you use, try not to spend more than two minutes on any one question.

You may find a topic is covered in several consecutive questions. In this case, be sure all your answers are similar and seem to fit together. It might be helpful to use the previous answers to validate each new set of choices. Another option is to check the next question because sometimes the answer, or a strong hint to one question, is the stem of the following question. Remember, when reading multiple-choice responses, the correct answer may be the most comprehensive choice—the one that combines several of the other answers or includes more details.

If the exam contains true/false questions, remember that statements containing absolute terms, like *never, always,* and *only,* will usually be false. Very little of medicine, or life itself, is absolute. Statements that contain words like *maybe* or *sometimes* tend to be true.

The scientific part of test building is putting all the information into questions, and it is an art form in the way the questions are put together to evaluate you. The key is to read each question carefully—try not to scan because you miss important key words like *incorrect* or *not* that would cause you to waste time or, more important, miss the answer. Remember your all-important "three Ps": be prudent, pace yourself, and use patience.

WRAPPING UP

You know how people say to go with your first hunch? Well, they're right. Your brain makes immediate connections based on stored information and your experience. Don't be afraid that the answer is wrong just because you didn't go through all the usual steps of logic. Research shows that first impressions tend to be correct.

It's okay to choose the same letter answer two or three times in a row. The answers are put into a question at random, so it could be that the same letter shows up as being correct up to five times. Don't change your answer if you have chosen the same letter more than once.

You have done the best you can by participating in class, practicing your skills, and reading your material. Trying to teach yourself the curriculum at the last minute just won't work, and ultimately your patients will suffer. Trust yourself and you abilities. Practice some of the tips in this section as your proceed through this book, and in the days before the exam, remember to eat well, exercise, and get plenty of sleep.

KEYS TO SUCCESS ACROSS THE BOARDS

- Study, Review, and Practice
- Keep a positive, confident attitude
- Follow all directions on the examination
- Do your best

Good luck!

You are encouraged to visit http://www.prenhall. com/success for additional tips on studying, test taking, and other keys to success. At this stage of your education and career, you will find these tips helpful.

Foundations of the EMT-Intermediate

unit objectives

Questions in this unit relate to DOT Objectives 1-1.1 to 1-1.48. The objectives are listed in the Appendix.

DIRECTIONS
Each of the questions or incomplete statements below is followed by suggested answers or completions. Select the **one answer** that is best in each case.

1. Most EMT-Intermediates are injured
   A. while lifting patients.
   B. by animals at the scene.
   C. by angry bystanders.
   D. at crime scenes.

2. Which of the following elements of physical fitness is the most important to the EMT-Intermediate?
   A. cardiovascular endurance
   B. muscular strength
   C. flexibility
   D. all of the above

3. Your target heart rate is best described as
   A. your ideal resting heart rate.
   B. your optimum heart rate during exercise.
   C. your ideal heart rate during a cardiovascular workout.
   D. 50% of your resting heart rate.

4. Isometric exercise is defined as exercise performed against
   A. stable resistance.
   B. increasing resistance.
   C. no resistance.
   D. the range of motion.

5. Which of the following statements most accurately describes the EMT-Intermediate?
   A. EMT-Intermediates function independently with their own license.
   B. EMT-Intermediates may function only under the direction of an EMS system's medical director.
   C. EMT-Intermediate credentialing or licensing is unnecessary in some states and provinces.
   D. EMT-Intermediates are not required to function under protocols.

6. Which of the following is **not** an example of a daily recommended food?
   A. whole-wheat bread
   B. an orange
   C. a cup of caffeinated coffee
   D. a glass of 2% milk

7. Which of the following exercises is no longer considered safe and effective?
   A. sit-ups
   B. abdominal crunches
   C. bench presses
   D. isometrics

8. _____ have the longest incubation periods.
   A. Whooping cough (pertussis) and German measles (rubella)
   B. Hepatitis and tuberculosis
   C. Influenza and pneumonia
   D. Chicken pox (varicella) and meningitis

9. You are about to assist a mother in delivering her baby at her home. Which of the following body substance isolation items is **not** considered necessary?
   A. gown
   B. gloves
   C. eyewear
   D. HEPA mask

10. Which of the following is considered the most important infection control practice for the EMT-Intermediate?

    A. wearing latex gloves

    B. wearing protective eyewear

    C. washing your hands

    D. disposing of needles appropriately

11. You have just finished a cardiac arrest call and have a contaminated laryngoscope blade to clean. Which of the following procedures is **not** recommended?

    A. sterilizing it with pressurized steam

    B. using a germicidal chemical cleaning agent

    C. soaking it in a bleach solution

    D. sterilizing it by radiation

12. When using a bleach solution to disinfect a backboard, the recommended mix is 1 part bleach to _____ part(s) water.

    A. 1

    B. 10

    C. 100

    D. 1000

13. You just brought in a patient with tuberculosis, but you were unaware that the patient was infected. According to the Ryan White Act, the medical facility must notify your designated infection control officer within _____ hours.

    A. 24

    B. 48

    C. 8

    D. 72

14. Your patient has just been notified he has terminal, inoperable cancer. He refuses to believe the diagnosis and goes about his business in a normal fashion, avoiding all conversation on the subject. He is in which stage of the grieving process?

    A. bargaining

    B. depression

    C. anger

    D. denial

15. Another cancer patient yells at you for asking him questions and appears aggravated even to have to deal with you. During the call, you cannot do anything to please him. Which stage of grief does he appear to be in?

    A. denial

    B. anger

    C. depression

    D. acceptance

16. Another cancer patient appears sad and withdrawn and will not communicate with you or his family. Which stage of grief does this demonstrate?

    A. denial

    B. anger

    C. depression

    D. acceptance

17. If your cancer patient appears to have realized his fate and to have achieved a reasonable level of comfort with the anticipated outcome, he may be in what stage of grief?

    A. denial

    B. anger

    C. depression

    D. acceptance

18. When informing someone of the death of a loved one, you should use the term

    A. expired.

    B. passed away.

    C. dead.

    D. none of the above

19. Which of the following physiological responses occurs during the alarm stage of stress?
    A. heart rate and blood pressure fall
    B. pupils constrict
    C. hormones are released from the adrenal medulla
    D. digestion increases

20. Which of the following best describes the resistance stage of stress?
    A. The victim is beginning to cope.
    B. Vital signs return to normal.
    C. Resistance to the stressor becomes stronger.
    D. all of the above

21. When your coping mechanisms no longer buffer job stressors, which can compromise both your personal health and your well-being, you are said to suffer from
    A. posttraumatic stress disorder.
    B. burnout.
    C. anxiety.
    D. demobilization.

22. Which of the following is **not** a warning sign or physical symptom of stress?
    A. heart palpitations
    B. GI distress
    C. increased salivation
    D. chest pain

23. A mental health professional should screen EMS personnel for abnormal stress-related symptoms within _____ after a critical incident.
    A. 2 months
    B. 4 months
    C. 6 months
    D. 8 months

24. The type of EMS system in which various levels of responders are dispatched to calls depending on the severity of the situation is known as a
    A. multilevel system.
    B. standard system.
    C. call screening system.
    D. tiered system.

25. State EMS agencies are usually responsible for all of the following except
    A. contracting local medical directors.
    B. recommending EMS legislation.
    C. licensing and certifying field personnel.
    D. enforcing statewide EMS regulations.

26. Who has the ultimate authority in all patient care–related issues in a local EMS system?
    A. state EMS director
    B. system medical director
    C. chief EMT-Intermediate on duty
    D. local EMS coordinator

27. Which of the following is an example of direct or online medical direction?
    A. developing protocols and standing orders
    B. consulting with the physician by radio during an emergency call
    C. designing continuing quality improvement activities
    D. conducting chart reviews

28. EMT-Intermediate field interventions that may be completed before contacting the medical direction physician are known as
    A. online medical direction orders.
    B. the 4 "Ts."
    C. intervener physician protocols.
    D. written protocol or offline orders.

29. Which of the following is an important area in which to educate the public?
    A. how to easily access the EMS system
    B. how to initiate basic life support procedures
    C. how to recognize a medical emergency
    D. all of the above

30. Which of the following is a component of a modern E-911 system?
    A. instant callback capabilities
    B. automatic location identification
    C. instant routing of the call
    D. all of the above

31. Which of the following is a nationally recognized level of EMT?
    A. EMT–Critical Care
    B. EMT–Ambulance
    C. EMT–Intermediate
    D. EMT–Cardiac Technician

32. The process by which an agency or association grants recognition to an individual who has met its qualifications is known as
    A. licensure.
    B. certification.
    C. reciprocity.
    D. censure.

33. The process by which a government agency grants permission to engage in a given occupation to an individual who has attained the degree of competency required to ensure the public's protection is known as
    A. licensure.
    B. certification.
    C. reciprocity.
    D. censure.

34. The process by which an agency grants credentials to an individual who has comparable credentials from another agency is known as
    A. licensure.
    B. certification.
    C. reciprocity.
    D. consensus.

35. The KKK standards deal with
    A. ambulance safety and design.
    B. minimum standard medical protocols.
    C. training and education of field personnel.
    D. air evacuation of trauma victims.

36. Hospital categorization is important because
    A. not every patient can afford every hospital.
    B. receiving facilities have varying capabilities.
    C. not all patients can be transported to the appropriate facility.
    D. it is impossible to match patient needs with hospital resources.

37. Quality assurance differs from quality improvement in that
    A. quality assurance deals with patient perceptions of quality.
    B. quality improvement is an objective look at clinical care.
    C. quality assurance is often viewed as punitive and negative.
    D. quality improvement does not elicit customer satisfaction information.

38. Research in EMS is important in order to
    A. justify future funding allocations.
    B. scientifically evaluate EMT-Intermediate care.
    C. weigh the benefits versus the risks of certain prehospital treatments.
    D. all of the above

39. Your number one priority during an emergency response is
    A. patient care.
    B. personal gratification.
    C. insurance information.
    D. safety.

40. You respond to a major automobile collision involving multiple patients. Which of the following patients would receive priority-1 transport?
    A. 45-year-old with no vital signs
    B. 6-year-old with lower-leg fracture and normal vital signs
    C. 25-year-old with abdominal bruising and signs of shock
    D. 68-year-old with mild respiratory distress and seat belt burns

41. When confronted with a serious unfamiliar medical situation that is not clearly outlined in your local protocols, you should
    A. improvise ALS procedures.
    B. contact medical direction for guidance.
    C. transport the patient BLS.
    D. none of the above

42. To receive optimum care, your critical trauma patient should be transported to which of the following facilities?
    A. Level I trauma center
    B. Level II trauma center
    C. Level III trauma center
    D. the closest hospital, regardless of the designation

43. You have a critical burn patient. The nearest rural hospital is 10 minutes away. The burn center is 45 minutes away. Your patient's HMO, per the family, directs you to take him to another facility that is 30 minutes away but that does not have burn treatment capabilities. On what should you base your transport decision?
    A. the needs of this patient
    B. knowledge of the capabilities of the hospitals in question
    C. advice from your medical direction physician
    D. all of the above

44. The rules that govern the conduct of members of a particular group or profession are called
    A. ethics.
    B. morals.
    C. standards.
    D. principles.

45. Professionalism is exhibited by all of the following **except**
    A. setting high standards.
    B. seeking self-improvement.
    C. earning the respect of your peers.
    D. aiming for the minimum standard.

46. On learning that he has made a mistake, the professional will
    A. blame someone else.
    B. accept the responsibility.
    C. blame the equipment.
    D. request a new partner.

47. Placing yourself in the shoes of the patient is practicing
    A. sympathy.
    B. integrity.
    C. empathy.
    D. diplomacy.

48. You have not placed a traction splint on a patient since your last refresher class 2 years ago. On your next call, your patient has an isolated midshaft femur fracture and requires traction. You fumble with the splint but manage to apply it with some discomfort to your patient. How could this have been avoided?

    A. Practice with the splint during down time.

    B. Have your partner apply it.

    C. Transport the patient with a fixation splint.

    D. Use blankets and straps to stabilize the leg.

49. The study of the factors that influence the frequency, distribution, and causes of injury, disease, and other health-related events in a population is called

    A. holography.

    B. epidemiology.

    C. pathophysiology.

    D. demographics.

50. In a lawsuit based on the wrongful death of a 50-year-old man, a jury might assess damages based on that man's loss of _____ years as a wage earner.

    A. 40

    B. 20

    C. 15

    D. 10

51. Components of an injury-surveillance program might include

    A. injury risk.

    B. teachable moments.

    C. primary prevention.

    D. all of the above

52. Homicide and rape are examples of wrongs against society and are tried in

    A. criminal court.

    B. tort court.

    C. civil court.

    D. none of the above

53. Which of the following is an example of a tort case?

    A. divorce

    B. suicide

    C. contract dispute

    D. malpractice

54. A "Medical Practice Act"

    A. defines the scope of practice for allied health care professionals.

    B. is a national standard for allied health care professionals.

    C. outlines ethical behavior guidelines for medical paraprofessionals.

    D. is unnecessary in states that license their EMT-Intermediates.

55. If, after you question an order from medical direction that you feel is inappropriate, the physician still wants you to carry it out, you should

    A. carry the order out as directed.

    B. refuse the order and document the incident.

    C. transport the patient BLS.

    D. call another hospital.

56. Laws that protect health care workers from liability in the event they stop and render roadside care are known as

    A. Good Samaritan laws.

    B. *res ipsa loquitor* laws.

    C. Ryan White laws.

    D. negligence laws.

57. Negligence is defined as
    A. bringing a lawsuit involving no physical harm.
    B. deviating from the standard of care.
    C. failing to prove proximate cause.
    D. all of the above

58. Which of the following is **not** a necessary component of a successful negligence suit?
    A. duty to act
    B. breach of duty
    C. proximate cause
    D. unlawful consent

59. Which of the following would be considered a breach of duty?
    A. malfeasance
    B. misfeasance
    C. nonfeasance
    D. all of the above

60. You are on the scene of an automobile crash and are taking a quick report of the crash from a police officer when you suddenly notice that your EMT partner just pulled a driver out of the window without any regard for immobilization. In this case, you could be held liable under which doctrine?
    A. delegation of authority
    B. proximate liability
    C. borrowed servant
    D. You are not responsible for the actions of this EMT.

61. All medical records are confidential. Under which of the following circumstances can a patient's medical record be released?
    A. a court order or subpoena
    B. third-party billing requirements
    C. patient consent
    D. all of the above

62. Stating on the air that "We've got Joe Jones again, and he's drunk and obnoxious as usual" could place the EMT-Intermediate in danger of being liable for
    A. assault.
    B. battery.
    C. libel.
    D. slander.

63. Writing on the run sheet that a certain patient "probably has AIDS from deviant homosexual activity" could place the EMT-Intermediate in danger of being sued for
    A. assault.
    B. defamation of character.
    C. libel.
    D. slander.

64. Informed consent means
    A. the adult patient is mentally competent.
    B. the patient understands the treatment and the risks.
    C. the patient agrees to the treatment.
    D. all of the above.

65. Which of the following would **not** fall under the concept of implied consent?
    A. an unconscious diabetic in insulin shock
    B. a 5-year-old in anaphylactic shock with no parent present
    C. a mentally retarded person with bilateral fractured femurs
    D. a diabetic who awakens following 50% dextrose therapy and refuses transport

66. Who—other than the patient—is required to give informed consent for an emancipated minor?
    A. parent
    B. legal guardian
    C. no one
    D. police officer

67. If your diabetic patient awakens following dextrose therapy and now absolutely refuses transport to the hospital, even after speaking with your medical direction physician on the phone, what should you do?

A. Have the patient sign a release form and document the incident thoroughly.

B. Transport the patient against his wishes.

C. Have the patient placed in custody by the police and transport.

D. Leave and return with a court order to transport.

68. Failure to formally transfer the patient to medical staff in the emergency department could place the EMT-Intermediate in danger of being held liable for

A. false imprisonment.

B. unlawful consent.

C. abandonment.

D. patient endangerment.

69. Threatening to defibrillate a patient if he does not quiet down could place the EMT-Intermediate in danger of being held liable for

A. assault.

B. battery.

C. libel.

D. slander.

70. Starting an IV on a competent patient who absolutely refuses one could place the EMT-Intermediate in danger of being held liable for

A. assault.

B. battery.

C. libel.

D. slander.

71. Transporting a patient to the hospital against his will could place the EMT-Intermediate in danger of being held liable for

A. false imprisonment.

B. kidnapping.

C. unlawful consent.

D. assault and battery.

72. If a question arises concerning the validity of advance directives, such as "do not resuscitate" orders or "living wills," the EMT-Intermediate should

A. contact the medical direction physican.

B. ignore all such orders and run the code.

C. accept and honor all such orders.

D. run a "slow code" in these cases.

73. Which of the following statements is true concerning prehospital documentation?

A. If you do not write it down, you did not do it.

B. A well-documented run sheet can be your best defense in court.

C. Intentional alterations of the run sheet are considered admissions of guilt.

D. all of the above

74. An EMT-Intermediate's best defense against potential legal liability is

A. purchasing medical malpractice insurance.

B. documenting as little as possible on the run sheet.

C. relying on Good Samaritan immunity.

D. practicing excellent prehospital care.

75. The rules or standards that govern the behavior of members of a particular group or profession are known as

A. morals.

B. laws.

C. ethics.

D. consequences.

76. Social, religious, or personal standards of right and wrong are known as
    A. morals.
    B. laws.
    C. ethics.
    D. consequences.

77. Your patient is a 56-year-old competent female who refuses all treatment and transport after falling on the sidewalk and twisting her ankle. You abide by her wishes and allow her to refuse your care. This is an example of
    A. nonmaleficence.
    B. autonomy.
    C. ethical relativism.
    D. justice.

78. After an emergency run, you wonder whether you should have initiated advanced life support procedures. As you review the circumstances, you wonder, if asked, how you will defend your actions to your medical director. This is known as the _____ test.
    A. relevance.
    B. universalizability.
    C. interpersonal justifiability.
    D. impartiality.

79. Which of the following statements is true regarding advance directives?
    A. Always follow the family's wishes.
    B. Accept verbal DNR orders from other health care providers.
    C. When in doubt, resuscitate.
    D. Never accept a prehospital advance directive.

80. Which of the following would normally receive the highest-priority care in a multiple-patient incident?
    A. a visiting president
    B. a critically injured soldier in war

C. the least injured person in a motor vehicle collision
D. a visiting movie star

Scenario

Questions 81 and 82 refer to the following scenario:

You are called to treat a gunman who was shot by police after assaulting an elderly woman and her young granddaughter. The patient suffers an unexpected cardiac arrest in your care.

81. Based on this scenario, choose the statement that is most correct.
    A. Failure to treat the patient to the best of your ability violates the Fair Treatment Act.
    B. Neglecting to treat the patient appropriately is considered illegal.
    C. Neglecting to treat the patient appropriately can make you liable for his death.
    D. None of the above is correct.

82. Your failure to treat the gunman appropriately may also be considered
    A. unethical.
    B. legal.
    C. appropriate.
    D. righteous.

83. The best method to ensure that you are acting ethically is to
    A. know the laws governing EMS in your state.
    B. avoid performing illegal acts while providing care.
    C. place the patient's welfare above everything but your own safety.
    D. become emotionally attached to each patient as if he or she was a member of your own family.

84. You have just completed a long-distance transfer of a patient to a hospital in another state. You have just left the hospital when you come across a woman standing at the curb who is feverishly waving you down. You stop your ambulance and get out and find an elderly man on the front lawn in cardiac arrest. You get your equipment out of the ambulance and begin resuscitation, including defibrillation and IV therapy. Your act of resuscitating this patient would be considered

A. illegal and unethical.

B. illegal but ethical.

C. legal and ethical.

D. legal but unethical.

85. While at the scene of a mass casualty, an EMT-Intermediate refuses to serve as the communications officer because he wants to be where the action is. His behavior would be considered

A. unethical.

B. illegal.

C. unprofessional.

D. respectful.

86. Your partner states that his EMT-Intermediate card expired 2 weeks ago. However, he continues to function without telling his superiors that his certification has lapsed because he really needs the money and his family can't afford to go without a paycheck. Your partner's act is

A. illegal.

B. ethical.

C. professional.

D. justifiable.

87. How would you best describe protocols?

A. Protocols allow you to treat the patient any way you deem necessary.

B. Protocols are suggestions of how you could possibly treat your patient.

C. Protocols are sets of policies that only paramedics follow, so they are not important to you as an EMT-Intermediate.

D. Protocols are guidelines that provide a standardized emergency care plan for patient treatment.

88. What is your most important responsibility once you arrive at the receiving facility?

A. to complete a prehospital care report

B. to drop off the patient so you can get ready for your next call

C. to relay patient information to the first orderly you see

D. to transfer the care of the patient to appropriate medical personnel and relay the patient information and treatment

89. Under which emergency situation should you be most concerned with transport time to the hospital?

A. an unresponsive patient from an overdose

B. an unresponsive patient with blunt abdominal trauma

C. a responsive patient complaining of chest pain

D. a responsive patient with an open tibia fracture

90. You have initiated an IV on an alert and oriented 38-year-old male whose chief complaint is general malaise. The patient informs you that he wishes to be transported to a facility where his family doctor is located. However, this facility is out of your jurisdiction. What would be the best way to handle this situation?

    A. Transport the patient to the out of jurisdiction facility.

    B. Transport the patient to a local facility because of the initiation of the IV.

    C. Contact the patient's family doctor for permission to transport to requested hospital.

    D. Contact the medical direction physician for advice.

91. Earlier in the day you transported an unresponsive female patient to a local facility for hyperpyrexia. During dinner, you suddenly realize that you did not inform the emergency department staff that the patient was on Coumadin. What would you do in this situation?

    A. No action is necessary because the medication has nothing to do with hyperpyrexia.

    B. Inform the emergency department physician immediately.

    C. Inform the emergency department ward clerk.

    D. Your written documentation will adequately cover this omission.

92. Returning from lunch, you and your partner come across a vehicle that has sheared a utility pole. On the roadway, there is one patient next to the car. The patient appears severely dyspneic with an active arterial bleed from the left thigh. What would be your initial action?

    A. control the major bleeding

    B. perform a scene size-up

    C. establish and maintain an airway

    D. stabilize the vehicle

93. Which of the following best describes online medical direction?

    A. Prehospital providers communicate by radio with a physician regarding patient treatment.

    B. Prehospital providers follow written protocols.

    C. Prehospital providers communicate with the emergency department's staff to notify them of the patient's arrival.

    D. Prehospital providers notify the physician of this patient's condition while en route to the emergency department.

94. Because the nursing staff at the hospital is busy, you provide the oral report to and transfer care to a nurse's aide. This action may be interpreted as

    A. assault.

    B. criminal malfeasance.

    C. negligence.

    D. abandonment.

95. A man tells you he is a physician and questions the treatment you are providing. The man asks you to perform and administer a larger dose of a drug that you consider to be inappropriate. You should

    A. ask that the medical direction physician's authority be transferred to the on-scene physician.

    B. deny any orders and contact the medical direction physician for patient care authority.

    C. ask that the medical direction physician's authority be transferred to the on-scene physician if proper identification is provided.

    D. if unsure, make all management decisions with input from both physicians.

96. Guidelines that are used when providing emergency care are called
    A. protocols.
    B. emergency care standards.
    C. treatment management plan.
    D. online orders.

97. Which statement best describes the relationship between the EMT-Intermediate and the medical direction physician?
    A. The EMT-Intermediate functions independently on his own certification or license.
    B. Care provided is solely the responsibility of the physician.
    C. The physician provides the legal right for the EMT-Intermediate to function.
    D. The responsibility for care provided rests solely with the EMT-Intermediate.

98. Which general statement best describes the difference in the prehospital management of trauma versus medical patients?
    A. Trauma patients require rapid transport; medical patients are typically transported after stabilization.
    B. Medical patients require rapid transport; trauma patients are transported after stabilization.
    C. All trauma and medical patients are transported rapidly.
    D. All trauma and medical patients are stabilized prior to transport.

99. To be effective, medical direction must have official and clearly defined authority over all aspects of the delivery of prehospital emergency care because
    A. protocols cannot be developed to cover every possible emergency situation.
    B. public safety can be ensured only if EMS providers receive close supervision.
    C. very few who require assistance from EMS are found in situations where a physician is present.
    D. all prehospital care provided is done so under the medical director's control.

100. Communication with a base hospital physician for treatment orders is also known as
    A. off-line medical direction.
    B. physician-directed care.
    C. online medical direction.
    D. standing orders.

101. Which of the following should be the priority on arrival at a car crash?
    A. Ascertain if the patient is conscious or unconscious.
    B. Assess the patient for possible life threats.
    C. Examine the scene for hazards.
    D. Determine if the fire department can gain access into the vehicle.

102. An example of an action based on an off-line order is
    A. initiating an IV line on a trauma patient prior to reporting the condition to the physician.
    B. contacting the medical direction and asking permission to initiate the trauma protocol.
    C. requesting a trauma team on a patient involved in a shooting.
    D. contacting dispatch for a helicopter for medical evacuation.

103. What should you do when a physician on-scene orders you to administer medication not included in your protocol?

    A. Follow the on-scene physician's order as long as he signs your EMS report.

    B. Have the on-scene physician speak with your medical direction regarding patient care.

    C. Instruct the on-scene physician to leave the scene or be arrested.

    D. Ask the physician to provide proof of his identity.

104. Development of treatment protocols should be guided by all of the following **except**

    A. the EMS director(s) and provider.

    B. state laws.

    C. the medical director(s).

    D. billing department.

105. Earlier in the shift you transported a 58-year-old male patient with chest pain. Later that day you take another patient to the same emergency department. While there, you inquire about the diagnosis and condition of the 58-year-old chest pain patient since both you and your partner did not believe the chest pain was caused by a myocardial infarction. Your activity is considered

    A. a method of performing quality assurance and continuous quality improvement.

    B. illegal and unethical.

    C. unprofessional since you are not permitted to discuss the case of another patient.

    D. a breach of the laws of confidentiality.

106. Which of the following best describes your responsibilities once you have delivered the patient to the emergency department?

    A. You are not responsible for the patient once you are in the emergency department.

    B. It is necessary that you provide an oral and written report to ensure a continuum of care in the emergency department.

    C. You do not need to provide an oral report to the emergency department staff since all the information will be contained within your EMS report.

    D. It is not necessary to report any additional findings while en route to the hospital because the physician will conduct his own physical exam on the patient.

107. You and your partner are treating a 57-year-old male who is complaining of difficulty breathing. You have the patient on a nonrebreather mask at 15 lpm and normal saline running at TKO. En route to the hospital, you pass a motor vehicle accident where a BLS unit is on-scene and has requested your assistance for their critical patient. You have the BLS crew transport your patient while you provide emergency care to the trauma patient. Your action can be considered to be

    A. ethical.

    B. failure of duty to act.

    C. proximate cause treatment.

    D. abandonment.

108. You are treating a 14-year-old boy with evidence of abdominal trauma and a tender rigid abdomen. Currently, he is alert and oriented and is refusing treatment and transport. The boy's 16-year-old brother states that his parents are at work and would not want him treated. You should

    A. provide emergency care and transport the patient.

    B. have the patient sign a refusal form and leave the scene.

    C. have the brother transport the patient.

    D. contact the parents for permission to provide emergency care.

109. You are called to the scene of an attempted suicide and find a behaviorally unstable and violent patient who is a potential threat to himself and others. Medical direction has indicated it is necessary to transport the patient. How should you best respond to the situation?

    A. Contact medical direction for an order for a sedative.

    B. Restrain the patient by using whatever means necessary.

    C. Use reasonable force to secure the patient.

    D. Leave the scene.

110. You have decided to provide positive pressure ventilation (PPV) to a COPD patient who is conscious, but in acute respiratory failure. You attempt to explain the procedure to the patient in order to obtain consent, but the patient does not seem to fully understand. You should

    A. continue emergency care and provide the positive pressure ventilation.

    B. stop emergency care until you get verbal consent.

    C. gain expressed consent prior to any invasive procedures.

    D. Informed consent is not necessary or applied to emergency medical care.

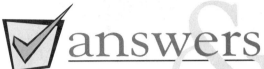

answers & rationales

Following each rationale, you will find a reference to the corresponding objective in the DOT National Standard EMT-Intermediate curriculum. An asterisk denotes material that is supplemental to the DOT curriculum. Page numbers after a rationale indicate where the question topic may be discussed in the Brady text *Intermediate Emergency Care* (Bledsoe, Porter, Cherry).

1.

A. Most EMT-Intermediates are injured while they are lifting because of poor biomechanics and poor physical conditioning. Embarking on a lifelong program of reasonable physical fitness will increase your chances for a long EMS career. (1-1.14a) (IEC p. 30)

2.

D. Cardiovascular endurance (aerobic capacity), muscular strength, and flexibility are equally important elements in any program of physical fitness for EMT-Intermediates. Some type of aerobic training, such as jogging, swimming, biking, or even walking briskly, is essential to build up enough endurance to work long shifts in the streets. Strength conditioning, such as weightlifting, is important to be able to carry patients and the multitude of equipment up and down flights of stairs. Flexibility exercises, such as stretching, are important in avoiding pulled muscles and ensure a full range of motion of your joints in the variety of movements you will perform during a shift. (1-1.14a) (IEC p. 28)

3.

C. Your target heart rate is the rate at which you receive the maximum aerobic benefit while exercising. You can approximate yours by subtracting your age from 220. Then subtract your resting heart rate from this number. Finally, multiply this number by 0.7 and add it to your resting heart rate to calculate your target heart rate. Try to maintain this rate while running, walking, biking, or swimming for at least 20–30 minutes a few times per week. (1-1.14a) (IEC p. 29)

4.

A. Isometric exercise is active exercise performed against a stable, or immobile, resistance. You simply contract your muscle against an immovable resistance. (1-1.14a) (IEC p. 29)

5.

B. EMT-Intermediates receive credentialing or licensing from a state or provincial agency. While all EMT-Intermediates must be certified or licensed, they may not practice independently. They may function only under the license and direction of an EMS system's medical director. (1-1.11) (IEC p. 29)

6.

C. The major food groups include breads and grains, vegetables, fruits, dairy products, and meat/fish. You should minimize your intake of fat, salt, sugar, cholesterol, and caffeine. Instead of a piece of apple pie, try an apple. (1-1.14a) (IEC p. 29)

7.

A. The old-fashioned sit-up is no longer considered a beneficial exercise because of the abnormal stress it puts on your lumbar spine. To get that "six-pack" look, do abdominal crunches, which target only the rectus abdominus muscles. A variation on the basic crunch is to twist gently to either side during the crunch to target the oblique muscles. A strong abdominal section helps stabilize the spine, especially during lifting. (1-1.14a) (IEC p. 29)

8.

B. The incubation period is the time between contact with a disease organism and the appearance of the first symptoms. Tuberculosis (2–6 weeks), hepatitis B and C (weeks or months), and AIDS (months or years) have long incubation periods, so you may not experience symptoms of such diseases for a long time following your exposure. EMT-Intermediates are at high risk for disease exposure. Consider the blood and body fluids of all patients as potentially dangerous and take the necessary body substance isolation precautions. (1-1.17) (IEC p. 33)

9.

D. You are trying to avoid body fluids that you should suspect are infectious. Splashing during childbirth is common. Gloves, protective eyewear, masks, and gowns are all reasonable protective measures to take. A HEPA (high-efficiency particulate air) or N-95 mask is unnecessary unless your patient also has confirmed or suspected tuberculosis. (1-1.15) (IEC pp. 33–34)

10.

C. While gloves, protective eyewear, and proper needle disposal are all essential components of a reasonable infection control policy, simply washing your hands is considered the most important. Not everyone knows how to do it properly. First, lather well with soap and water. Then scrub for at least 15 seconds, making sure to get underneath your fingernails (ideally with a brush). Then point your hands down while you rinse so that the soap and water run away from your body. Finally dry your hands on a clean towel. It sounds simple, but sometimes the simplest things are the most effective. (1-1.15) (IEC p. 34)

11.

C. Soaking in a bleach solution is appropriate for disinfecting objects that have come in direct contact with a patient's intact skin. For items such as a laryngoscope, which is inserted into your patient's mouth and is covered with oral secretions, this is ineffective and inappropriate. Sterilization by heat, steam, or radiation is recommended for killing all microorganisms on an object. However, since these methods are all impractical in the field, there are EPA-approved solutions for sterilization you can use. (1-1.15) (IEC p. 35)

12.

B. The recommended bleach solution mix is 1 part bleach to 10 parts water. (1-1.15) (IEC p. 35)

13.

B. According to the Ryan White Act, the medical facility must notify your infection control officer that your patient had tuberculosis within 48 hours. Your officer or supervisor should notify you that you have been exposed, and your employer must arrange for you to be evaluated and followed up by a physician or other appropriate health care professional. This also pertains to occupational exposure to AIDS, hepatitis, diphtheria, meningitis, plague, hemorrhagic fever, and rabies. (1-1.17) (IEC p. 36)

14.

D. The patient in denial exhibits the inability or refusal to believe the reality of the event. It is a defense mechanism that can last for hours, days, weeks, or even months. During this stage, the person puts off dealing with the inevitable event. (1-1.63) (IEC p. 37)

15.

B. Often patients or their families will aim their anger at you. This rage is just a frustration related to their inability to control the situation. Just remember to remain calm; do not take it personally, and allow them to vent their feelings. Quite often this is all they need, it is inexpensive, and you are providing the best care possible—comfort, understanding, and compassion. (1-1.63) (IEC p. 37)

16.

C. People who despair at their fate and misfortune may enter the depression stage. During this stage, they withdraw into their private world and may choose not to communicate with you or even their closest and most intimate friends and loved ones. During this stage, provide reassurance and gentle guidance. (1-1.63) (IEC p. 37)

17.

D. In the end, grieving people generally come to accept their situation as inevitable. They realize, even while others may still be angry or depressed, that their fate has been cast. They appear to have achieved a reasonable level of comfort with the anticipated outcome. In these cases, the family may need your support more than the patient. (1-1.63) (IEC p. 37)

18.

C. When informing someone of the death of a loved one, help him work through the denial stage by using the word "dead." Avoid euphemisms such as expired, passed away, or moved on. Recognize that the family will cope with death in much the same manner as they deal with everyday stressors. (1-1.63) (IEC pp. 37–39)

19.

C. During the alarm stage, the body prepares to defend itself against a perceived stressor by initiating the "fight or flight" response. This dates back to prehistoric times, when man needed all his abilities to fight or run away from the saber-toothed tiger. As the body responds to stress, the endocrine system releases epinephrine and norepinephrine. These hormones cause increases in pulse and blood pressure (to deliver more oxygenated blood to vital organs), dilated pupils (to improve vision), excessive perspiration (to decrease body temperature), increased muscle tension (to anticipate increased muscle use), and increased blood glucose levels (to supply fuel to vital tissues). (1-1.14a) (IEC p. 40)

20.

D. The resistance stage begins as the victim adapts to the stressor. It is brought on by the use of various coping mechanisms. Vital signs return to normal. As adaptation develops, resistance to the particular stressor increases. (1-1.14a) (IEC p. 40)

21.

B. Many an EMT-Intermediate career has been prematurely ended because of burnout. When the coping mechanisms no longer keep you afloat, burnout is inevitable. EMT-Intermediates need to develop interests outside of EMS and cultivate strong relationships and support to help them withstand the many and varied stressors of EMT-Intermediate life. (1-1.14a) (IEC p. 41)

22.

C. Many of the physiological reactions to stress are mediated by the sympathetic nervous system. Stress triggers an increase in sympathetic tone by releasing norepinephrine and epinephrine. Examples of signs and symptoms are heart palpitations, GI distress, and chest pain. Sympathetic stimulation causes decreased secretion from the salivary glands, resulting in dry mouth. (1-1.14a) (IEC p. 42)

23.

A. Following a critical incident, a mental health professional should screen EMS personnel for abnormal stress-related symptoms within 2 months. (1-1.14a) (IEC p. 44)

24.

D. A "tiered" system is one in which basic life support first responders are dispatched unless advanced life support is needed. In that case, both are simultaneously dispatched to the emergency, and the first responders initiate care until the higher level arrives. (1-1.1) (IEC p. 7)

25.

A. State EMS agencies are typically responsible for allocating funding to local systems, recommending legislation concerning the prehospital practice of medicine, licensing and certifying field providers, enforcing all state EMS regulations, and appointing regional advisory councils. Hiring a local system medical director is the responsibility of the local EMS administrative agency. (1-1.3) (IEC p. 10)

26.

B. The local EMS system medical director is the ultimate authority in all patient care–related issues in the local EMS system. All prehospital patient care activities are extensions of this physician's license. Only a physician is licensed to practice medicine. This doctrine is known as "delegation of authority." (1-1.1) (IEC p. 10)

27.

B. Direct or online medical direction exists when prehospital providers communicate directly with the physician at a medical direction or resource hospital. The physician's direction is usually based on established protocols for managing specific problems. This physician assumes responsibility and gives treatment orders for patients. Direct medical direction physicians should be experienced in emergency medicine. (1-1.11) (IEC p. 11)

28.

D. EMT-Intermediate field interventions that may be completed before contacting the medical direction physician are known as written protocol, offline orders, or standing orders. These orders are established by indirect medical direction prior to the emergency call. They allow EMT-Intermediates to perform certain procedures without a direct order from the base station physician. (1-1.11) (IEC p. 11)

29.

D. The public is an essential but often overlooked component of an EMS system. An EMS system should have a plan for educating the public about recognizing an emergency situation, accessing the EMS system, and initiating basic life support procedures. (1-1.1) (IEC p. 12)

30.

D. The basic emergency telephone service is a service that enables the caller to dial three digits, 911, to reach a single public safety answering point. Enhanced 911 (E-911) provides automatic location identification of the caller, instant routing of the call to the appropriate emergency service agency, and instant callback capabilities if the caller hangs up too soon. (1-1.1) (IEC p. 12)

31.

C. The National Registry of EMTs recognizes and the U.S. Department of Transportation develops training curricula for three levels of field providers: EMT-Basic, EMT-Intermediate, and EMT–Paramedic. There exist, however, approximately 30 various levels of field providers nationwide. (1-1.3) (IEC pp. 14–15)

32.

B. Certification is the process by which an agency or association grants recognition to an individual who has met its qualifications. It is not a license to practice but rather a statement that a person has fulfilled predetermined requirements. Each EMT-Intermediate must maintain current certification by following the guidelines established by the certifying agency. (1-1.3, 1-1.27) (IEC p. 14)

33.

A. A license is permission to engage in a given occupation. A government agency grants licensure to individuals who have attained the degree of competency required to ensure the public's protection. A state grants licenses to teachers, physicians, nurses, and barbers. Some states also license their EMT-Intermediates. (1-1.13, 1-1.27) (IEC p. 14)

34.

C. Reciprocity is the process by which an agency grants automatic certification or licensure to an individual who has comparable credentials from another agency. Some states grant automatic EMT-Intermediate certification to persons who hold an EMT-Intermediate card from another state. Others grant certification to individuals who are nationally registered. (1-1.3, 1-1.27) (IEC p. 14)

35.

A. In 1974, responding to a request from the U.S. Department of Transportation, the General Services Administration developed the KKK standards, which established federal specifications for ambulances. The original guidelines and the subsequent revisions are aimed at improving ambulance design and safety features. (1-1.1) (IEC p. 16)

36.

B. Since all hospitals are not equal in terms of emergency and support service capabilities, hospital categorization is an important function of an EMS system. It identifies the readiness and capability of a hospital and its staff to receive and effectively treat emergency patients. Categorization resulted from the realization that patients have varying degrees of illness and injury and that receiving facilities have varying capabilities to provide initial or definitive care. (1-1.1) (IEC pp. 16–17)

37.

C. Quality assurance programs are primarily designed to maintain continuous monitoring and measurement of the quality of clinical care delivered. They emphasize evaluation of response times, adherence to protocols, patient survival, and other indicators. They are often viewed as punitive and negative. (1-1.14) (IEC p. 18)

38.

D. In order to provide a scientific basis for prehospital EMS, a formal, ongoing research program is an essential component of the system. Research is necessary to justify future funding allocations, to scientifically evaluate EMT-Intermediate care, and to weigh the benefits versus the risks of certain prehospital treatments. (1-1.10) (IEC p. 19)

39.

D. Always remember that the number one priority during any emergency response is your personal safety. You can do your patient no good if you become a victim yourself. Never let your guard down because the most placid and safe scene can instantly become deadly. (1-1.64) (IEC p. 22)

40.

C. Priority-1, or immediate, transport is for patients who require definitive care that you cannot provide on the scene. The patient with signs of shock and abdominal bruising probably has an intraabdominal hemorrhage. He needs surgery and whole-blood replacement, neither of which you can provide. In his case, perform a rapid trauma assessment while you prepare for immediate transport. Perform all other assessments and treatments en route to the hospital. (1-1.1) (IEC p. 17)

41.

B. You will eventually encounter an unfamiliar situation that confuses you. In these cases, your best resource is the medical direction physician, who is there to help you sort out the problem and guide your care. (1-1.11) (IEC p. 11)

42.

A. Receiving facilities are designated by the level of care they can provide. The American College of Surgeons categorizes trauma centers by levels. A Level I trauma center provides the highest level of care. (1-1.1) (IEC p. 17)

43.

D. As an EMT-Intermediate, you will be confronted with situations that call for quick decision making under pressure. Your patient's very life may depend on your decision. You can base that decision on knowledge, experience, your patient's best interest, and guidance from your medical direction physician. (1-1.1) (IEC p. 22)

44.

A. Ethics are the rules of conduct that govern members of a particular group or profession. Examples of ethical codes for EMS include the EMT Code of Ethics and the EMT Oath. They are not laws or morals but rather guidelines for the behavior expected from professionals. (1-1.1) (IEC p. 69)

45.

D. Professionalism describes the conduct or qualities that characterize a practitioner in a particular field or occupation. Professionals take pride in their work and earn the respect of their peers by the way they conduct daily business. They are the role models who set high standards for themselves and their colleagues. The professional EMT-Intermediate promotes only excellent patient care. (1-1.16) (IEC pp. 24–25)

46.

B. When a professional makes a mistake, he does only three things: He admits it, he learns from it, and he tries never to repeat it. Professionals accept the responsibility for their actions and do their best to place their patients' best interest first, not their egos. Professionals don't complain, blame others, or make excuses for poor performance. (1-1.17) (IEC p. 25)

47.

C. By identifying with your patient's situation and trying to understand his feelings, you are practicing empathy. You can show empathy by being supportive and reassuring; having a calm, compassionate demeanor; and demonstrating respect for others. (1-1.68) (IEC p. 26)

48.

A. Professional EMT-Intermediates spend the vast majority of their time preparing for the next emergency call. Being an EMT-Intermediate means accepting the responsibility of being the leader in the prehospital phase of emergency medical care. Leaders understand that performance requires preparation. The end of the training program marks only the beginning of the EMT-Intermediate's education. Any skill erodes when not used. The key to confidence on the scene is competence. The key to competence is practice. (1-1.4) (IEC p. 25)

49.

B. The study of the factors that influence the frequency, distribution, and causes of injury, disease, and other health-related events in a population is known as epidemiology. Many injuries result from interaction with potential hazards and can be predicted. Studying these factors is the first step in prevention. (1-1.19) (IEC p. 46)

50.

C. The "years of productive life" calculation is made by subtracting the deceased's age from 65. In this case, $65 - 50 = 15$. (1-1.19) (IEC p. 46)

51.

D. As medical professionals, EMT-Intermediates should take part in an injury-surveillance program. This involves identifying potential injury risks, maintaining related injury statistics, teaching prevention to patients and others immediately following an incident, and developing prevention programs to keep injuries from occurring. (1-1.19) (IEC p. 46)

52.

A. Criminal law deals with crimes against society and their punishments. Criminal litigations are legal actions taken by the state against the offending individual. Homicide and rape are examples of criminal wrongs. To convict requires proof beyond a reasonable doubt. (1-1.46) (IEC p. 53)

53.

D. Tort law, a branch of civil law, deals with civil wrongs committed by one individual against another. A medical malpractice suit is an example of a tort action against an EMT-Intermediate. Unlike in a criminal case, only a preponderance of evidence (50% + 1) is needed to win the case. (1-1.46) (IEC p. 53)

54.

A. A "Medical Practice Act" is specific state legislation that defines the scope of practice and role of the EMT-Intermediate and other allied health care professionals. It establishes the requirements for those who will be allowed to practice and identifies certification and licensing procedures. Medical practice acts differ from state to state. (1-1.30) (IEC p. 54)

55.

B. As an EMT-Intermediate, you practice under the license of the physician giving you

orders. However, you are still held responsible for your own actions. In this case, if you are sure the order is contraindicated and potentially harmful to your patient, you must refuse the order and document the incident thoroughly. (1-1.13) (IEC p. 54)

56.

A. Laws that protect off-duty health care workers from liability in the event they stop and render roadside care are known as Good Samaritan laws. A person is immune from liability for assisting at the scene of a medical emergency if he acts in good faith, is not grossly negligent, and does not accept payment for services. Unfortunately, "grossly negligent" is a subjective term, and the plaintiff's attorney will portray the EMT-Intermediate as such. A jury of nonmedical civilians will listen to testimony and decide the outcome. In many cases, the Good Samaritan defense has not held up in court. (1-1.36) (IEC p. 55)

57.

B. Negligence is defined as deviating from accepted standards of care. In medicine, negligence is synonymous with malpractice. EMT-Intermediates can be negligent by not performing to the standard of care (failure to immobilize the spine), by performing beyond their training and certification (any skill not approved by the local medical director), or by performing at a substandard level (unrecognized esophageal intubation with a tracheal tube). (1-1.29) (IEC p. 56)

58.

D. To win a negligence case, the plaintiff's attorney must prove that an EMT-Intermediate's breach of duty caused harm to the patient. Once again, in a tort case, only a preponderance of evidence is needed to win. (1-1.32) (IEC pp. 56–57)

59.

D. Breach of duty also means deviating from the standard of care. It can take the form of malfeasance (performing a wrongful act, such as assaulting your patient), misfeasance (performing improperly, such as failing to recognize an esophageal intubation), or nonfeasance (failing to perform an indicated procedure, such as immobilizing the spine). (1-1.29) (IEC p. 57)

60.

C. As an EMT-Intermediate, one of your responsibilities is supervising the actions of other EMS providers—in this case, your EMT partner. You may be liable for any negligent act he commits under the borrowed servant doctrine. (1-1.35) (IEC p. 59)

61.

D. It is true that all medical records are confidential. But there are special circumstances in which the release of medical information is not only practical but also essential. These include patient consent, when other medical providers need to know, a subpoena, and third-party billing requirements. (1-1.37) (IEC p. 60)

62.

D. Slander is the act of injuring a person's character, name, or reputation by false or malicious spoken words. Information

transmitted over the radio should be limited to essential matters of patient care. Such a medical report should never contain the patient's name or the EMT-Intermediate's subjective opinions. (1-1.29) (IEC p. 61)

63.

C. Libel is the act of injuring a person's character, name, or reputation by false or malicious writings. Allegations of libel can be avoided by respecting the patient's confidentiality. The medical record should be accurate and confidential; slang and labels should be avoided. Never write anything on the run report that could be construed as libel. (1-1.29) (IEC p. 61)

64.

D. Informed consent must be obtained from every conscious, mentally competent adult before treatment can be started. To give informed consent, the adult patient must be mentally competent, understand the treatment and the risks, and agree to be treated. (1-1.29) (IEC pp. 61–62)

65.

D. With implied consent, it is assumed that the patient would want lifesaving treatment if he were able to provide expressed consent. If the patient becomes competent, expressed consent must be attained to continue treatment. (1-1.29) (IEC p. 62)

66.

C. An emancipated minor is considered an adult and can give informed consent. This is a person under 18 years old who is married, pregnant, a parent, a member of the armed forces, or financially independent and living away from home. (1-1.29) (IEC p. 62)

also could be a criminal or a civil offense. (1-1.29) (IEC p. 65)

67.

A. Competent patients have the right to be left alone. This patient, now awake and competent, has every legal right to refuse your help. Respect his wishes but document that you informed him of the dangers of refusing help and make sure he understands the risks involved in refusing. (1-1.38) (IEC pp. 63–64)

68.

C. Abandonment is the termination of the EMT-Intermediate–patient relationship without assuring continuation of the care. EMT-Intermediates should not initiate care and then arbitrarily discontinue it. Physically leaving a patient unattended on an emergency department stretcher may be grounds for abandonment if the patient's condition deteriorates. (1-1.29) (IEC p. 64)

69.

A. Assault is defined as unlawfully placing a person in apprehension of immediate bodily harm without his consent. Threatening to defibrillate a patient if he does not quiet down could place an EMT-Intermediate in danger of being sued for assault. Assault can be either a criminal or a civil offense. (1-1.29) (IEC p. 65)

70.

B. Battery is the unlawful touching of another individual without his consent. Starting an IV on a competent patient who absolutely refuses one could place the EMT-Intermediate in danger of being sued for battery. Battery

71.

A. Everyone has the right to be left alone. False imprisonment is defined as unlawful and unjustifiable detention. Transporting a patient to the hospital against his will could constitute false imprisonment. In these cases, EMT-Intermediates should ensure that the transportation is medically justified. (1-1.29) (IEC p. 65)

72.

A. When questions concerning the validity of "do not resuscitate" orders or "living wills" arise in the field, EMT-Intermediates should contact the medical direction physician. EMT-Intermediates do not have the legal authority and are not in the position to evaluate the validity of such documents. (1-1.41) (IEC pp. 66–67)

73.

D. A complete, well-written run report is an EMT-Intermediate's best protection in a malpractice proceeding. To the court, observations and treatments not documented on the run report were not performed. The medical record should never be altered because this may amount to an admission of guilt by the EMT-Intermediate. (1-1.43) (IEC pp. 68–69)

74.

D. An EMT-Intermediate's best defense against potential legal liability is practicing the highest quality of patient care, which includes good documentation. (1-1.35) (IEC p. 52)

75.

C. The rules or standards that govern the behavior of members of a particular group or profession are known as ethics. Every profession has a set of ethics developed by that profession. General ethical guidelines for EMS providers include the EMT Oath and the EMT Code of Ethics. (1-1.1) (IEC p. 69)

76.

A. Social, religious, or personal standards of right and wrong are known as morals. Just as ethical standards guide your actions as an EMT-Intermediate, so will your own personal morals. (1-1.46) (IEC p. 69)

77.

B. A competent adult has the right to be left alone. Respecting the patient's right allows the patient to practice autonomy. Just remember to follow your medical director's guidelines for refusal of care and document the incident thoroughly. (1-1.72) (IEC p. 71)

78.

C. Asking whether you can defend or justify your actions to others is using the interpersonal justifiability test. Soliciting other opinions helps an EMT-Intermediate navigate through the sometimes murky waters of emergency medicine. (1-1.25) (IEC p. 73)

79.

C. Whenever you doubt the validity of an advance directive, resuscitate the patient. During a crisis, an EMT-Intermediate is not trained to judge the validity of a legal document. (1-1.41) (IEC pp. 67, 74)

80.

A. "Triage" is a French word meaning "to sort." Triaging medical care is a necessity fraught with different rules for different situations. For example, in civilian life the most injured and salvageable patient gets the highest priority. In war, the least injured soldier gets the highest priority in order to return him to the fighting. A visiting dignitary, such as the president or vice president, immediately receives special treatment because of his importance. (1-1.25) (IEC p. 76)

81.

C. Regardless of your impression of the patient as a person or as a member of society, you cannot allow your prejudices or opinions to influence your care. As such, failure to treat the patient to the best of your ability can make you liable for his death. The Fair Treatment Act has nothing to do with prehospital care, and the degree of legality in not following standing orders for treatment is not the cause of your liability. (1-1.25) (IEC p. 52)

82.

A. Not treating him to the best of your ability because you have developed an opinion about him is considered unethical. EMTs cannot prejudge patients. Following your protocols and treating the patient to the best of your ability will be deemed appropriate, legal, and ethical. (1-1.25) (IEC p. 77)

83.

C. Ethical activity involves placing the patient's welfare above everything but your own safety. Knowing the laws of your state may prevent you from performing illegal acts but not necessarily unethical acts. As an EMT-Intermediate, you must not become emotionally attached to your patient; rather, maintain a detached concern for him or her. (1-1.25) (IEC pp. 27, 70–71)

84.

B. Stopping and assisting the elderly man is considered ethical behavior. However, providing care at an advanced level out of your certification or licensure jurisdiction, in this case another state, is considered illegal. (1-1.46) (IEC p. 77)

85.

C. Refusing to serve as the communications officer is an unprofessional act. It does not constitute illegal or unethical behavior since he is not refusing to deliver care to the injured patients. (1-1.6) (IEC p. 27)

86.

A. It is imperative to keep your certification or license current while practicing prehospital care. If your certification or license should lapse and you continue to function as an EMT-Intermediate, you are acting illegally. It is your legal, ethical, and professional responsibility to keep your certifications and licensure current. (1-1.46) (IEC pp. 14, 55)

87.

D. Protocols are important for the EMT-Intermediate. They provide a basis for medical care and a standardized approach to the patient. (1-1.11) (IEC p. 11)

88.

D. Your responsibility to your patient does not end until you transfer care to appropriate medical personnel (doctor or nurse) at the hospital. The EMT-Intermediate must report the patient's status, the treatment that was initiated, and any response to the prehospital treatment. (1-1.29) (IEC pp. 64–65)

89.

B. Certain prehospital emergencies, specifically trauma, can be managed only in the hospital's emergency department or operating suite. As such, resuscitation measures for major trauma patients must be initiated in the field or during transport with rapid movement of the patient to an appropriate medical facility. Recognizing the differing philosophies between treating medical and trauma patients in the prehospital environment by the EMT-Intermediate is pivotal in decreasing morbidity and mortality from trauma. (1-1.1) (IEC pp. 65–66)

90.

D. Contact the medical direction physician for advice. As an EMT-Intermediate, you practice under the control of the medical director who has delegated authority to other medical direction physicians. Therefore, you must contact the medical direction physician for advice and permission to transport this patient to another facility. Transporting this patient to the out-of-jurisdiction facility without the advisement of medical direction would be a blatant violation of the physician–EMT-Intermediate relationship— especially if something detrimental happened en route. Transporting the patient to the local facility may be unnecessary, depending on the decision of the medical direction physician. In this situation, you are not accountable to the family doctor. (1-1.11) (IEC pp. 65–66)

91.

B. The patient care continuum begins when treatment is initiated in the field and extends into the emergency department. This continuum is made possible by effective communication between prehospital personnel and the emergency department staff. Failure to communicate breaks this continuum and ultimately compromises patient care. The omission in relaying the medication history can affect the way a patient is treated or evaluated in the emergency department and quite possibly ultimate patient outcome. The emergency department physician is directly responsible for the general welfare of the patient. In this sense, merely contacting the emergency department clerk is not the best selection. Direct communication with the emergency department physician would be the best way to resolve this oversight. (1-1.6) (IEC p. 23)

92.

B. Your initial responsibility on the scene lies in sizing up the incident, determining what resources will be needed, and ensuring that the scene is safe prior to entry. In this situation, you must locate any potential hazards and identify the number and severity of patients so additional resources can be dispatched. (1-1.6) (IEC p. 22)

93.

A. Online medical direction requires you to communicate directly with the physician by radio, phone, or other communicating devices. (1-1.11) (IEC pp. 64–65)

94.

D. Anytime you relinquish patient care to personnel with less training than yourself, you are abandoning your patient. Negligence is a deviation from accepted standards of care recognized by law. (1-1.29) (IEC pp. 64–65)

95.

B. In this scenario, care and direct communication with the medical direction physician is imperative. The management decisions are to be provided by the medical direction physician. If care is provided by a physician prior to arrival of the EMT-Intermediate and medical direction communications are not established, do the following: Make sure you look at proper identification. Ensure that the physician will accept responsibility and document the care as required by the local system. If the treatment is different than that established by the system, the physician should accompany (in the ambulance) the patient to the hospital. If the physician does not agree to these terms, the medical direction physician regains responsibility for patient care. (1-1.13) (IEC p. 11)

96.

A. Protocols provide guidelines that facilitate delivery of emergency care. Standing orders allow specific interventions to be carried out without direct medical direction. Usually standing orders describe the specific delivery of emergency care. The protocol could include off-line orders that are written standard or online orders that require you to contact medical direction for permission to perform specific care. Standing orders are used when medical direction cannot be contacted. (1-1.11) (IEC p. 10)

97.

C. The EMT-Intermediate's legal right to function is derived from the medical direction physician. Care provided by the EMT-Intermediate is considered an extension of the medical direction physician. In practice, the responsibilities are shared. (1-1.11) (IEC p. 29)

98.

A. The critical trauma patient requires rapid transport. Surgery is often required to manage the trauma patient's condition. The quicker the patient's traumatic injury is identified and bleeding is stopped, the greater the chance the patient will survive. In general, medical patients are typically provided more on-scene stabilization prior to transport. Not all patients are transported rapidly, and not all patients are stabilized prior to transport. (1-1.1) (IEC p. 22)

99.

D. All prehospital care provided is done so under the medical director's authority. Therefore, in order to be effective, medical direction must have official and clearly defined authority over all aspects of the delivery of prehospital emergency care. (1-1.11) (IEC p. 10)

100.

C. Direct communication with a base hospital physician for treatment orders during an emergency call is known as online medical direction. (1-1.12) (IEC p. 11)

101.

C. All the answers listed must be accomplished by the EMT-Intermediate on the scene of a car crash. The order, however, is important. The first thing that must be done is ensuring the safety of you and your crew as well as other rescue personnel. (1-1.) (IEC p. 22)

102.

A. Protocols and standing orders are the guidelines provided by the medical director governing patient care. If you carry out treatment based on written guidelines, it is an example of off-line medical direction. If the protocol requires you to first consult the medical director prior to providing care, this is an example of online medical direction. Initiating an IV line prior to physician contact would be authorized by an off-line order. (1-1.12) (IEC p. 11)

103.

B. Whenever a physician is on scene and wants to influence your treatment, it is best to have that physician speak directly to the medical direction physician regarding patient care options. This is done so that optimal patient care can be discussed between the physicians (often the on-scene physician does not know your standing orders). The on-scene physician must also agree to travel with you to the hospital in the ambulance if he or she decides to assume responsibility for patient care and continue to direct patient care. (1-1.13) (IEC p. 11)

104.

D. All the named individuals should be part of the decision-making process in development or revision of standing orders except for the billing department. The medical aspect of the provision of emergency medical services is not influenced by the billing department or any insurance providers. (1-1.11) (IEC p. 11)

105.

A. One method of continuous quality improvement that EMT-Intermediates are encouraged to perform is a follow-up on the patients whom they have treated. You can compare your field impression with the official diagnosis and determine if your field treatment was correct and accurate. This is not a breach of confidentially since it involves the patient whom you cared for and transported. (1-1.14) (IEC p. 18)

106.

B. Your care for the patient does not stop when you step foot into the emergency department. An orderly transfer of care must be established so that the continuum of care from the prehospital setting to the hospital environment is ensured. Both your oral and your written reports are important in establishing the continuum of care for the patient. Leaving the patient in the emergency department without a proper transfer of care to an equally or higher-trained medical professional may constitute abandonment. (1-1.29) (IEC pp. 64–65)

107.

D. In this case, advanced life support care was initiated; consequently, turning care over to a BLS unit would be abandonment. EMS personnel must remain with the patient until the patient is under the care of other EMS

personnel of equal or greater training. (1-1.29) (IEC p. 64)

108.

A. The child should be treated under the doctrine of implied consent. The EMT-Intermediate has the responsibility to treat the child because of the possible life threat. Neither child is old enough to sign a refusal. Attempts to contact the parents should be delegated to law enforcement at the scene or by the emergency department staff. (1-1.29) (IEC p. 62)

109.

C. Reasonable force may be used to restrain a violent patient. However, not all mental health laws allow patients to be transported and hospitalized against their will. EMT-Intermediates need to be familiar with their jurisdictions. Police authorization may not always be necessary, but it is a definite legal advantage. (1-1.40) (IEC p. 65)

110.

A. Implied consent is used to provide emergency care for patients with altered mental states, or those who are unresponsive or who cannot make a rational decision. (1-1.29) (IEC p. 62)

UNIT

2

Overview of Human Systems

unit objectives

Questions in this unit relate to DOT objectives 1-2.1 to 1-2.66. The objectives are listed in the Appendix.

DIRECTIONS Each of the questions or incomplete statements below is followed by suggested answers or completions. Select the **one answer** that is best in each case.

1. The basic unit of life is the
   A. nucleus.
   B. tissue.
   C. organ.
   D. cell.

2. The three main components of a cell are the
   A. cell membrane, cytokine, and nucleus.
   B. cell membrane, nucleus, and organelles.
   C. cytoplasm, organelles, and nucleus.
   D. organelles, cytoplasm, and cell membrane.

Match the following cellular terms with their respective definitions:

3. _____ nucleus
4. _____ cytosol
5. _____ golgi
6. _____ mitochondrion
7. _____ lysosome
8. _____ peroxisome
9. _____ phagocyte

   A. scavenger cell
   B. packages enzymes and mucus
   C. clear liquid portion of cytoplasm
   D. neutralizes alcohol and toxins
   E. energy factory
   F. contains DNA
   G. contains digestive enzymes

10. The structure that surrounds the cell and protects it from the outer environment is the
    A. membrane.
    B. organelle.
    C. mitochondrion.
    D. cytoplasm.

11. The skin, mucous membranes, and intestinal tract lining are examples of
    A. muscle tissue.
    B. connective tissue.
    C. nerve tissue.
    D. epithelial tissue.

12. The only muscle tissue that can contract without external stimulation is
    A. cardiac muscle.
    B. smooth muscle.
    C. skeletal muscle.
    D. connective muscle.

13. Bones, cartilage, and fat are examples of
    A. epithelia.
    B. organelles.
    C. connective tissue.
    D. organ systems.

14. The type of muscle found in the inner lining of hollow organs is
    A. skeletal muscle.
    B. epithelial muscle.
    C. smooth muscle.
    D. connective muscle.

15. The natural tendency of the body to maintain a constant, stable internal environment is called
    A. osmosis.
    B. organism stability.
    C. hemostasis.
    D. homeostasis.

16. Ductless glands that secrete their hormones directly into the bloodstream are called _____ glands.
    A. lipophilic
    B. endocrine
    C. exocrine
    D. paracrine

17. _____ respond to changes in arterial PCO_2 levels.
    A. Baroreceptors
    B. Neuroreceptors
    C. Chemoreceptors
    D. Alpha receptors

18. _____ respond to changes in blood pressure.
    A. Baroreceptors
    B. Neuroreceptors
    C. Chemoreceptors
    D. Alpha receptors

19. As your blood pressure falls, your body initiates a series of mechanisms to increase it. These mechanisms then begin to subside as your blood pressure returns to normal. This process is known as a(n)
    A. positive feedback loop.
    B. enhanced compensatory mechanism.
    C. pathological homeopathic episode.
    D. negative feedback loop.

20. Which of the following statements is true regarding anaerobic metabolism?
    A. The cells cease to metabolize glucose.
    B. There is a marked increase in ATP production.
    C. The sodium-potassium pumps increase their rates.
    D. The cells metabolize glucose without oxygen.

21. Water makes up approximately _____ of total body weight.
    A. 30%
    B. 60%
    C. 80%
    D. none of the above

22. Where is most of this water is found?
    A. between the cells
    B. in the blood vessels
    C. in the cells
    D. none of the above

23. As we age, our total body water
    A. increases.
    B. decreases.
    C. stays the same.
    D. varies with the individual.

24. All of the following happen when your fluid levels drop **except**
    A. ADH is secreted.
    B. the kidneys reabsorb sodium.
    C. more urine is excreted.
    D. water shifts into the intravascular compartment.

25. All of the following are signs of dehydration **except**
    A. poor skin turgor.
    B. sacral edema.
    C. sunken fontanels.
    D. tachycardia.

26. Dehydrated patients should receive
    A. an isotonic solution.
    B. lactated Ringer's.
    C. normal saline.
    D. all of the above

27. A positively charged ion is called a(n)
    A. cation.
    B. anion.
    C. colloid.
    D. crystalloid.

28. The chief extracellular cation that regulates fluid distribution is
    A. bicarbonate.
    B. sodium.
    C. potassium.
    D. magnesium.

29. The chief intracellular cation that aids in electrical impulse transmission is
    A. magnesium.
    B. sodium.
    C. potassium.
    D. calcium.

30. The cation that plays a major role in muscle contraction is
    A. bicarbonate.
    B. sodium.
    C. potassium.
    D. calcium.

31. The principal buffer of the acid-base system is
    A. bicarbonate.
    B. sodium.
    C. potassium.
    D. magnesium.

32. Electrolytes are measured in
    A. mg/kg.
    B. mEq/L.
    C. mEq/dl.
    D. mcg/L.

33. The movement of water through a semipermeable membrane from an area of low solute concentration toward an area of high solute concentration is called
    A. diffusion.
    B. facilitated diffusion.
    C. active transport.
    D. osmosis.

34. Infusing a hypotonic solution into the bloodstream causes water to move
    A. into the cells.
    B. into the blood vessel.
    C. out of the cells.
    D. none of the above

35. The movement of solute particles through a semipermeable membrane from an area of high solute concentration toward an area of low solute concentration is called
    A. diffusion.
    B. facilitated diffusion.
    C. active transport.
    D. osmosis.

36. Infusing a hypertonic solution into a blood vessel will cause all of the following to happen **except**
    A. an osmotic gradient toward the vein.
    B. a fluid shift into the blood vessel.
    C. an increase in blood pressure.
    D. a decrease in intravascular blood volume.

37. A solution with the same osmolarity as blood plasma is said to be
    A. hypotonic.
    B. hypertonic.
    C. isotonic.
    D. none of the above

38. In a freshwater drowning, what happens as water enters the pulmonary capillaries?
    A. It remains in the capillaries.
    B. It quickly diffuses into the cells.
    C. It draws additional fluid into the blood vessel.
    D. none of the above

39. Sodium is transported out of the cell against the gradient in a process called
    A. facilitated diffusion.
    B. facilitated transport.
    C. passive diffusion.
    D. active transport.

40. The insulin/glucose relationship is an example of
    A. facilitated diffusion.
    B. facilitated transport.
    C. passive diffusion.
    D. active transport.

41. Oncotic force is created by _____ in the intravascular space.
    A. cations
    B. sodium ions
    C. plasma proteins
    D. potassium ions

42. Filtration is caused by
    A. oncotic force.
    B. sodium and potassium ions.
    C. plasma proteins.
    D. hydrostatic pressure.

43. Which of the following can cause tissue edema?
    A. increased oncotic force
    B. decreased hydrostatic pressure
    C. decreased capillary permeability
    D. lymphatic channel obstruction

44. Osmoreceptors are located in the _____.
    A. medulla
    B. aortic arch
    C. hypothalamus
    D. pituitary

45. The majority of blood volume consists of
    A. red blood cells.
    B. plasma.
    C. platelets.
    D. white blood cells.

46. The percentage of red blood cells in the blood is called
    A. homeostasis.
    B. hematocrit.
    C. hemoglobin.
    D. hematoma.

47. Red blood cells make up what percentage of total blood volume in the healthy adult?
    A. 20
    B. 45
    C. 55
    D. 60

48. The normal pH for the human blood is
    A. 7.0–8.0
    B. 7.35–7.45
    C. 7.3
    D. 7.5

49. The fastest mechanism for correcting the body's acid-base abnormalities is the
    A. respiratory system.
    B. renal system.
    C. buffer system.
    D. none of the above

50. A patient with a pH of 7.2 and a $PaCO_2$ of 52 torr is in a state of
    A. respiratory acidosis.
    B. respiratory alkalosis.
    C. metabolic acidosis.
    D. metabolic alkalosis.

51. A probable cause of the patient's condition in question 50 is
    A. near drowning.
    B. amphetamine drug overdose.
    C. antacid ingestion.
    D. excessive vomiting.

52. The reasons behind the pH and $PaCO_2$ abnormalities in the patient in question 50 include
    A. an increase in carbon dioxide elimination.
    B. an increase in bicarbonate concentration.
    C. a decrease in carbon dioxide retention.
    D. none of the above

53. Immediate management of the patient in question 50 with this condition includes
    A. coaching the patient to breathe slower.
    B. administering sodium bicarbonate.
    C. ventilating with positive pressure.
    D. none of the above

54. Which of the following is true regarding a patient in alkalosis?
    A. The pH is abnormally low.
    B. The hydrogen ion concentration is abnormally high.
    C. There are no bicarbonate ions present.
    D. none of the above

55. Management of a patient in respiratory alkalosis includes
    A. hyperventilating.
    B. coaching and reassuring.

C. breathing into a paper bag.
D. administering sodium bicarbonate.

56. Which of the following factors does **not** affect the heart's stroke volume?
    A. heart rate
    B. preload
    C. afterload
    D. contractile force

57. Stroke volume could be increased by all of the following **except**
    A. increasing venous return.
    B. increasing contractile force.
    C. decreasing afterload.
    D. promoting venodilation.

58. The amount of blood pumped from the heart in one contraction is called
    A. preload.
    B. afterload.
    C. stroke volume.
    D. tidal volume.

59. Which of the following statements best illustrates the Starling's law of the heart?
    A. The greater the afterload, the greater the stroke volume.
    B. The less the stroke volume, the less the afterload.
    C. The greater the preload, the greater the cardiac contractile force.
    D. The less the preload, the greater the afterload.

60. In order to decrease the workload on the heart in a patient with CHF, you should
    A. place the patient in the Trendelenberg position.
    B. administer a drug that dilates the veins.
    C. administer a fluid challenge.
    D. hyperventilate the patient.

61. The amount of blood pumped by the heart in 1 minute is called
    A. minute volume.
    B. stroke volume.
    C. cardiac output.
    D. contractile volume.

62. The amount of resistance against which the heart must pump in order to eject blood is called
    A. stroke volume.
    B. end-diastolic volume.
    C. afterload.
    D. pulse pressure.

63. Baroreceptors constantly monitor for changes in
    A. oxygen levels.
    B. carbon dioxide levels.
    C. heart rate.
    D. blood pressure.

64. A decrease in the baroreceptors' stretch causes all of the following **except**
    A. peripheral vasodilation.
    B. increased cardiac output.
    C. increased heart rate.
    D. bronchodilation.

65. Flow through a blood vessel is dependent on
    A. vessel diameter.
    B. fluid viscosity.
    C. vessel length.
    D. all of the above

66. The greatest change in peripheral resistance occurs in the
    A. aorta.
    B. arteries.
    C. arterioles.
    D. capillaries.

67. Which of the following is a component of the "Fick principle"?
    A. adequate FiO_2
    B. adequate hematocrit
    C. adequate diffusion of gases
    D. all of the above

68. Anaerobic metabolism results in which of the following?
    A. inefficient energy
    B. increased pyruvic acid formation
    C. glycolysis
    D. all of the above

69. The first stage of glucose breakdown is known as
    A. the Krebs cycle.
    B. the citric acid cycle.
    C. glycolysis.
    D. aerobic metabolism.

70. The second stage of glucose breakdown is known as
    A. the Krebs cycle.
    B. progressive metabolism.
    C. glycolysis.
    D. anaerobic metabolism.

71. Which of the following happens during the shock state?
    A. The Krebs cycle produces increased energy.
    B. Glycolysis creates pyruvic acid.
    C. Pyruvic acid degrades into lactic acid.
    D. B and C

72. Which of the following is **not** a catecholamine?
    A. norepinephrine
    B. adrenalin
    C. cortisol
    D. epinephrine

Match the following physiological effects with their respective adrenergic receptors:

73. _____ peripheral vasoconstriction

74. _____ increased heart rate

75. _____ increased diaphoresis

76. _____ bronchodilation

77. _____ increased cardiac contractions

78. _____ vasodilation

    A. alpha 1
    B. alpha 2
    C. beta 1
    D. beta 2

79. Which of the following best illustrates a major function of smooth muscle?
    A. formation of the heart
    B. maintenance of blood pressure
    C. connect bone to bone
    D. move the skeleton

80. You are assessing a patient who has been slashed with a knife on the back of the hand over the middle of the metacarpals. The wound is very deep, and the patient complains of great difficulty in moving his index and middle fingers. Which of the following structures do you suspect to be damaged?
    A. tendons
    B. ligaments
    C. cartilage
    D. ulna and radius

81. Skeletal muscles promote the primary movement of the human body through which of the following actions?
    A. relaxation
    B. voluntary stretching
    C. involuntary stretching
    D. contraction

82. Which of the following illustrates a prime function of the muscular system?
    A. provides the body with structure
    B. prevents internal fluid loss
    C. moves the skeletal bones
    D. provides for the storage of fat

83. You are assessing a 23-year-old male who states that he twisted his left knee while playing football. Assessment reveals ecchymosis and edema in the area of the injury. Which of the following choices best represents the most appropriate management of this injury?
    A. application of a pressure bandage
    B. immobilization of the extremity
    C. application of ice only
    D. transport in a position of comfort

84. Within the human body, the kidneys function to
    A. form feces.
    B. cleanse blood plasma of waste.
    C. regulate body temperature.
    D. absorb glucose from the blood.

85. A patient has been struck in the back with a baseball bat. On assessment, you note an obvious fracture to the twelfth rib along the midscapular line on the left side. Which of the following organs would you suspect may possibly be injured?
    A. bladder
    B. stomach
    C. liver
    D. kidney

86. Urine moves through the urinary system in which order?
    A. ureter, kidney, urethra, bladder
    B. kidney, urethra, bladder, ureter
    C. kidney, ureter, bladder, urethra
    D. urethra, kidney, bladder, ureter

87. Which of the following choices best describes location of the urinary bladder?
    A. pelvic cavity, posterior to the pubic bone
    B. abdominal cavity, adjacent to the gallbladder
    C. pelvic cavity, posterior to the vertebrae
    D. abdominal cavity, directly behind the umbilicus

88. Which of the following would the EMT-Intermediate be most likely to observe in acute renal failure?
    A. vomiting of blood
    B. decreased urinary output
    C. blood in the stool
    D. increased urinary output

89. The production of sperm and secretion of hormones is the function of the
    A. penis.
    B. scrotum.
    C. testes.
    D. vas deferens.

90. The primary male sex hormone is
    A. gonadtropin.
    B. testosterone.
    C. estrogen.
    D. luteinizing hormone.

91. The female reproductive structures are the ovaries, fallopian tubes, uterus, and
    A. vagina.
    B. estrogen.
    C. ova.
    D. bladder.

92. The primary female sex hormone is
    A. estrogen.
    B. testosterone.
    C. gonadotropin.
    D. luteinizing hormone.

93. Which organ is responsible for the exchange of oxygen and nutrients between maternal and fetal circulation?
    A. endometrium.
    B. vagina.
    C. uterus.
    D. placenta.

94. The endocrine organ known as the "master gland" is the
    A. pancreas.
    B. pituitary.
    C. thymus.
    D. thyroid.

95. The hormone that enhances uterine contraction and stimulates milk production in the mammary glands is
    A. follicle-stimulating hormone.
    B. human growth hormone.
    C. vasopressin.
    D. oxytocin.

96. Hormones produced by the medulla of the adrenal glands
    A. increase blood pressure by increasing heart rate and strength of contraction and constricting peripheral blood vessels.
    B. maintain blood pressure and force of contraction by slowing heart rate and dilating peripheral blood vessels.
    C. produce bronchoconstriction, increase the rate of digestion, decrease blood glucose levels, and inhibit metabolism.
    D. produce pupillary constriction, increase the rate of digestion, slow heart rate, and dilate peripheral blood vessels.

97. Which of the following pairs of hormones secreted by the pancreas work in opposition to each other?

    A. glucagon and somatostatin

    B. pancreatic polypeptide and insulin

    C. glucagon and insulin

    D. insulin and somatostatin

98. Diabetes mellitus is a common metabolic disorder that occurs as a result of

    A. excessive production of insulin.

    B. excessive production of glucagon.

    C. inadequate production of insulin.

    D. inadequate production of glucagon.

99. The chamber of the heart that receives deoxygenated blood from the body is the

    A. left atrium.

    B. right ventricle.

    C. left ventricle.

    D. right atrium.

100. The chordae tendonae are located

    A. on the ventricular side of the AV valves.

    B. on the ventricular side of the aortic and pulmonic valve.

    C. outside the epicardium, supporting the heart in the pericardial sac.

    D. on the atrial side of the mitral valve.

101. Which of the following is **not** a property of myocardial cells?

    A. conductivity

    B. reactivity

    C. automaticity

    D. contractility

102. Which of the following statements best represents blood flow through the heart?

    A. left atrium, left ventricle, lungs, right atrium, right ventricle

    B. right atrium, right ventricle, lungs, left atrium, left ventricle

    C. right atrium, left atrium, lungs, left ventricle

    D. right atrium, right ventricle, lungs, left ventricle, aorta

103. A significant increase in the heart rate above 160 beats per minute will potentially

    A. decrease cardiac output.

    B. lower oxygen requirements of the heart.

    C. increase stroke volume.

    D. result in increased coronary artery perfusion.

104. If a patient receives a medication to increase the force of myocardial contraction, this will affect primarily

    A. heart rate.

    B. stroke volume.

    C. peripheral vascular resistance.

    D. none of the above

105. The primary pacemaker of the heart is the

    A. sinoatrial node.

    B. intraatrial pathways.

    C. atrioventricular node.

    D. bundle of His.

106. Which of the following usually has no effect on heart rate?

    A. increased sympathetic tone

    B. increased parasympathetic tone

    C. lowered dopaminergic tone

    D. enhanced vagal tone

107. If a drug increases the force of ventricular contraction, it would be termed a positive _____ agent.

    A. chronotropic

    B. dromotropic

    C. inotropic

    D. isotropic

108. Which of the following heart valves would be responsible for causing pulmonary edema if it allows regurgitation of blood?

A. tricuspid

B. pulmonic

C. mitral

D. aortic

109. Which of the following organs should **not** be categorized as part of the gastrointestinal system?

A. pancreas

B. stomach

C. rectum

D. adrenal glands

110. The purpose of the pancreas is to

A. act as both an exocrine and an endocrine gland.

B. release stored glycogen back into the bloodstream.

C. produce bile for the small intestine.

D. release estrogen into the bloodstream.

111. After clearing the stomach, food passes into the

A. jejunum.

B. duodenum.

C. ileum.

D. ascending colon.

112. Food is propelled along the course of the small and large intestines by the rhythmic contraction waves known as

A. peristalsis.

B. paresis.

C. portal waves.

D. muscular intropy.

113. The role of the gallbladder is to

A. produce bile.

B. house urine until it is removed by the body.

C. store bile until needed.

D. none of the above

114. When the protective mucosal lining of the stomach is lost, the acids of the stomach start to erode the stomach wall. This is called

A. gastritis.

B. gastric ulcers.

C. diverticulitis.

D. appendicitis.

115. If a perforation were to occur in the proximal end of the small intestines, the abdominal pain would best be characterized as

A. "dull," with a gradual onset.

B. "heavy," with a rapid onset.

C. "burning," with a rapid onset.

D. "crampy," with a slow onset.

116. Organs of the abdominal cavity are catagorized as

A. hollow, solid, and movable.

B. vascular, solid, and hollow.

C. fibrous, movable, and immovable.

D. hollow, solid, and striated.

117. Rupture of which of the following abdominal structures would produce the fastest onset of hypoperfusion?

A. descending aorta

B. portal vein

C. spleen

D. liver

118. A person can live normally without which one of the following gastrointestinal organs?

A. esophagus

B. jejunum

C. kidneys

D. appendix

119. Which of the following is **not** a function of the skeletal system?

A. protection

B. support

C. mobility

D. reflexes

120. Another EMT-Intermediate tells you that a patient in a car accident has a possible fracture to the zygomatic arch. You would suspect that

A. it involves the chin.

B. the patient may also have a black eye (periorbital ecchymosis).

C. the patient will need endotracheal intubation.

D. the patient has a lower-extremity fracture.

121. Which of the following bones is **not** one found in the cranium?

A. parietal

B. temporal

C. acromion

D. frontal

122. The atlas and axis are part of

A. the vertebral column.

B. the pelvis.

C. the thoracic rib cage.

D. the ankle joint.

123. Which of the following bones is **not** known as a long bone?

A. fibula

B. femur

C. humerus

D. sacrum

124. An injury to the metacarpals may affect the ability to

A. walk.

B. write.

C. chew.

D. bend over.

125. Which of the following helps create smooth, pain-free movement?

A. articular cartilage

B. parietal fluid

C. greater omentum

D. arthroid discs

126. The vertebrae that must support the most weight are the

A. cervical.

B. thoracic.

C. lumbar.

D. coccyx.

127. With a fracture of the humerus, what blood vessel may also be damaged?

A. radial artery

B. brachial artery

C. iliac artery

D. ulnar artery

128. The thoracic ribs offer protection to all the following organs **except** the

A. lungs.

B. diaphragm.

C. heart.

D. descending aorta.

129. Which of the following is primarily responsible for preventing the collapse of the alveoli?

A. visceral pleura

B. surfactant

C. parenchyma

D. pleural fluid

130. The posterior wall of the trachea is composed of

A. cartilagenous rings.

B. branches of the terminal bronchioles.

C. lung parenchyma.

D. smooth muscle.

131. The bronchi enter the lungs at the point known as the pulmonary _____.

A. hilum

B. pleura

C. carina

D. hyoid

132. Gas exchange can occur in all of the following areas **except**

A. alveoli.

B. alveolar ducts.

C. pleura.

D. terminal bronchioles.

133. The cricothyroid membrane is located

A. inferior to the thyroid cartilage and superior to the cricoid cartilage.

B. superior to the thyroid cartilage and inferior to the hyoid bone.

C. lateral to the cricoid and posterior to the trachea.

D. inferior to the cricoid and superior to the thyroid cartilage.

134. The Hering-Breuer reflex is responsible for

A. monitoring blood flow through the pulmonary capillaries.

B. preventing overexpansion of the lungs.

C. decreasing respiratory rate due to increases in PaO_2.

D. increasing myocardial contractility.

135. The majority of carbon dioxide is transported in the blood

A. attached to hemoglobin.

B. dissolved in plasma.

C. as bicarbonate.

D. on the surface of the red blood cell.

136. Which of the following structures is primarily responsible for controlling expiration?

A. apneustic center

B. medullary chemoreceptors

C. cerebellar center

D. pneumotaxic center

137. The amount of dead space associated with ventilation in the adult male is approximately

A. 500 ml.

B. 350 ml.

C. 150 ml.

D. 50 ml.

138. You have your patient on a nonrebreather mask at 15 lpm. You estimate the percentage of oxygen to be 95%. When you call in to the hospital, medical direction asks what the FiO_2 is. Which of the following would represent the FiO_2 in this patient?

A. 95

B. 1

C. .5

D. .95

139. A patient involved in a motor vehicle crash is unable to move his right lower extremity. He can feel both pain and light touch. The structure that was most likely injured is the

A. cerebellum.

B. efferent nerve tract.

C. parasympathetic nervous system.

D. afferent nerve tract.

140. A patient faints while standing in line at the grocery store. The physician at the emergency department states that peripheral pooling caused her to faint. Which of the following is most likely responsible for the vasodilation leading to the fainting episode?

    A. efferent nerve tracts

    B. somatic nervous system

    C. vagus nerve

    D. cerebrum

141. What is acetylcholine?

    A. the primary neurotransmitter of the parasympathetic nervous system

    B. a drug used to reduce edema in a spinal cord injured patient

    C. the substance found postganglionically in the sympathetic nervous system

    D. a substance that increases the heart rate and contraction

142. A patient has apparently suffered a head injury. He has no fine motor coordination and is unable to maintain a posture. He most likely injured the

    A. cerebrum.

    B. medulla oblongata.

    C. mesencephalon.

    D. cerebellum.

143. A patient has a fixed and dilated pupil. He most likely has an injury to which cranial nerve?

    A. first

    B. third

    C. fifth

    D. tenth

144. A hematoma that forms above the outer most layer of the meninges and below the skull is known as a(n)

    A. subarachnoid hematoma.

    B. epidural hematoma.

    C. subdural hematoma.

    D. intracerebral hematoma.

145. A person who was struck in the head has difficulty speaking. He has most likely suffered an injury to what portion of the brain?

    A. occipital lobe

    B. frontal lobe

    C. parietal lobe

    D. temporal lobe

146. The patient suffering from hypoglycemia typically presents with tachycardia; pale, cool, and clammy skin; and anxiousness. This is most likely caused by stimulation of the

    A. parasympathetic nervous system.

    B. cerebellum.

    C. sympathetic nervous system.

    D. cerebrum.

147. Which part of the brain houses the hypothalamus?

    A. cerebrum

    B. diencephalon

    C. mesencephalon

    D. medulla

148. Which of the following responses would result from stimulation of an adrenergic fiber?

    A. decreased heart rate

    B. constricted pupil

    C. increase in gastric motility

    D. vasoconstriction

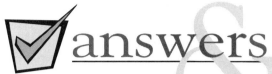

answers & rationales

Following each rationale, you will find a reference to the corresponding objective in the DOT National Standard EMT-Intermediate curriculum. An asterisk denotes material that is supplemental to the DOT curriculum. Page numbers after a rationale indicate where the question topic may be discussed in the Brady text *Intermediate Emergency Care* (Bledsoe, Porter, Cherry).

1.

D. The basic unit of life is the cell. It contains all the necessary components to turn essential nutrients into energy and to carry on essential life functions. (1-2.2) (IEC p. 83)

2.

D. The three main components of a cell are the cell membrane (semipermeable outer covering), the cytoplasm (thick, viscous fluid), and the organelles (inner structures). (1-2.2) (IEC p. 84)

Matching (1-2.2) (IEC pp. 84–85, 106)

3.   F   nucleus
4.   C   cytosol
5.   B   golgi
6.   E   mitochondrion
7.   G   lysosome
8.   D   peroxisome
9.   A   phagocyte

10.

A. The cell membrane is a semipermeable structure that surrounds the cell and protects it from the outer environment. (1-2.2) (IEC p. 84)

11.

D. Epithelial tissue lines body surfaces and protects the body. Certain types of epithelial tissue perform specialized functions, such as secretion, absorption, diffusion, and filtration. (1-2.12) (IEC p. 85)

12.

A. Cardiac muscle tissue is found only within the heart. It has the unique capability of spontaneous contraction without external stimulation. This property is called automaticity. (1-2.12) (IEC p. 85)

13.

C. Connective tissue is the most abundant tissue in the body. It provides support, connection, and insulation. (1-2.12) (IEC p. 86)

14.

C. The type of muscle found in the inner lining of hollow organs, such as the intestines, airways, and blood vessels, is called smooth muscle. It is generally under the control of the involuntary or autonomic component of the central nervous system. (1-2.18) (IEC p. 86)

15.

D. The natural tendency of the body to maintain a constant, stable internal environment is called homeostasis. The EMT-Intermediate should understand this process in order to recognize how the body attempts to correct underlying problems. (1-2.3) (IEC p. 87)

16.

B. Endocrine glands are ductless and secrete their hormones directly into the circulatory system. Examples include the pancreas, pituitary gland, thyroid, parathyroid, adrenal gland, and gonads. Glands that release their secretion into the epithelial surfaces of the body are called exocrine glands. Examples of these secretions are mucus, sweat, and saliva. (1-2.27) (IEC p. 87)

17.

C. As the name suggests, chemoreceptors respond to changes in chemistry. Our chemoreceptors, located in the medulla, the carotid arteries, and the aortic arch, sense changes in pH, PO_2, and PCO_2. (1-2.58) (IEC p. 87)

18.

A. As the name suggests, baroreceptors respond to changes in pressure in our circulatory system. They are located in the carotid sinus and the aortic arch. They are stretch-sensitive receptors that stretch with increased pressure in the blood vessel. (1-2.49) (IEC p. 87)

19.

D. A negative feedback loop occurs when the body attempts to reverse, or compensate for, a pathophysiological process. In this example, the body tries to increase blood pressure through a series of compensatory mechanisms until the pressure returns to normal, similar to a thermostat that triggers the furnace to turn on when the temperature drops below your setting. (1-2.49) (IEC p. 88)

20.

D. During anaerobic metabolism, the cells continue to do their jobs but without an adequate oxygen supply. The result is a marked decrease in ATP production and an increase of harmful acids. If oxygen is applied in time, the condition is reversible. If not, it is irreversible, and cell death is imminent. (1-2.64) (IEC p. 647)

21.

B. Water is the most abundant substance in the human body. In fact, it accounts for approximately 60% of total body weight. (1-2.62) (IEC p. 89)

22.

C. Approximately 75% of total body water (TBW) is found within the intracellular compartment. This compartment is found inside the body's cells. Refer to the following chart. (1-2.60) (IEC p. 89)

Compartment	Percentage of TBW	Volume in 70-kg Adult
Intracellular fluid	75.0	31.50 L
Extracellular fluid	25.0	10.50 L
Interstitial fluid	17.5	7.35 L
Intravascular fluid	7.5	3.15 L

23.

B. As we age, our TBW decreases. Refer to the following chart. (1-2.62) (IEC p. 904)

Age	TBW
Infant	75–80%
1 year	70–75%
Late childhood	65–70%
Early adulthood	65–70% males
	60–65% females
Late adulthood	45–55%

24.

C. When your fluid levels drop, the pituitary gland at the base of the brain secrets ADH, or antidiuretic hormone. ADH causes the kidneys to reabsorb more water back into the bloodstream and excrete less urine. (1-2.65) (IEC p. 91)

25.

B. Clinically, the dehydrated patient exhibits dry mucous membranes and poor skin turgor. As the dehydration becomes more severe, the pulse will quicken, and the blood pressure will drop. In infants, the anterior fontanel may be sunken. (1-2.62) (IEC p. 92)

26.

D. Treatment for dehydration is fluid replacement. Since you cannot determine electrolyte deficits in the field, you should use isotonic solutions, such as normal saline or lactated Ringer's. For mild to moderate dehydration, run the infusion at 100–200 ml per hour. (1-2.62) (IEC p. 92)

27.

A. Electrolytes are substances that dissociate into charged particles when placed in water. Ions with a positive charge are called cations. (1-2.62) (IEC p. 93)

28.

B. Sodium is the most prevalent cation in the extracellular fluid. It plays a major role in regulating the distribution of water. (1-2.63) (IEC p. 94)

29.

C. Potassium is the most prevalent cation in the intracellular fluid. It plays an important role in the transmission of electrical impulses. (1-2.63) (IEC p. 94)

30.

D. Calcium has many physiological functions. It plays a major role in muscular contraction as well as nerve impulse transmission. (1-2.63) (IEC p. 94)

31.

A. Bicarbonate is the principal buffer of the body. It neutralizes the highly acidic hydrogen ion and other organic acids. (1-2.63) (IEC p. 94)

32.

B. Electrolytes are usually measured in milliequivalents per liter (mEq/L). (1-2.63) (IEC p. 94)

33.

D. Osmosis is the movement of water across a semipermeable membrane from an area of lesser solute concentration to an area of greater solute concentration. This movement occurs until the solute concentrations on both sides are equal. (1-2.9) (IEC p. 95)

34.

A. Infusing a hypotonic solution into the bloodstream causes water to move from the bloodstream into the cells. This occurs because water tends to move from areas of low solute concentration, which in this case will be the bloodstream, toward areas of higher solute concentration, which in this case will be the interstitial spaces and cells. (1-2.61) (IEC pp. 94–95)

35.

A. Diffusion is the movement of solutes from an area of greater concentration to an area of lesser concentration. This movement occurs until the solute concentrations on both sides are equal. (1-2.9) (IEC p. 95)

36.

D. Infusing a hypertonic solution into a blood vessel will cause an osmotic gradient, which shifts water into the blood vessel. This will cause an increase in blood pressure. (1-2.61) (IEC pp. 94–95)

37.

C. A solution with the same osmolarity as blood plasma is isotonic. Isotonicity is a state in which solutions on opposite sides of a semipermeable membrane have equal concentrations. (1-2.61) (IEC p. 94)

38.

B. In a freshwater drowning, water enters the pulmonary capillaries and quickly diffuses into the cells. This occurs because freshwater is hypotonic. (1-2.61) (IEC p. 1073)

39.

D. Sodium is transported out of the cell by a process called active transport. Active transport is a biochemical process in which substances use energy to move across the cell membrane against the normal gradient. Active transport is faster than diffusion, but it requires the expenditure of energy. (1-2.9) (IEC p. 95)

40.

A. The insulin/glucose relationship is an example of facilitated diffusion. Facilitated diffusion is a biochemical process in which a substance is selectively transported across a membrane using helper proteins and requires energy. (1-2.9) (IEC p. 96)

41.

C. Oncotic force or pressure is caused by the presence of plasma proteins in the blood, which make the blood hypertonic and draw water into the bloodstream. This is the principal force that returns water to the blood from the capillary beds following cellular respiration. (1-2.61) (IEC p. 97)

42.

D. While oncotic force pulls water into the intravascular space, hydrostatic pressure forces water out. This process, known as filtration, is caused by the pressure increase in the arteries during systole. Normally, these opposing processes equal out. When they do not, the result is tissue edema or poor turgor. (1-2.61) (IEC p. 97)

43.

D. Tissue edema is caused by an increase in hydrostatic pressure, a decrease in oncotic force, increased capillary permeability, or a blocked lymph channel. In these cases, water remains in the interstitial spaces and cannot be absorbed into circulation. (1-2.61) (IEC p. 97)

44.

C. Osmoreceptors, located in the hypothalamus, monitor for changes in the osmolarity of the blood. When the blood has less fluid, the osmoreceptors stimulate the release of antidiuretic hormone (ADH), which stimulates water reabsorption in the kidneys. (1-2.65)

45.

B. Plasma makes up approximately 55% of the total blood volume. It consists of 92% water, 6–7% proteins, and a small portion containing electrolytes, lipids, enzymes, clotting factors, glucose, and other dissolved substances. (1-2.31) (IEC p. 104)

46.

B. The percentage of blood occupied by red blood cells is referred to as the hematocrit. Normal hematocrit in the healthy person is approximately 45%. (1-2.31) (IEC p. 106)

47.

B. Red blood cells account for approximately 45% of the total blood volume. This percentage is known as the patient's hematocrit. (1-2.31) (IEC p. 106)

48.

B. The normal pH for the human blood is 7.35–7.45. (1-2.66) (IEC p. 97)

49.

C. There are three major mechanisms to remove acids from the body. The fastest mechanism is often referred to as the buffer system, or the bicarbonate buffer system. This system works in seconds. (1-2.63) (IEC p. 98)

50.

A. A patient with a pH of 7.2 and a $PaCO_2$ of 52 torr is in a state of respiratory acidosis. (1-2.66)

51.

A. A probable cause of this patient's condition could be a near drowning. Respiratory acidosis is caused by the retention of carbon dioxide. This can result from impaired ventilation due to problems occurring in either the lungs or the respiratory center of the brain. (1-2.64) (IEC p. 1072)

52.

D. The reasons behind this patient's pH and $PaCO_2$ levels include a decrease in carbon dioxide elimination and an increase in carbon dioxide retention. (1-2.64) (IEC p. 100)

53.

C. Immediate management of the patient in respiratory acidosis is aimed at improving ventilation and oxygenation. Vigorously ventilate this patient with positive pressure and 100% oxygen. (1-2.64)

54.

D. Alkalosis is a state in which the patient's hydrogen ion concentration is abnormally low and the pH high. (1-2.66) (IEC p. 97)

55.

B. Management of a patient in respiratory alkalosis is aimed at helping the patient retain carbon dioxide. Respiratory alkalosis results from the excessive elimination of carbon dioxide. This can occur with anxiety or after climbing to a high altitude. It can also occur as a compensatory mechanism in shock and a variety of other serious hypoxic conditions. For this reason, withholding oxygen from this patient could prove to be a fatal mistake. Simply place your patient on a rebreather mask with 10–15 lpm of oxygen flow and coach him to breathe slowly. (1-2.64)

56.

A. The amount of blood ejected by the heart at one contraction is referred to as the stroke volume. Stroke volume is determined by preload, afterload, and contractile force. (1-2.53) (IEC p. 196)

57.

D. Stroke volume could be increased by increasing the venous return, by increasing the contractile force of the heart, and by decreasing the afterload. (1-2.42) (IEC pp. 196–197)

58.

C. The amount of blood pumped from the heart in one contraction is called stroke volume. It is measured in ml. Normal stroke volume in the healthy adult at rest is 60–100 ml. (1-2.42) (IEC p. 196)

59.

C. The greater the volume of the preload is, the more the ventricles are stretched. The greater the stretch, up to a certain point, the greater the subsequent cardiac contraction. This is referred to as the Starling's law of the heart. It is also called the Frank Starling mechanism in honor of the physiologists Frank and Starling who identified the mechanism. (1-2.42) (IEC p. 197)

60.

B. For a patient in severe congestive heart failure (CHF), you want to decrease the workload on the heart by decreasing preload. You could accomplish this by administering drugs such as nitroglycerin and furosemide, which dilate the veins. Dilating the veins causes pooling of blood on the venous side and decreases preload. (1-2.42) (IEC pp. 197–198)

61.

C. The amount of blood pumped by the heart in 1 minute is called cardiac output. Cardiac output is calculated by stroke volume times heart rate. (1-2.42) (IEC p. 198)

62.

C. The amount of resistance against which the heart must pump is called afterload. The heart must overcome this resistance in order to eject blood. Afterload is determined by the degree of peripheral vascular resistance. Peripheral resistance is determined by the degree of vasoconstriction present on the arterial side. (1-2.42) (IEC p. 197)

63.

D. Baroreceptors are located in the carotid bodies and the arch of the aorta. These stretch receptors closely monitor blood pressure by the amount of stretch. (1-2.49) (IEC p. 198)

64.

A. Baroreceptors are stretch receptors that stretch with increased pressure. When they detect reduced flow and pressure, they send messages to the brain to stimulate the sympathetic nervous system. This results in increased heart rate and cardiac output to increase circulation and bronchodilation. (1-2.42) (IEC p. 198)

65.

D. Blood flow through a blood vessel is determined by peripheral resistance and pressure within the system. Peripheral resistance is defined as resistance to blood flow and is dependent on three factors: the length of the vessel, the diameter of the vessel, and blood viscosity. (1-2.44) (IEC p. 198)

66.

C. There is very little resistance to blood flow through the aorta and arteries. A significant change in peripheral resistance occurs at the arteriole level. This is because the inside diameter of the arteriole is much smaller compared to the aorta and arteries. Additionally, the arteriole has a pronounced ability to change its diameter as much as fivefold in response to local tissue needs and autonomic nervous system signals. (1-2.44) (IEC p. 199)

67.

D. The movement and utilization of oxygen in the body depend on the following conditions: an adequate concentration of inspired oxygen, appropriate movement of oxygen across the alveolar-capillary membrane into the bloodstream, an adequate number of red blood cells to carry the oxygen, proper tissue perfusion, and efficient off-loading of oxygen at the tissue level. These conditions are collectively known as the Fick principle. (1-2.56, 1-2.57) (IEC pp. 199–200)

68.

D. During periods of inadequate tissue perfusion, cell metabolism switches from an aerobic to an anaerobic mode. Results of this process are inefficient energy, an increase in pyruvic acid formation, and glycolysis. (1-2.11) (IEC p. 647)

69.

C. The first stage of glucose breakdown is known as glycolysis, which does not require oxygen and creates pyruvic acid. This stage is anaerobic. (1-2.11)

70.

A. The second stage of glucose metabolism is the Krebs cycle. During this stage, oxygen degrades the pyruvic acid into carbon dioxide and water and releases energy in the form of ATP (adenosine triphosphate). (1-2.11)

71.

D. During the shock state, the absence of oxygen for cellular metabolism results in glycolysis, which creates pyruvic acid. The pyruvic acid degrades into lactic acid, reducing oxygen transport by red blood cells and furthering cell hypoxia. (1-2.11)

72.

C. The hormones epinephrine (adrenalin) and norepinephrine (noradrenalin) are known as catecholamines. Catecholamines stimulate the alpha and beta receptors of the sympathetic nervous system. (1-2.30) (IEC pp. 188, 197)

Matching (1-2.30) (IEC p. 171)

73. **A** Peripheral vasoconstriction
74. **C** Increased heart rate
75. **A** Increased diaphoresis
76. **D** Bronchodilation
77. **C** Increased cardiac contractions
78. **D** Vasodilation

79.

B. Smooth muscle is contained within many internal organs. Through contraction, smooth muscle can bring about changes in size (pupils) or promote movement (digestion). Smooth muscle is found in the arterioles and functions to change the size of the lumen and thus regulates blood pressure. When the smooth muscle contracts, the lumen decreases in size and the blood pressure increases. Conversely, when the lumen increase in size, the blood pressure is decreased. The structure of the heart is formed by cardiac muscle. Ligaments are responsible for connecting bone to bone.

Skeletal muscle is responsible for promoting the movement of the skeleton, not smooth muscle. (1-2.18) (IEC p. 130)

80.

A. In light of the mechanism, location, and complaint of difficulty in moving the fingers, the EMT-Intermediate should consider a possible injury to the tendons that link the phalanges to the muscles in the forearm. Tendons connect muscle to bone. If the tendons on the back of the hand are severed, the link that provides for finger movement is greatly diminished or lost altogether. Ligaments join bone to bone at joints. (1-2.17) (IEC p. 133)

81.

D. For skeletal muscle to facilitate movement, the individual muscle fibers must contract. When muscle fibers contract, they shorten and exert a pulling motion, thereby initiating movement. Skeletal muscles cannot promote movement by a pushing motion, for when they push, relaxation occurs. (1-2.18) (IEC p. 130)

82.

C. A prime function of the human muscular system is to provide movement via the manipulation of the skeletal bones. The bones do not move themselves but rely on the skeletal muscles. Therefore, the skeletal system provides the body with structure, and the muscular system provides the movement. Internal fluid loss is more a function of the skin rather than the skeletal muscle, and fat is stored by adipose tissue and not the actual muscle cells. (1-2.17) (IEC pp. 130, 133)

83.

B. Because field distinguishment of strains, sprains, dislocation, and fractures is difficult, appropriate EMT-Intermediate treatment would include the "worst-case scenario," assumption of a fracture and subsequent immobilization. Immobilizing a knee in the position found can effectively be accomplished with a vacuum splint or a soft splint such as a pillow and tape. In this situation, compression bandages are ill advised in that they do not allow for outward expansion of edema. Restricting this naturally occurring injury response could cause inward compression of blood vessels and nerve fibers and a general worsening of the situation. Application of ice is appropriate in the management of the edema but does not represent overall best choice since the injury demands immobilization also. The same holds true for transporting in a position of comfort. (*)

84.

B. Within the human body, the kidneys serve to cleanse waste products from the blood. The hypothalamus regulates body temperature, while glucose absorption and feces production generally occur in the gastrointestinal system. (1-2.59, 1-2.62) (IEC p. 221)

85.

D. Based on anatomical location, the EMT-Intermediate must suspect possible damage to the left kidney. The kidneys are located in the retroperitoneal cavity between the twelfth thoracic and third lumbar vertebrae. Any blunt trauma to the back with an associated rib fracture must raise the index of suspicion as to kidney involvement. The bladder is located in the pelvic cavity and would not be affected by a blow to the back. Also, the liver is located on the right side of the peritoneal cavity, not the left. The stomach is also located in the peritoneal cavity but in front of the kidneys. (1-2.6) (IEC p. 218)

86.

C. From the internal to external environment, urine must pass through the kidney, ureter, bladder, and urethra. (1-2.62) (IEC p. 219)

87.

A. The urinary bladder is located low in the pelvic cavity, directly behind the pubic bone. The vertebral column lies posterior to the bladder. The urinary bladder is not located in the abdominal cavity. (1-2.6) (IEC p. 219)

88.

B. Kidneys facilitate the formation of urine. Acute renal failure would cause a decrease in the formation and output of urine. An increase in urinary output would not be noted. Vomiting of blood and blood in the stool arise from the intestinal tract and are not directly related to acute renal failure. (1-2.63) (IEC p. 221)

89.

C. In the male reproductive system, the testes are responsible for the production of sperm and the secretion of hormones. (*) (IEC p. 230)

90.

B. Testosterone is synthesized from cholesterol in the testes and is the primary hormone of the male reproductive system. (*)

91.

A. The female reproductive structures are the ovaries, fallopian tubes, uterus, and vagina. (*) (IEC p. 224)

92.

A. The primary female sex hormone is estrogen. (1-2.28) (IEC p. 228)

93.

D. The placenta is the organ responsible for the exchange of oxygen and nutrients between maternal and fetal circulation. (*)

94.

B. The pituitary gland is the endocrine organ known as the "master gland" because it secretes several hormones that control other endocrine glands. (1-2.27) (IEC p. 178)

95.

D. Oxytocin is the hormone that enhances uterine contraction and stimulates milk production in the mammary glands. It is secreted by the posterior pituitary gland. (1-2.28) (IEC p. 178)

96.

A. Epinephrine and norepinephrine are sympathomimetic hormones produced by the medulla of the adrenal glands. Their effects include increasing blood pressure by increasing heart rate, increasing strength of contraction, and constricting peripheral blood vessels. (1-2.30) (IEC p. 181)

97.

C. Although the interactions of the pancreatic hormones are not completely understood, glucagon and insulin work in opposition to each other. Glucagon increases the blood glucose level by releasing glucose stores in the liver, while insulin decreases it by aiding its entry into the cells. (1-2.29) (IEC p. 180)

98.

C. Inadequate production of insulin causes diabetes mellitus. It is a common metabolic disorder leading to a chronic elevation in blood glucose levels. (1-2.29) (IEC p. 949)

99.

D. The right atrium receives deoxygenated blood from the body by way of the superior and inferior vena cava. The blood is then moved to the right ventricle by atrial contraction and gravity. The right ventricle perfuses the blood through the lungs for oxygenation. After being received by the left atrium and delivered to the left ventricle, it is pumped to the body. (1-2.47) (IEC p. 186)

100.

A. Chordae tendonae are fibrous structures that are attached to papillary muscles in the ventricles. Their purpose is to prevent regurgitation of blood into the atria that would occur if the AV valves were allowed to invert during ventricular contraction. There are no such structures in the atria or on the semilunar valves. (1-2.37) (IEC p. 185)

101.

B. The cardiac cells have four special properties that are unique to the cells of the heart. These properties are conductivity, the ability to propagate an electrical impulse from cell to cell; automaticity, the ability to initiate its own impulse; contractility, the ability to contract when stimulated; and excitability, the ability to respond to an impulse. (1-2.18, 1-2.39) (IEC p. 192)

102.

B. Blood flow through the heart starts at the right atrium and then proceeds through the right ventricle and pulmonary arteries to the lungs. Blood returns from the lungs via the pulmonary veins and enters the left atrium, which delivers it to the left ventricle and then to the aorta. (1-2.39) (IEC p. 186)

103.

A. The heart uses the diastole phase for filling, which in turn provides the preload for the ventricles. In situations of extreme tachycardia, the diastolic period is so short that there is ineffective filling, which subsequently drops ventricular stroke volume. The increased heart rate will increase O_2 requirements of the heart and diminish coronary artery perfusion since they are perfused during the diastolic phase. (1-2.42) (IEC p. 860)

104.

B. A drug that makes the heart contract more forcefully, also known as a positive inotropic agent, will increase the stroke volume of the heart. This increase in stroke volume also increases cardiac output. To increase the rate, one would have to administer a sympathomimetic or parasympatholytic. An increase in systemic vascular resistance is achieved by giving an alpha-stimulating drug. (1-2.42) (IEC pp. 189, 197-198)

105.

A. The primary pacemaker of the heart is the sinoatrial, or SA, node. It has an intrinsic

discharge rate of 60 to 100 beats per minute. The intraatrial pathways only distribute the discharge wave for uniform atrial contraction. The AV node is the secondary pacemaker with a discharge rate of 40 to 60 beats per minute. The bundle of His transmits the impulse from the AV node to the bundle branches. (1-2.39) (IEC p. 192)

106.

C. Dopaminergic receptors are in the renal vessels and mesenteric vasculature. Stimulation or blockage of these sites will influence the degree of constriction or dilation they experience. Influencing either the sympathetic or the parasympathetic (vagal) nervous system will alter the heart rate. (1-2.43) (IEC p. 171)

107.

C. Inotropic agents increase the force of contraction in the ventricles. A positive dromotropic agent increases conduction velocity, and a chronotropic agent increases heart rate. Isotropic is a fabricated term. (1-2.43) (IEC p. 189)

108.

C. The mitral valve, also known as the bicuspid valve, is located between the left ventricle and left atrium. It is under the greatest amount of strain caused by pressures generated during left-ventricular contraction. In some patients, this valve progressively fails, allowing regurgitation of blood into the left atrium, increasing hydrostatic pressure in the pulmonary veins and eventually leading to pulmonary edema. (1-2.37) (IEC p. 185)

109.

D. The adrenal glands sit atop each kidney and release hormones into the bloodstream from autonomic stimulation. The pancreas secretes certain digestive enzymes. The stomach helps with the digestion of food. The rectum is part of the distal GI tract leading to elimination of fecal material from the body. (1-2.59) (IEC pp. 216–218)

110.

A. The pancreas is a gland with two major purposes. It creates hormones for the body to help regulate glucose levels (endocrine role), and it also produces digestive enzymes for the body (exocrine role). The liver stores glycogen, not the pancreas, and bile is produced by the liver. Estrogen is a female hormone secreted by the ovaries. (1-2.29) (IEC p. 180)

111.

B. From the stomach, food passes into the small intestine for continued digestion and absorption of necessary contents. The small intestine is comprised of three parts (in order): duodenum, jejunum, and ileum. The ascending colon is a portion of the large intestine. (1-2.59) (IEC pp. 216–217)

112.

A. The wavelike contractions that result in the propulsion of food through the alimentary tract are known as peristalsis. Paresis is weakness of voluntary muscle, and portal waves does not mean anything. Muscular intropy would refer to stimulation or contraction of a muscle. (1-2.59) (IEC p. 216)

113.

C. The gallbladder is located inferior to the liver and stores bile created by the liver. The urinary bladder stores urine until it is eliminated from the body. (1-2.59) (IEC p. 218)

114.

B. Gastric ulceration occurs when the hydrochloric acid of the stomach erodes the mucosal lining of the stomach wall. This can be severe enough to cause gastric hemorrhaging. Gastritis may present with similar discomfort as gastric ulceration, but it refers specifically to inflammation of the mucosal lining. Diverticulitis is an inward pouching of intestinal tissue, usually located in the large intestine, and is a common cause of hematochezia. (1-2.59) (IEC pp. 216, 1040–1041)

115.

C. The small intestine is usually acidic because of the hydrochloric acid that comes from the stomach during the digestion process. If perforation should occur, the low pH of the contents usually causes immediate pain of a burning characteristic as the acid acts on the other abdominal structures. (1-2.59) (IEC p. 1037)

116.

B. Organs of the abdominal cavity can be categorized into hollow organs (stomach, intestines, gallbladder, etc.), solid organs (spleen, liver, pancreas), or vascular organs (vena cava, aorta). This categorization is useful because organs in the same category typically have similar presentations should an injury occur. (1-2.6) (IEC pp. 213–214, 634)

117.

A. The descending aorta, also called the abdominal aorta, is a vascular structure that provides arterial blood to the abdominal organs and lower extremities. Should a rupture occur, it can cause massive hemorrhaging, as the blood will exit the aorta under systolic pressure. This will produce the fastest onset of hypoperfusion of the structures listed. (1-2.6) (IEC p. 214)

118.

D. The appendix is a structure located at the junction of the small and large intestine in the right lower quadrant. It is not uncommon for it to be removed when it ruptures or becomes inflamed, and it has no effect on quality of life. (1-2.6) (IEC pp. 1037–1038)

119.

D. The skeletal system provides three very important functions: support, protection to organs within certain cavities (e.g., the cranium or thoracic cavity), and motion in conjunction with muscles. It does not play a role in reflex arcs. These are a function of the nervous system. (1-2.14) (IEC p. 113)

120.

B. The zygomatic arch is commonly known as the cheekbone. Given its location, a fracture of the zygomatic arch may also result in small hemorrhages into the soft tissue around the eye and result in a black eye. The bone in the chin is known as the mandible. Intubation needs and lower-extremity findings may be present if it is significant

trauma but is not dependent on zygomatic fractures. (1-2.14) (IEC pp. 135–139)

121.

C. The cranium is created by the fusion of numerous bones. The major bones are the frontal bone, the temporal bones, the occipital bone, and the parietal bones. The acromion is the process located at the junction of the scapula and clavicle. (1-2.14) (IEC p. 135)

122.

A. The atlas is the first cervical vertebra, and it supports the skull. It allows the rotation movement characteristic to the head. The second cervical vertebra is known as the axis, and it has a protrusion, the ondontoid process, which projects into the atlas and allows the vertebrae to remain aligned. Both are part of the vertebral column. (1-2.14) (IEC p. 148)

123.

D. The sacrum is a bone that is part of the pelvic structure and is considered to be an irregular bone. The other three bones are considered long bones. (1-2.15) (IEC p. 115)

124.

B. Metacarpals are the smaller bones of the hands. An injury here would most likely result in an inability to use the fingers or to write. The metatarsals are small foot bones, injury of which could cause an inability to walk. Damage to the mandible can cause an inability to chew. Vertebral damage could result in an inability to bend over. (1-2.14) (IEC p. 118)

125.

A. The articular surface is a smooth cartilage that overlays the point where two bones move over each other. This greatly reduces friction and pain associated with bones rubbing. Synovial fluid is a lubricating fluid present in the joint capsules. The greater omentum is a lining in the abdominal cavity that helps protect the abdominal contents. (1-2.14) (IEC p. 116)

126.

C. The lumbar vertebrae have the largest body section, which is the portion that supports weight. (1-2.14) (IEC p. 150)

127.

B. The brachial artery travels along the humerus. Alongside every bone is a nerve, artery, and vein. In most locations in the body, the name of the bone is also the name of the artery; for example, the radial artery runs alongside the radius. (1-2.47) (IEC p. 194)

128.

D. The sternum, ribs, and thoracic vertebrae provide protection to the lungs, heart, and diaphragm along with other thoracic structures. They do not, however, protect the descending aorta since it travels through the abdominal cavity—beyond the level of the ribs. (1-2.14) (IEC pp. 151–153)

129.

B. Surfactant is a lipoprotein that decreases the surface tension of the alveoli and prevents collapse. (1-2.53) (IEC p. 205)

130.

D. The posterior wall of the trachea is comprised only of smooth muscle. The anterior and lateral aspects are supported by cartilagenous structures. (1-2.18) (IEC p. 204)

131.

A. The pulmonary hilum is the point where the bronchi enter the lungs. (1-2.18) (IEC p. 204)

132.

C. Gas exchange will occur primarily in the alveoli; however, minimal exchange may occur in the alveolar ducts and terminal bronchioles. No gas exchange occurs in the pleura. (1-2.56, I-2.57) (IEC p. 204)

133.

A. The cricothyroid membrane is located inferior to the thyroid cartilage and superior to the cricoid cartilage. (1-2.5) (IEC p. 203)

134.

B. The Hering-Breuer reflex is responsible for preventing overexpansion of the lungs. Stretch fibers located in the lungs send impulses to the medulla to regulate the volume of air taken into the lungs. (1-2.58) (IEC p. 211)

135.

C. About 66% of the circulating carbon dioxide is transported in the form of bicarbonate (HCO_3). To a much lesser extent, CO_2 is transported dissolved in plasma and attached to hemoglobin. (1-2.57) (IEC p. 210)

136.

D. The pneumotaxic center, located in the pons, is responsible for controlling expiration. The apneustic center, also located in the pons, is the backup to stimulate breathing if the respiratory center in the medulla should fail. (1-2.58) (IEC p. 211)

137.

C. The amount of dead space associated with ventilation is about 150 ml in the adult male patient. Thus, 350 ml of the typical tidal volume of 500 ml are used in gas exchange. (1-2.55) (IEC p. 212)

138.

D. FiO_2 is the fraction of inspired oxygen. The FiO_2 is 0.95 if the patient is breathing in 95% oxygen. An FiO_2 of 1.0 represents a patient breathing 100% oxygen. (1-2.57) (IEC p. 210)

139.

B. Efferent nerve tracts transmit impulses from the brain to muscle and control motor function. (1-2.19) (IEC p. 156)

140.

C. The parasympathetic nervous system affects vasodilation. About 75% of the parasympathetic nervous impulses are carried by the vagus nerve. (1-2.19) (IEC pp. 155, 1029)

141.

A. Acetylcholine is the neurotransmitter of the parasympathetic nervous system. The neurotransmitter of the sympathetic nervous system is norepinephrine. (1-2.23) (IEC p. 172)

142.

D. The cerebellum is responsible for controlling fine motor movement, coordination, posture, and equilibrium. (1-2.24) (IEC p. 160)

143.

B. The third cranial nerve (occulomotor nerve) controls the pupillary response. (1-2.26) (IEC p. 167)

144.

B. The space between the dura mater, the outermost layer of the meninges, and the skull is called the epidural space. A collection of blood in this space is called an epidural hematoma. (1-2.25) (IEC p. 158)

145.

D. The temporal lobe area controls speech. The parietal lobe controls sensory function, the occipital lobe controls vision, and the frontal lobe controls personality and motor function. (1-2.24) (IEC p. 160)

146.

C. The sympathetic nervous system, known as the "fight or flight" response, will increase heart rate and cause the skin to become pale, cool, and clammy in the hypoglycemic patient. This is a response from the secretion and circulation of epinephrine. (1-2.26) (IEC pp. 168–171)

147.

B. The hypothalamus, thalamus, and limbic system are all housed in the diencephalon. (1-2.24) (IEC p. 160)

148.

D. An adrenergic fiber is usually associated with the sympathetic nervous system. Vasoconstriction is a sympathetic nervous system response. (1-2.26) (IEC p. 171)

UNIT

3 Emergency Pharmacology

unit objectives

Questions in this unit relate to DOT objectives 1-3.1 to 1-3.19. The objectives are listed in the Appendix.

DIRECTIONS Each of the questions or incomplete statements below is followed by suggested answers or completions. Select the **one answer** that is best in each case.

1. Furosemide and diazepam are examples of
   A. chemical names.
   B. trade names.
   C. brand names.
   D. generic names.

2. Lasix® and Valium® are examples of
   A. trade names.
   B. chemical names.
   C. official names.
   D. generic names.

3. Atropine and digitalis are examples of drugs derived from
   A. plants.
   B. minerals.
   C. animals.
   D. synthetics.

4. Insulin is an example of a drug derived from
   A. plants.
   B. minerals.
   C. animals.
   D. synthetics.

5. Calcium chloride and magnesium sulfate are examples of drugs derived from
   A. plants.
   B. minerals.
   C. animals.
   D. synthetics.

6. The first drug legislation in the United States was the
   A. Narcotics Act.
   B. Pure Food and Drug Act.
   C. Federal Food, Drug, and Cosmetic Act.
   D. Durham-Humphrey Amendment.

7. The Federal Food, Drug, and Cosmetic Act of 1938 requires that
   A. all ingredients be placed on the label.
   B. all opium by-products be classified according to schedules.
   C. all prescriptions be filled within 72 hours.
   D. all of the above

8. The Harrison Narcotic Act of 1915 regulates the sale of
   A. cocaine.
   B. morphine.
   C. all drugs.
   D. barbiturates and amphetamines.

9. The Controlled Substances Act of 1970 establishes
   A. schedules for abusive drugs.
   B. time limits for filling prescriptions.
   C. prohibitions on refills for classified drugs.
   D. all of the above

10. Examples of Schedule I drugs, which have a high abuse potential and no medically acceptable medical indications, are
    A. diazepam and methadone.
    B. heroin and LSD.
    C. Vicodin and phenobarbital.
    D. cocaine and opium.

11. Examples of Schedule II drugs, which have a high abuse potential but accepted medical indications, are
    A. mescaline and lorazepam.
    B. heroin and codeine.
    C. cocaine and morphine.
    D. diazepam and phenobarbital.

12. Examples of Schedule III drugs, which have a lower abuse potential than Schedule I and II drugs and have accepted medical indications, are
    A. Vicodin and Tylenol with codeine.
    B. heroin and morphine.
    C. diazepam and lorazepam.
    D. none of the above

13. Examples of Schedule IV drugs, which have a low abuse potential and accepted medical indications, are
    A. morphine and codeine.
    B. phenobarbital and lorazepam.
    C. Vicodin and Tylenol with codeine.
    D. heroin and LSD.

14. Which of the following statements is true regarding over-the-counter drugs?
    A. They are usually a higher dose than their prescribed counterparts.
    B. They still require a physician's order to administer in the field.
    C. They present a higher risk to patients taking them.
    D. all of the above

15. Adenosine is administered into the bloodstream, is distributed to all body regions, and is rapidly metabolized by red blood cells. This information is known as its
    A. bioequivalence.
    B. bioassay.
    C. pharmacokinetics.
    D. pharmacodynamics.

16. Which of the following statements is **false** regarding the administration of drugs to a pregnant woman?
    A. Her altered anatomy and physiology may alter the drug's pharmacokinetics.
    B. The drug may pass through the placenta and reach the fetus.
    C. Therapeutic levels for the mother may be toxic levels for the fetus.
    D. All drugs are considered contraindicated for the pregnant woman.

17. Why do infants and young children pose special considerations when dosing drugs?
    A. They have a higher free drug availability than adults.
    B. They have a much greater proportion of extracellular fluid.
    C. They have overdeveloped blood-brain barriers.
    D. The newborn's metabolic rate is much higher than an adult's.

18. Which of the following statements is true regarding drug administration to geriatric patients?
    A. Depressed liver function may alter biotransformation.
    B. Their gastric motility increases with age.
    C. Compromised renal function may increase elimination.
    D. all of the above

19. You administer epinephrine 1:1000 subcutaneously to a patient in severe anaphylactic shock. Which of the following statements is true?
    A. The drug probably will be readily absorbed into the bloodstream.
    B. Subcutaneous blood flow during the shock state is increased.
    C. Capillary bed shutdown may impede drug absorption.
    D. none of the above

20. Which of the following affects a drug's rate of absorption?
    A. its concentration
    B. its pH
    C. its solubility
    D. all of the above

21. You administer via IV a lidocaine bolus of 1 mg/kg followed by a 2-mg/min IV drip. The initial bolus is called the _____ dose, and the drip is called the _____ dose.
    A. initial, follow-up
    B. loading, maintenance
    C. preceding, following
    D. large, small

22. In order to cross the blood-brain barrier or the placenta barrier, a drug should be
    A. ionized.
    B. lipid soluble.
    C. protein bound.
    D. all of the above

23. Which organ(s) is/are responsible for the majority of the biotransformation process?
    A. liver
    B. kidneys
    C. intestines
    D. lungs

24. Renal excretion of drugs can be affected by
    A. glomerular filtration.
    B. blood pressure.
    C. change in the urine pH.
    D. all of the above

25. Which of the following is a **not** an enteral route?
    A. rectal
    B. buccal
    C. umbilical
    D. sublingual

Match the following liquid drug forms with their respective definitions:

26. _____ tincture
27. _____ suspension
28. _____ emulsion
29. _____ spirit
30. _____ elixer

    A. alcohol and water solvent with flavorings
    B. volatile drug in alcohol
    C. extracted with alcohol
    D. oily solvent
    E. preparation that precipitates when left alone

31. The force of attraction between a drug and a receptor is known as
    A. agonism.
    B. antagonism.
    C. affinity.
    D. efficacy.

32. A drug's ability to produce the expected response is known as
    A. agonism.
    B. antagonism.
    C. affinity.
    D. efficacy.

33. Which of the following statements is true regarding the drug/receptor response?
    A. Drugs can inhibit a cell's normal function.
    B. Drugs can stimulate a cell's normal function.
    C. Drugs can impart a new function to a cell.
    D. A and B

34. Drugs that bind to a receptor and produce a response are known as
    A. antagonists.
    B. agonists.
    C. biotransformers.
    D. lytics.

35. Drugs that bind to a receptor and block a response are known as
    A. antagonists.
    B. agonists.
    C. inhibitors.
    D. mimetics.

36. Repeating boluses of lidocaine until the desired effect is reached is an example of
    A. synergism.
    B. potentiation.
    C. cumulative action.
    D. agonism.

37. A patient who once took 5 mg of diazepam each day now requires 10 mg. This is an example of
    A. potentiation.
    B. tolerance.
    C. becoming refractory.
    D. untoward effect.

38. An individual reaction to a drug that is unusually different from that normally seen is called a(n)
    A. hypersensitivity.
    B. idiosyncrasy.

C. adverse reaction.
D. untoward effect.

39. Drugs with a low therapeutic index
    A. are difficult to titrate.
    B. have a narrow therapeutic range.
    C. are easy to overdose.
    D. all of the above

40. Drugs that relieve the sensation of pain are known as
    A. anesthetics.
    B. analgesics.
    C. neuroleptics.
    D. anxiolytics.

41. Morphine is an example of a(n)
    A. narcotic analgesic.
    B. opioid antagonist.
    C. opioid agonist/antagonist.
    D. nonopioid analgesic.

42. Besides pain relief, which of the following is an indication for using morphine?
    A. hypotension
    B. respiratory failure
    C. pulmonary edema
    D. COPD

43. Ibuprofen is an example of a(n)
    A. nonsteroidal antiinflammatory drug.
    B. nonopioid analgesic.
    C. antipyretic.
    D. all of the above

44. Which of the following drugs would you use to treat a heroin overdose?
    A. morphine
    B. diazepam
    C. naloxone
    D. nalbuphine

45. The space between two nerve cells is called a
    A. neuroeffector junction.
    B. neurotransmitter junction.
    C. synapse.
    D. neuron.

Match the neurotransmitters with their respective uses:

46. _____ sympathetic preganglionic
47. _____ sympathetic postganglionic
48. _____ parasympathetic preganglionic
49. _____ parasympathetic postganglionic

    A. acetylcholine
    B. norepinephrine

50. The parasympathetic nervous system is responsible for
    A. custodial functions.
    B. resting heart rate.
    C. digestion.
    D. all of the above

51. The parasympathetic nervous system exerts its control via
    A. several cranial nerves.
    B. three thoracic nerves.
    C. some lumbar nerves.
    D. all of the above

52. When stimulated, parasympathetic receptors cause
    A. decreased salivation.
    B. pupil dilation.
    C. increased heart rate.
    D. none of the above

53. Medications that stimulate the parasympathetic nervous system are called
    A. anticholinergics.
    B. parasympatholytics.

    C. parasympathomimetics.
    D. cholinergic antagonists.

54. Classic effects of cholinergic medications include
    A. increased salivation.
    B. decreased gastric motility.
    C. dry mucous membranes.
    D. constipation.

55. Acetylcholine is degraded by
    A. monoamine oxidase.
    B. cholinesterase.
    C. neostigmine.
    D. cholinesterase inhibitors.

56. Which of the following drugs is a direct-acting cholinergic?
    A. physostigmine (Antilirium)
    B. neostigmine (Prostigmine)
    C. echothiophate (Phospholine Iodide)
    D. bethanechol (Urecholine)

57. Which of the following drugs is a reversible cholinesterase inhibitor?
    A. physostigmine (Antilirium)
    B. sarin
    C. echothiophate (Phospholine Iodide)
    D. bethanechol (Urecholine)

58. Treatment for toxic cholinergic exposure, such as nerve gas, includes
    A. atropine.
    B. pralidoxime.
    C. Protopam.
    D. all of the above

59. Atropine is classified as a
    A. nicotinic agonist.
    B. nicotinic antagonist.
    C. muscarinic agonist.
    D. muscarinic antagonist.

60. The sympathetic nervous system is responsible for
    A. vegetative functions.
    B. custodial functions.
    C. "feeding and breeding."
    D. the stress response.

61. Sympathetic fibers arise from
    A. several sacral nerves.
    B. T1–L2.
    C. cranial nerves III–X.
    D. the midbrain.

62. When stimulated, the sympathetic nervous system causes all of the following physiological responses **except**
    A. pupil dilation.
    B. peripheral vasodilation.
    C. increased cardiac contractions.
    D. increased heart rate.

Match the following adrenergic receptors with their respective functions:

63. _____ alpha 1
64. _____ alpha 2
65. _____ beta 1
66. _____ beta 2
67. _____ dopaminergic

    A. renal artery dilator
    B. arteriole and bronchial dilator
    C. peripheral vasoconstrictor
    D. increased chronotropy and inotropy
    E. presynaptic inhibition

68. An alpha 1 agonist works by
    A. dilating bronchial smooth muscle.
    B. dilating arterioles.
    C. causing massive fluid shifts.
    D. constricting peripheral vessels.

69. Which of the following diuretics works in the loop of Henle?
    A. furosemide (Lasix)
    B. hydrochlorothiazide (HydroDIURIL)
    C. spironolactone (Aldactone)
    D. mannitol (Osmitrol)

70. Which of the following is a side effect of administering furosemide too quickly?
    A. vasoconstriction
    B. reflex bradycardia
    C. tinnitis and deafness
    D. hyperkalemia

71. An alpha 1 antagonist reduces blood pressure by
    A. causing direct vasoconstriction.
    B. reducing peripheral vascular resistance.
    C. reducing the intrinsic firing rate of the SA node.
    D. increasing angiotension conversion.

72. Nitroglycerin is administered to patients suffering from angina because it
    A. lowers the heart rate.
    B. increases preload.
    C. dilates coronary arteries.
    D. all of the above

73. Aspirin is classified as a(n)
    A. antiplatelet.
    B. anticoagulant.
    C. antihyperlipidemic.
    D. thrombolytic.

74. After administering a nitroglycerin tablet sublingually, a patient complains of a bitter, burning sensation under his tongue. Your next course of action would be to
    A. explain to the patient that this is normal.
    B. instruct the patient to immediately chew and swallow the tablet.

C. give the patient approximately 8 ounces of water.

D. instruct the patient to immediately spit the tablet out.

75. You are examining a 45-year-old male who complains of substernal chest pain. The patient states that after onset, he took two unprescribed nitroglycerin tablets he found in a friend's medicine cabinet. What action would be appropriate in reference to the nitroglycerin?
    A. Examine the nitroglycerin and container.
    B. Instruct the patient to swallow a third tablet from the container.
    C. Contact the physician whose name is on the container.
    D. Instruct the patient to take another nitroglycerin tablet from the container.

76. Select the proper route and dosage for a single administration of nitroglycerin.
    A. sublingual spray at 4 mg/spray
    B. sublingual tablet at 0.4 mg/tablet
    C. sublingual spray at 4 g/spray
    D. sublingual tablet at 1/100 g/tablet

77. Which of the following is the most appropriate order of treatment for a patient with chest pain who has never taken nitroglycerin before?
    A. nitroglycerin, IV
    B. IV, nitroglycerin, oxygen
    C. IV, nitroglycerin
    D. oxygen, IV, nitroglycerin

78. You are assessing a patient involved in a motor vehicle accident. The patient suffered blunt trauma to the chest and abdomen and is complaining of substernal chest pain that radiates to the left shoulder. The patient is anxious and presents with vital signs of BP 108/58, HR 136, RR 32, and skin that is cool and diaphoretic. Appropriate management of this patient would include
    A. oxygen, full immobilization, IV, nitroglycerin.
    B. oxygen, IV, transport.
    C. oxygen, full immobilization, IV.
    D. oxygen, full immobilization, nitroglycerin, IV.

79. In which of the following would the administration of nitroglycerin be beneficial?
    A. shock
    B. seizures
    C. congestive heart failure
    D. allergic reactions

80. Which of the following represents a possible adverse reaction to nitroglycerin?
    A. bronchial constriction
    B. hypertension
    C. tachycardia
    D. pupillary constriction

81. Which of the following best describes the mechanism by which nitroglycerin reduces chest pain?
    A. decreasing cardiac workload
    B. increase in cardiac contractility
    C. constriction of the coronary arteries
    D. dilation of the bronchioles

82. Which of the following best describes why a nitroglycerin tablet is administered sublingually?
    A. to avoid gastric irritation
    B. to discourage possible vomiting
    C. to avoid aspiration of the tablet
    D. to promote rapid absorption

83. You are assessing a 60-year-old male whose chief complaint is substernal chest pain accompanied by shortness of breath and diaphoresis. The patient has a history of cardiac problems and presents with vital signs of BP 86/72, HR 68, RR 24. Appropriate management of this individual would consist of
    A. oxygen, IV of normal saline.
    B. oxygen, IV, nitroglycerin 0.4 mg.
    C. oxygen, IV, nitroglycerin 0.2 mg.
    D. oxygen, nitroglycerin 4 mg.

84. Which of the following best describes the action of diazepam in seizure control?
    A. It inhibits seizure activity by depressing the medulla.
    B. It suppresses the spread of seizure activity through the motor cortex.
    C. It prevents seizures by activating the parasympathetic nervous system.
    D. It is a potent central nervous system stimulant that prevents the formation of seizures.

85. To manage an adult patient in status epilepticus, the dosage of diazepam is
    A. 1–5 mg IV.
    B. 5–10 mg IV.
    C. 10–15 mg IV.
    D. 15–20 mg IV.

86. Identify the correct drug class for diazepam.
    A. antidepressants
    B. depressants
    C. narcotics
    D. benzodiazepine

87. When administering diazepam intravenously, it should be given slowly to
    A. minimize venous irritation.
    B. speed up the action of the drug.

    C. avoid hypersensitivity reactions.
    D. prevent accidental overdose.

88. Diazepam would be indicated in all of the following situations **except**
    A. acute anxiety states.
    B. status epilepticus.
    C. unconsciousness of unknown origin.
    D. major motor seizures.

89. After administering diazepam to your patient, you observe that he is drowsy and that his blood pressure and respiratory rate have slightly decreased. You know that this occurred because
    A. he is hypersensitive to the medication.
    B. he received an accidental overdose.
    C. these are common side effects of this drug.
    D. you administered the medication too slowly.

90. Your pediatric patient is in status epilepticus. What is the correct dosage of diazepam in this situation?
    A. 0.1–0.3 mg/kg
    B. 0.5–2 mg/kg
    C. 2–6 mg
    D. 5–10 mg

91. Diazepam should not be mixed with other drugs because it may cause
    A. a severe hypersensitivity reaction.
    B. an accidental overdose.
    C. precipitation within the IV line or vein.
    D. drowsiness.

92. The preferred route for the emergency administration of diazepam is
    A. oral.
    B. sublingual.

C. intramuscular.

D. intravenous.

93. Diazepam is used as a premedication for cardioversion primarily because it

A. calms the patient and depresses the central nervous system.

B. reduces anxiety and diminishes the patient's recall.

C. relaxes skeletal muscles and prevents pain after the procedure.

D. is relatively short acting and does not cause hypersensitivity.

94. Which of the following most accurately describes the effect of 50% dextrose?

A. causes a decrease in the patient's blood pressure

B. raises the blood glucose level

C. promotes bronchodilation

D. causes peripheral vasoconstriction

95. 50% dextrose is administered to manage

A. hypoglycemia.

B. seizures.

C. head injury.

D. hypertension.

96. A major contraindication to the administration of 50% dextrose is

A. acute renal failure.

B. acute stroke.

C. seizures.

D. tachycardia.

97. The proper dose of 50% dextrose in the adult patient is

A. 20 mg.

B. 25 g.

C. 1 mg/kg.

D. none of the above

98. What is the major risk associated with the administration of 50% dextrose?

A. tachycardia

B. respiratory hypoventilation

C. tissue necrosis with extravation

D. lowered blood pressure

99. Thiamine is known more commonly as a

A. drug for headaches.

B. muscle relaxer.

C. vitamin.

D. hormone.

100. The mechanism of action for thiamine is to

A. increase the transfer of glucose into cells.

B. allow sugar to last longer for cellular metabolism.

C. increase sugar absorption from the small intestine.

D. increase the energy gained from the metabolism of sugar.

101. Thiamine can be administered by

A. IV push and IM.

B. SQ injection.

C. IM injection and rectally.

D. IV only.

102. The appropriate dose of thiamine in the prehospital environment is

A. 100 mg.

B. 1 mg/kg.

C. 10 g.

D. none of the above

103. What is the major contraindication associated with the administration of thiamine?

A. hypoglycemia

B. hypotension

C. hypovolemia

D. hypersensitivity

104. Which of the following best describes the mechanism of action of epinephrine?

A. stimulates the sympathetic nervous system

B. stimulates the parasympathetic nervous system

C. blocks the central nervous system

D. reduces peripheral vascular resistance

105. The property that makes epinephrine most desirable in cardiac arrest is

A. beta 1 stimulation.

B. beta 2 stimulation.

C. alpha stimulation.

D. dopaminergic stimulation.

106. What is the preferred concentration and route for epinephrine in cardiac arrest?

A. 1:1000 concentration via IM or SQ administration

B. 1:10,000 concentration via IVP

C. 1:1,000 concentration via IVP or endotracheally

D. 1:10,000 concentration via IM or SQ

107. What is the initial dose for epinephrine in cardiac arrest?

A. 10 mcg

B. 1 mcg

C. 1 mg

D. 10 mg

108. All of the following are potential side effects of epinephrine **except**

A. palpitations.

B. bradycardia.

C. hypertension.

D. pallor.

109. Which of the following drugs can adsorb poisons that have been ingested?

A. ipecac

B. procardia

C. activated charcoal

D. oral glucose

110. The dose of activated charcoal for an adult patient is

A. 50 g.

B. 50 mg.

C. 5 oz.

D. 1 mg/kg.

111. An indication for the administration of Benadryl is

A. anaphylaxis.

B. coma of unknown origin.

C. nausea and vomiting.

D. asthma attacks.

112. The usual adult dose of Benadryl is

A. 5 mg/kg.

B. 50 mg/kg.

C. 50 mg.

D. 5 g.

113. The mechanism of action for Benadryl is to

A. block histamine release.

B. block histamine receptors.

C. block beta receptor sites.

D. block alpha receptor sites.

114. Which of the following is **not** a beta 2–specific drug that can be administered by a nebulizer?

A. Ventolin

B. Bronkosol

C. Alupent

D. Somophyllin

115. A beta 2 drug is considered a
    A. sympathetic agonist.
    B. parasympathetic agonist.
    C. sympathetic antagonist.
    D. parasympathetic antagonist.

116. What is the primary action of a beta 2 drug?
    A. vasodilation
    B. increased heart rate
    C. bronchodilation
    D. positive inotropy

117. The proper dose for Albuterol is
    A. 3.0 mg in 3 ml of normal saline.
    B. 2.5 mg in 2.5 ml of normal saline.
    C. 1.0 mg in 5 ml of normal saline.
    D. 0.5 mg in 2.5 ml of normal saline.

118. The primary indication for the use of a beta 2–specific drug is
    A. congestive heart failure.
    B. pneumonia.
    C. bronchoconstriction.
    D. myocardial infarction.

119. Which of the following drugs would be used in the management of the hypoglycemic patient?
    A. Albuterol
    B. glycogen
    C. glucagon
    D. Inderal

120. Which of the following would be an indication for the use of glucagon?
    A. patient who overdosed on propranolol
    B. patient with an altered mental status and a blood glucose level of 240 mg/dl

C. patient with an altered mental status from ingestion of diazepam
    D. liver failure associated with acetominophen overdose

121. Glucagon can best be described as a(n)
    A. drug made up of glucose.
    B. hormone secreted by the alpha cells in the pancreas.
    C. antiarrythmic agent to control PVCs.
    D. drug used to reverse thiamine deficiency.

122. Which of the following best describes the mechanism of action of glucagon?
    A. The glucose contained within the drug raises the blood glucose level.
    B. It decreases the inotropic and chronotropic properties of the heart.
    C. It stimulates an increase in insulin production and secretion, allowing the glucose to enter the cells.
    D. It stimulates the liver to convert glycogen stores into free glucose.

123. You are managing a hypoglycemic patient and are unable to establish an IV. What would be the correct dose for glucagon?
    A. 0.25 mg
    B. 0.5 mg
    C. 1.0 mg
    D. 2.5 mg

124. Naloxone is classified as a
    A. narcotic agonist.
    B. central nervous system stimulant.
    C. narcotic antagonist.
    D. benzodiazepine antagonist.

125. On which of the following drugs would Narcan have no effect?

A. Demerol

B. Fentanyl

C. Nubain

D. Valium

126. When administering Narcan, which of the following criteria could be used to determine when the appropriate dose has been reached?

A. The patient becomes alert and combative.

B. The respiratory depression has been reversed.

C. The patient's blood increases by 10 mm Hg.

D. The pupils dilate from a constricted state.

127. What would be considered a contraindication for use of Narcan?

A. a patient who has had a bad reaction to it before

B. if the patient has ingested alcohol with the narcotic agent

C. if the drug ingested or injected is a synthetic narcotic

D. if the patient is comatose from the drug overdose

128. From your history, you gather that the unresponsive patient has ingested a large number of Darvon pills and drank a fifth of whiskey. The proper dose of Narcan in this case would be

A. 1 mg IV.

B. 2 mg ET.

C. 5 mg IV.

D. 25 mg ET.

129. Which of the following is a first-line drug in the treatment of ventricular dysrhythmias?

A. magnesium sulfate

B. atropine

C. lidocaine

D. adeosine

130. You have administered a bolus of lidocaine to a patient experiencing ventricular tachycardia. The lidocaine abolished the ventricular tachycardia. Your next action should be to

A. start an infusion of lidocaine at 2 mg/min.

B. administer a second bolus at 1.5 mg/kg.

C. monitor the patient and rebolus with lidocaine at 0.5 mg/kg if any ectopy occurs.

D. increase the oxygen and continue to monitor the patient.

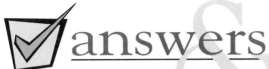

answers & rationales

Following each rationale, you will find a reference to the corresponding objective in the DOT National Standard EMT-Intermediate curriculum. An asterisk denotes material that is supplemental to the DOT curriculum. Page numbers after a rationale indicate where the question topic may be discussed in the Brady text *Intermediate Emergency Care* (Bledsoe, Porter, Cherry).

1.

D. Furosemide and diazepam are examples of generic names. The generic name is the name usually given to a drug by its first manufacturer and is an abbreviated version of the chemical name. (1-3.3) (IEC pp. 234–235)

2.

A. Lasix® and Valium® are examples of trade names. The trade name is a name given to a drug by each manufacturer. A medication may appear under several trade names if it is made by a number of manufacturers. (1-3.3) (IEC pp. 234–235)

3.

A. Atropine and digitalis are examples of drugs derived from plants. (1-3.4) (IEC p. 235)

4.

C. Insulin and Pitocin are examples of drugs derived from animals. (1-3.4) (IEC p. 235)

5.

B. Calcium chloride and magnesium sulfate are examples of drugs derived from minerals. (1-3.4) (IEC p. 235)

6.

B. In an effort to regulate and eliminate "snake-oil salesmen," Congress enacted the Pure Food and Drug Act in 1906 and named the U.S. Pharmacopoeia as the country's official source for drug information. (1-3.2) (IEC p. 236)

7.

A. The Federal Food, Drug, and Cosmetic Act of 1938 requires the names of all ingredients of foods and medications to be placed on the product label. It also requires that the labels state whether the ingredients are habit forming and what percentages of those drugs are present. (1-3.2) (IEC p. 236)

8.

B. The Harrison Narcotic Act of 1915 regulates the sale, importation, and manufacture of the opium plant and its derivatives. (1-3.2) (IEC p. 236)

9.

D. Since 1970, the government has regulated addictive medications through the Controlled Substances Act. This act classifies addictive medications into five schedules, prohibits the refilling of prescriptions for Schedule II drugs, and requires that the original prescription be filled within 72 hours. (1-3.3) (IEC p. 237)

10.

B. Schedule I drugs have a high abuse potential, and their use may lead to severe dependence. They have no accepted medical indications and are used for research, analysis, or instruction only. Examples include heroin, LSD, and mescaline. (1-3.5) (IEC p. 237)

11.

C. Schedule II drugs have a high abuse potential, and their use may lead to severe dependence. However, they have accepted medical indications. Examples include opium, cocaine, morphine, codeine, oxycodone, methadone, and secobarbital. (1-3.5) (IEC p. 237)

12.

A. Schedule III drugs have less abuse potential than Schedule I and II drugs, and their use may lead to moderate or low physical or high psychological dependence. However, they have accepted medical indications.

Examples include limited opioid amounts combined with noncontrolled substances, such as Vicodin and Tylenol with codeine. (1-3.5) (IEC p. 237)

13.

B. Schedule IV drugs have a low abuse potential compared to Schedule III drugs, and their use causes limited physical and psychological dependence. They have accepted medical indications. Examples include diazepam, lorazepam, and phenobarbital. (1-3.5) (IEC p. 237)

14.

B. Over-the-counter (OTC) medications are usually available in lower doses than their prescribed counterparts and present a lower risk for patients taking them. Most EMS systems require EMS providers to obtain a physician's order (written, verbal, or standing) to administer OTC drugs. (1-3.8) (IEC p. 237)

15.

C. A drug's pharmacokinetics refer to its absorption, distribution, metabolism, and excretion. EMT-Intermediates should be familiar with this information for all drugs they administer. For example, by knowing that adenosine is metabolized rapidly en route to the heart, you know you need to administer it rapidly into a vein close to the heart and flush the line immediately. (1-3.14) (IEC p. 242)

16.

D. Administering any drug to a pregnant woman is risky to both the mother and her unborn child. Even after birth, if she is nursing, she can transfer the drug's effects to her infant. There are, however, circumstances that demand the use of drugs for the health of the baby and mother. These include diabetes, hypertension, and seizure disorders. (1-3.7) (IEC pp. 239–240)

17.

A. Some drugs bind to plasma proteins in the blood. But not all the drug molecules bind. The ones that do not are available in the body to cause the desired or undesired effects. This is known as free drug availability. Since children under 1 year old have diminished plasma protein concentrations, these drugs have higher free drug availability. Because of this, you can expect to reach therapeutic and toxic effects at lower doses. (1-3.7) (IEC pp. 240–241)

18.

A. Most drugs are metabolized, or biotransformed, in the liver. If your patient has depressed liver function because of the aging process or a disease such as cirrhosis or hepatitis, you can expect drug action to be prolonged. (1-3.7) (IEC p. 241)

19.

C. During the shock state, blood flow to the peripheral blood vessels in the skin is blocked in order to preserve circulation to the vital organs. Administering a drug into the subcutaneous tissue during the shock state may result in decreased, if any, absorption. In severe anaphylaxis, epinephrine may be administered at a lower concentration (1:10,000) directly into a vein. (1-3.15) (IEC pp. 242–243)

20.

D. How well a drug is absorbed is determined by a number of factors. These include its concentration, pH, ionization, and solubility; the nature of the absorbing surface; and blood flow through the administration area. (1-3.15) (IEC pp. 242–243)

21.

B. A loading dose is administered to raise the blood levels of a drug quickly to a therapeutic level. A maintenance dose is administered to keep the blood levels in the therapeutic range. You would load your patient (in stable ventricular tachycardia) until the rhythm converts to sinus rhythm and then begin the drip to prevent a sudden recurrence. (1-3.15) (IEC p. 244)

22.

B. For a drug to cross the blood-brain barrier or the placenta barrier, it should be nonionized, lipid soluble, and non–protein bound. (1-3.15) (IEC p. 244)

23.

A. Most drugs are metabolized, or biotransformed, in the liver. Patients with preexisting liver disease can be expected to develop toxic blood levels of drugs at lower doses than do those with healthy livers. A good example of this is lidocaine. If you suspect your patient has an impaired liver, consider administering a reduced dose. (1-3.15) (IEC p. 244)

24.

D. Most drugs are excreted in the urine. Conditions that affect renal elimination include glomerular filtration, which is affected by blood pressure and blood flow; urine pH; and drugs that affect the ATP pumps. (1-3.15) (IEC p. 245)

25.

C. Enteral routes deliver medications by absorption through the GI tract. These include oral (PO), orogastric tube (OG), nasogastric tube (NG), sublingual (SL), buccal, and rectal (PR). (1-3.12) (IEC pp. 245–246)

Matching (1-3.10) (IEC pp. 246–247)

26.	C	tincture
27.	E	suspension
28.	D	emulsion
29.	B	spirit
30.	A	elixir

31.

C. Affinity is the force of attraction between a drug or other substance and a receptor. For example, the carbon monoxide molecule has an affinity for hemoglobin that is 210 times greater than the affinity of the oxygen molecule. The same holds true for drugs. The greater the affinity, the stronger the bond. (1-3.15) (IEC p. 247)

32.

D. Efficacy describes a drug's ability to produce a response. It is different from its ability to bind with the receptor. One drug may bind more easily, but another may cause a stronger response when bound. (1-3.15) (IEC p. 248)

33.

D. Drugs are not magical. They cannot alter a cell's function qualitatively, only quantitatively. They can either stimulate or inhibit a cell's normal physiological function. For example, acetylcholine will stimulate a smooth muscle cell to constrict, while albuterol will inhibit constriction (resulting in dilation). (1-3.15) (IEC p. 248)

34.

B. Drugs that bind to a receptor and produce a response are known as agonists. An example is epinephrine, which stimulates the alpha and beta receptors in the heart, blood vessels, and lower airways. (1-3.15) (IEC p. 248)

35.

A. Drugs that bind to a receptor and block a response are known as antagonists. An example is naloxone, which blocks the narcotic receptor sites. (1-3.15) (IEC p. 248)

36.

C. Repeating boluses of lidocaine until the desired effect is reached is an example of cumulative action. This occurs when a drug is administered in several doses, causing an increasing effect that is usually due to a buildup of the drug in the blood. (1-3.15) (IEC p. 250)

37.

B. A patient who requires a higher dose of the same medication to reach the desired effect is an example of tolerance. In order to produce the desired effect, you must increase the dose. (1-3.15) (IEC p. 249)

38.

B. An idiosyncrasy is an individual reaction to a drug that is unusually different from that normally seen. For example, antibiotics normally cause gastrointestinal distress. If antibiotics turn your hair green, this is an idiosyncrasy. (1-3.14) (IEC p. 249)

39.

D. Drugs with a low therapeutic index are difficult to titrate because they have a narrow therapeutic range. It is very easy to overdose patients on these types of drugs. (1-3.15) (IEC pp. 250–251)

40.

B. Analgesics are drugs that relieve the sensation of pain. There are basically two types of analgesics—narcotic analgesics (from the opioid plant) and nonnarcotic analgesics. (1-3.18)

41.

A. Morphine is a narcotic analgesic or narcotic agonist. It stimulates the release of pain-reducing peptides called endorphins, which reduce the sensation of pain. (1-3.18) (IEC p. 268)

42.

C. Morphine is prescribed for moderate to severe pain. In addition, its vasodilatory effects are beneficial in reducing the workload of the heart by causing venous pooling in the extremities. This effect helps rid the lungs of excess fluid in patients with pulmonary edema. (1-3.18) (IEC p. 268)

43.

D. Ibuprofen is classified as a nonopioid analgesic with antipyretic (fever-reducing) properties. It is in a subclass known as nonsteroidal anti-inflammatory drugs (NSAIDs). (1-3.18)

44.

C. Heroin is an opioid agonist. When overdosed, it causes severe respiratory depression, unconsciousness, and pinpoint pupils. To treat a heroin overdose, administer naloxone, a competitive opioid antagonist. The naloxone will compete with the heroin for the receptor sites and block the effects of the opioid—namely, respiratory depression. (1-3.18) (IEC p. 268)

45.

C. There is no physical connection between two nerve cells. Instead, there is a space called a synapse. The space between a nerve cell and the target organ it innervates is called a neuroeffector junction. A neurotransmitter is a chemical that conducts a nervous impulse across a synapse or neuroeffector junction. (1-3.1) (IEC p. 253)

Matching (1-3.1) (IEC p. 253)

46.	A	sympathetic preganglionic
47.	B	sympathetic postganglionic
48.	A	parasympathetic preganglionic
49.	A	parasympathetic postganglionic

50.

D. The parasympathetic nervous system controls primarily custodial or vegetative functions, such as digestion of food and resting heart rate. It is often referred to as the "feed or breed" aspect of the autonomic nervous system. (1-3.1) (IEC p. 252)

51.

D. The parasympathetic nervous system exerts its control via cranial nerves III (occulomotor), VII (facial), IX (glossopharyngeal), and X (vagus) and via sacral nerves S_2–S_4. (1-3.1) (IEC p. 173)

52.

D. When stimulated, the parasympathetic nervous system decreases the heart rate, promotes increased salivation, and causes pupillary constriction. (1-3.2) (IEC p. 253)

53.

C. Drugs that stimulate the parasympathetic nervous system are called parasympathomimetics. Drugs that antagonize the parasympathetic nervous system are called parasympatholytics or anticholinergics. (1-3.1) (IEC p. 253)

54.

A. A helpful mnemonic for remembering the side effects of cholinergic medications is "SLUDGE." SLUDGE stands for salivation, lacrimation, urination, defecation, gastric motility, and emesis. (1-3.1) (IEC p. 253)

55.

B. Acetylcholine is biodegraded by the enzyme cholinesterase. One of the common ways to prolong cholinergic effects is to administer drugs that inhibit the breakdown of acetylcholine by cholinesterase. (1-3.1) (IEC pp. 253–254)

56.

D. Bethanechol (Urecholine) is the prototype cholinergic medication that acts directly on ACh receptors, much like acetylcholine, except that it is not biodegraded by cholinesterase, resulting in a longer duration of action. (1-3.1) (IEC p. 253)

57.

A. The two common reversible cholinesterase inhibitors are physostigmine (Antilirium) and neostigmine (Prostigmine). Physostigmine (short acting) is used to treat anticholinergic overdoses. Neostigmine (long acting) is used to treat myasthenia gravis. Both inhibit the breakdown of acetylcholine by cholinesterase. (1-3.1) (IEC p. 254)

58.

D. Treatment for toxic cholinergic overdose, such as nerve gas or organophosphate insecticides, includes large doses of atropine and pralidoxime (Protopam, 2-Pam). Atropine competes for ACh receptor sites, while pralidixome encourages cholinesterase release. (1-3.1)

59.

D. Atropine is the prototype muscarinic antagonist. It binds with ACh receptors and blocks the effects of ACh on muscarinic sites. It is most often used to increase the heart rate in symptomatic bradycardia. (1-3.1) (IEC p. 254)

60.

D. In contrast to the parasympathetic, the sympathetic nervous system is our body's defense against extreme stress. Also known as the "fight or flight" response, the sympathetic storm readies our bodies to withstand perceived threats. (1-3.1) (IEC p. 252)

61.

B. Sympathetic nerve fibers arise from the spinal cord at the levels of T1–L2 and run along each side of the spinal column in special ganglionic "chains." In addition, collateral ganglia that innervate the abdominal organs are located in the abdominal cavity. (1-3.1) (IEC p. 173)

62.

B. When stimulated, the sympathetic nervous system causes pupillary dilation, an increase in heart rate, an increase in the force of cardiac contractions, peripheral vasoconstriction, and an increase in metabolic rate. All these reactions are designed to help us meet the challenge of a severe physical or psychological stressor. (1-3.1) (IEC p. 253)

Matching (1-3.1) (IEC pp. 256–257)

63.   C   alpha 1
64.   E   alpha 2
65.   D   beta 1
66.   B   beta 2
67.   A   dopaminergic

68.

D. Alpha 1 agonists cause peripheral vasoconstriction and mild bronchoconstriction. Drugs in this class include epinephrine, norepinephrine, phenylephrine, and ephedrine. They are used to raise blood pressure and decrease nasal congestion, and they are combined with local anesthetics to decrease systemic absorption. (1-3.1) (IEC p. 256)

69.

A. Loop diuretics block sodium reabsorption in the ascending loop of Henle, increasing the excretion of water. The most popular loop diuretic is furosemide (Lasix). (1-3.18) (IEC p. 266)

70.

C. Administering furosemide too rapidly may cause ototoxicity, resulting in tinnitis or deafness. (1-3.18)

71.

B. Alpha 1 receptors are located in the peripheral blood vessels. When stimulated, they cause profound vasoconstriction. When blocked, they reduce peripheral vascular resistance and lower the blood pressure. (1-3.1) (IEC p. 257)

72.

C. People with angina take nitroglycerin to cause vasodilation and to cause venous pooling. This reduces preload and the workload of the heart. It also dilates the coronary arteries, allowing more oxygenated blood to reach the myocardium. (1-3.18) (IEC p. 269)

73.

A. Aspirin is the prototype antiplatelet drug. It decreases the formation of platelet plugs by inhibiting cyclooxygenase, the enzyme needed for platelet aggregation. (1-3.18) (IEC p. 259)

74.

A. The burning or stinging sensation the patient may experience when taking nitroglycerin is considered normal and often indicates the potency of the tablet or spray. In this situation, the EMT-Intermediate should explain to the patient that this is a normal side effect with the medication and will pass in a few minutes. (1-3.18)

75.

A. The EMT-Intermediate must examine the nitroglycerin and container. More specifically, the condition and expiration date must be determined. Nitroglycerin tends to deteriorate rapidly after exposure to air and light and lose its efficacy after the medicine has expired. This may explain the failure of the nitroglycerin to alleviate this individual's chest pain. Instructing the patient to take another pill from the same container is inappropriate in that this medication has been prescribed for someone else. Contacting the physician whose name is on the container will do little for the patient. (1-3.18) (IEC pp. 238–239)

76.

B. Nitroglycerin can be administered by either sublingual tablet or sublingual spray. The correct dosage for a single dose would be 0.4 mg, or 1/150 grain. (1-3.18) (IEC p. 269)

77.

D. The correct order of intervention is best represented by oxygen, IV, nitroglycerin.

Oxygen is always a first-line drug in the management of chest pain. An IV should be established prior to the administration of the nitroglycerin for the patient who has never received the drug before, just in case the patient has an adverse reaction to the medication and requires immediate fluids and/or other medications. (1-3.18) (IEC pp. 269, 924)

78.

C. The most appropriate care for this patient is oxygen, full immobilization, IV en route, and no nitroglycerin. This patient appears to be in compensatory shock as indicated by the mechanism of injury and vital signs. Nitroglycerin and its vasodilation effect are contraindicated in the presence of shock. Also, there is no true indication for administration of nitroglycerin. (1-3.18) (IEC pp. 727–732, 768–769)

79.

C. Nitroglycerin may be beneficial to the patient suffering the effects of congestive heart failure. The nitroglycerin causes vasodilation, which can decrease the quantity of blood returning to the heart, and a decrease in peripheral vascular resistance. In congestive heart failure, there is more blood entering the heart than the heart can effectively pump. This results in pulmonary edema, associated respiratory distress, and hypoxia. (1-3.18) (IEC p. 269)

80.

C. Tachycardia may be a side effect of nitroglycerin. The vasodilatory aspects of nitroglycerin reduce the blood return to the myocardium and this results in a corresponding reduction in the cardiac output. Blood pressure is often decreased, and if it is lowered to the point of significant hypotension, the body will attempt to compensate with an increase in the heart rate. This is in an attempt to deliver more oxygenated blood to the cells. This is the reason that many authorities state that the systolic blood pressure should be lowered only 10% of its initial value. Bronchial constriction, hypertension, and pupillary constriction are not physiological side effects to the administration of nitroglycerin. (1-3.18) (IEC p. 269)

81.

A. Nitroglycerin is a smooth-muscle relaxant that reduces cardiac workload. During times of stress or exercise, the heart often needs more oxygen than narrowed coronary arteries can supply. Relaxing the peripheral arteries reduces resistance, and to some extent, dilating the coronary arteries increases coronary blood flow and perfusion to the ischemic cells. (1-3.18) (IEC p. 269)

82.

D. Because the underside of the tongue is rich in capillaries, sublingual administration of nitroglycerin tablets promotes rapid absorption and therefore fast drug action in the body. (1-3.18) (IEC pp. 269, 277)

83.

A. Appropriate management of this patient would include oxygen and a crystalloid IV. Nitroglycerin is contraindicated in this situation because of a state of hypotension. (1-3.18) (IEC pp. 269, 924)

84.

B. Diazepam is an effective agent to control seizure activity because it suppresses the spread of seizure activity through the motor cortex of the brain. (1-3.18) (IEC p. 264)

85.

B. To manage status epilepticus, the dosage of diazepam is 5–10 mg IV, titrated to effect. (1-3.18) (IEC p. 264)

86.

D. Diazepam is in the drug class known as benzodiazepines. (1-3.18) (IEC p. 264)

87.

A. When administering diazepam intravenously, it should be given slowly to minimize venous irritation and hypotension. (1-3.18)

88.

C. It would be inappropriate to give diazepam to manage an unconsciousness of unknown origin or one who is known to be hypersensitive. Diazepam is indicated for the management of acute anxiety states, status epilepticus, and major motor seizures. (1-3.18) (IEC p. 264)

89.

C. After administering diazepam, it is not unusual to observe drowsiness or decreases in your patient's blood pressure or respiratory rate. These are common side effects of this medication. (1-3.18) (IEC p. 264)

90.

A. The correct dosage of diazepam for the management of pediatric status epilepticus is

0.1–0.3 mg/kg. The maximum single dose for a child under the age of 5 years is 5 mg; the maximum single dose for a child over the age of 5 years is 10 mg. Pediatric doses are typically based on weight. (1-3.18)

91.

C. Diazepam should not be mixed with other drugs because it may cause possible precipitation in the IV line or in the vein. (1-3.18)

92.

D. The intravenous route is preferred for the emergency administration of diazepam. An alternative route of administration for pediatric patients is rectal. (1-3.18) (IEC pp. 264, 785)

93.

B. Diazepam is an effective premedication for cardioversion and other procedures because it reduces anxiety and diminishes the patient's recall. (1-3.18) (IEC pp. 264, 915)

94.

B. 50% dextrose is a drug that is sugar in a form that the body can immediately utilize. It should be used in situations where the patient presents with signs and symptoms of hypoglycemia. (1-3.18) (IEC p. 264)

95.

A. Since dextrose effectively raises the blood sugar level, it should be administered to those persons who have an altered mental status with a BGL level of (generally) less than 50 mg/dl. It can be used for unresponsiveness, but only if it is confirmed as hypoglycemia. (1-3.18) (IEC p. 264)

96.

B. The major contraindication of the administration of 50% dextrose is in a patient with increased intracranial pressure from a stroke or head trauma. In these persons, dextrose has been shown to increase intracranial pressure and worsen neurological outcomes. Only administer it to stroke or head-injured patients if hypoglycemia is confirmed. (1-3.18) (IEC pp. 264, 755, 1025)

97.

B. The correct dose for 50% dextrose in the hypoglycemic patient is 25 g. This usually comes packaged as 25 g in 50 ml of solution and is labeled as 50% dextrose in water. (1-3.18) (IEC p. 264)

98.

C. 50% dextrose is very hypertonic, and if it is administered in anything less than a patent IV line, extravation can occur. When this happens, tissue necrosis is often the result. (1-3.18) (IEC p. 264)

99.

C. Thiamine is known more commonly as vitamin B_1. It is necessary for the full mobilization of energy from sugar sources. It is not manufactured by the body, so thiamine must come from the diet. (1-3.18) (IEC pp. 755, 1019)

100.

D. Thiamine is a vitamin that is not made by the body but is necessary for the conversion of pyruvic acid into acetyl-coenzyme-A. Without this step, a large majority of energy available in glucose cannot be used. (1-3.18) (IEC pp. 755, 1019)

101.

A. The preferred route for thiamine administration is IV push. However, in the absence of an IV line, it can be administered deep IM. (1-3.18) (IEC p. 755)

102.

A. The dose for thiamine is 100 mg. It is the same dose regardless of whether it is administered IV push or intramuscularly. (1-3.18) (IEC pp. 755, 1019)

103.

D. In the emergency setting, there are no contraindications to the use of this drug with the exception of known hypersensitivity to the drug. (1-3.18)

104.

A. Epinephrine is a drug that stimulates adrenergic receptors. That classifies this drug as a sympathomimetic, one that stimulates the sympathetic nervous system. (1-3.18) (IEC pp. 265–266)

105.

C. Epinephrine stimulates alpha and beta sites equally. In cardiac arrest, however, it is the alpha effects that are most desirable. These alpha effects cause an increase in vasoconstriction, which will increase perfusion pressures generated during the administration of external chest compressions. (1-3.18) (IEC pp. 170–171, 197, 266)

106.

B. Epinephrine in cardiac arrest should be administered via IV push. When given IV push, 1 mg of 1:10,000 solution should be used. When given down the ET tube, the dose is increased 2–2.5 times. (1-3.18) (IEC p. 266)

107.

C. The initial IV push dose of epinephrine in cardiac arrest is 1 mg. It can be repeated every 3–5 minutes. (1-3.18)

108.

B. Since epinephrine is a drug that stimulates the sympathetic nervous system, the side effects will include palpitations, possible hypertension, nausea/vomiting, and tachycardia and pale skin. (1-3.18) (IEC pp. 265–266)

109.

C. Activated charcoal is a drug that, when administered soon after an ingestion poisoning, adsorbs (binds) the poison so that it can pass through the gastrointestinal tract in a whole form without being absorbed. The porous charcoal minimizes absorption into the body. Ipecac is an emetic agent, procardia is a calcium channel blocker, and oral glucose is for hypoglycemic emergencies. (1-3.18) (IEC p. 974)

110.

A. The correct adult dose of activated charcoal is 50–75 g. (1-3.18)

111.

A. Benadryl (diphenhydramine) is an antihistamine used to counteract the effects of histamine release. It is used in those instances when there is a large amount of histamine release within the body, such as anaphylaxis or allergic reactions. It is not warranted in a coma of unknown etiology and is contraindicated for asthma. (1-3.18) (IEC p. 265)

112.

C. The adult dose of Benadryl is 25–50 mg IV push or IM. Of the two routes, the IV administration is preferred. (1-3.18) (IEC p. 265)

113.

B. The major mechanism of action for Benadryl is the blockage of histamine receptor sites, thereby blocking histamine action. It cannot influence the amount of histamine released in response to the antigen. (1-3.18) (IEC p. 265)

114.

D. Somophyllin has beta 2 properties; however, it cannot be delivered by nebulizer. This drug is usually administered as an IV infusion. (1-3.18) (IEC pp. 261–262, 966)

115.

A. A beta 2 drug is considered a sympathetic agonist because it has beta 2 properties that mimic those of the sympathetic nervous system resulting in bronchodilation. An antagonist has properties that act against the sympathetic nervous system. Even though a parasympathetic antagonist, like atropine, would reverse bronchoconstriction, it does not contain beta 2 properties. (1-3.18) (IEC pp. 256–258, 261)

116.

C. The primary action of a beta 2 drug is bronchodilation. Some vascular smooth-muscle dilation will also result from beta 2 stimulation. An increased heart rate (chronotropic effect) and increased contractility of the myocardium (inotropic effect) occur from beta 1 properties. (1-3.18) (IEC pp. 257, 261–263)

117.

B. The proper dose of Albuterol is 2.5 mg mixed in 2.5 ml of normal saline for nebulization. The total amount mixed is 0.5 ml of a 0.5% solution. (1-3.18) (IEC p. 261)

118.

C. The primary indication for the use of a beta 2 specific drug is bronchoconstriction associated with bronchial asthma, emphysema, chronic bronchitis, and COPD. (1-3.18) (IEC pp. 257, 261–263)

119.

C. Glucagon is an alternative drug that can be used in the treatment of a patient who is hypoglycemic. It is a hormone that stimulates the conversion of liver glycogen to glucose, and conversion of noncarbohydrate substances into glucose, thereby raising the blood glucose level. It is only effective if glycogen stores are available. Intravenous 50% dextrose remains the number one drug of choice in the management of hypoglycemia. (1-3.18) (IEC p. 267)

120.

A. Glucagon is also used in the treatment of beta blocker overdose. Propranolol is a beta blocker. (1-3.18) (IEC p. 267)

121.

B. Glucagon is a protein hormone that is secreted by the alpha cells in the pancreas. It does not contain any glucose. (1-3.18) (IEC p. 267)

122.

D. Glucagon raises the blood glucose level by stimulating the conversion of glycogen, the stored form of glucose in the liver, back into free glucose that enters the blood and is available for use by the cells. This in turn raises the blood glucose level. (1-3.18) (IEC p. 267)

123.

C. The typical dose is 1.0 mg. Glucagon is normally administered as an IM injection in the hypoglycemic patient. If an IV was established, 50% dextrose should be administered and not glucagon. (1-3.18) (IEC p. 267)

124.

C. Naloxone is considered a narcotic antagonist. It competes for opiate binding sites or blocks the ability of the opiate or narcotic to bind at a receptor site. (1-3.18) (IEC p. 268)

125.

D. Narcan will not reverse the effects of benzodiazepines, like Valium. Demerol, Fentanyl, and Nubain are all narcotic substances. Narcan only will affect and block opiate derivatives or synthetic narcotics. (1-3.18) (IEC pp. 264, 267)

126.

B. As a general rule, the appropriate dose of Narcan is enough to reverse any respiratory depression or hypotension associated with the narcotic. It is not recommended that enough be given to completely arouse the patient because most patients become agitated and violent when completely responsive. (1-3.18) (IEC p. 268)

127.

A. The only contraindication to the use of Narcan is hypersensitivity to the drug. (1-3.18) (IEC p. 268)

128.

C. Darvon typically requires larger doses of Narcan to achieve a response. In this case, 5 mg of Narcan would be an appropriate dose to use to try to elicit a response from the patient. (1-3.18)

129.

C. Lidocaine is a drug used in the treatment of ventricular dysrhythmias. (1-3.18) (IEC p. 267)

130.

A. Once you have abolished the ectopy using a lidocaine bolus, it is necessary to maintain the therapeutic dose by starting an infusion. The infusion ranges from 2 mg/min to 4 mg/min. In this case, since only one dose of 1.0 mg/kg was administered, an infusion set at 2 mg/min is used. (1-3.18) (IEC p. 267)

UNIT 4

Venous Access and Medication Administration

unit objectives

Questions in this unit relate to DOT objectives 1-4.1 to 1-4.25. The objectives are listed in the Appendix.

DIRECTIONS

Each of the questions or incomplete statements below is followed by suggested answers or completions. Select the **one answer** that is best in each case.

1. Which of the following would you use to clean the skin prior to starting an IV?

   A. an antiseptic solution

   B. a disinfectant solution

   C. neither A nor B

   D. either A or B

2. Nitroglycerin patches are examples of _____ medications.

   A. intradermal

   B. transtracheal

   C. subcutaneous

   D. transdermal

Match the following percutaneous medication routes with their respective definitions:

   3. _____ sublingual

   4. _____ buccal

   5. _____ ocular

   6. _____ aural

   7. _____ nasal

   A. through the mucous membranes of the eye

   B. through the nares

   C. into the ear canal

   D. between the cheek and gums

   E. under the tongue

8. Your mother's eye drop prescription reads 2 gtts o.s. What does this mean?

   A. 2 drops each day

   B. 2 drops each eye

   C. 2 drops right eye

   D. 2 drops left eye

9. When setting up a nebulizer treatment, set the oxygen source at 1pm.

   A. 2–4

   B. 5–8

   C. 9–12

   D. 15

10. For patients with decreased tidal volumes, how would you administer a nebulized medication?

    A. Connect the nebulizer to a bag-valve-mask.

    B. Inject the medication down the ET tube.

    C. Spray the medication into the oral cavity.

    D. none of the above

11. Which of the following drugs can be administered directly down an endotracheal tube?

    A. sodium bicarbonate

    B. atropine

    C. diazepam (Valium)

    D. dopamine

12. Which of the following devices facilitates the use of a metered dose inhaler?

    A. endotracheal tube

    B. bag-valve-mask

    C. nebulizer

    D. spacer

13. Where do you measure the amount of liquid in a medicine cup?

    A. at the sides

    B. at the center

    C. at the highest level

    D. none of the above

14. A teaspoon holds _____ ml of liquid.
    A. 1
    B. 3
    C. 5
    D. 10

15. After administering a medication orally, follow it with at least _____ ounces of water to push the medication into the stomach.
    A. 4–8
    B. 10–15
    C. 1–3
    D. 16–20

16. Which of the following may **not** be administered via an orogastric tube?
    A. crushed time-release capsules
    B. crushed pills
    C. crushed tablets
    D. liquids

17. Which of the following statements regarding rectal administration is true?
    A. Absorption is usually slow.
    B. The drug is subject to hepatic alteration.
    C. The drug will not pass through the liver.
    D. Absorption time is unpredictable.

18. You are preparing to administer 3 cc of medication. Which size syringe would be most appropriate?
    A. 5 cc
    B. 3 cc
    C. 10 cc
    D. 20 cc

19. Which of the following is the largest-bore hypodermic needle?
    A. 27 gauge
    B. 25 gauge
    C. 19 gauge
    D. 18 gauge

20. You hold a glass vial containing a medication that reads 250 mg in 10 ml. What is the concentration?
    A. 4/1
    B. 10/1
    C. 25/1
    D. none of the above

21. An intradermal injection is administered at a _____ angle to the skin.
    A. 45°
    B. 90°
    C. 180°
    D. 10°

22. A subcutaneous injection is administered at a _____ angle to the skin.
    A. 45°
    B. 90°
    C. 180°
    D. 15°

23. An intramuscular injection is administered at a _____ angle to the skin.
    A. 45°
    B. 90°
    C. 180°
    D. 55°

24. You are ordered to administer 5 ml of a medication IM. You can safely administer this medication into all of the following muscles **except** the
    A. vastus lateralis.
    B. rectus femoris.
    C. deltoid.
    D. dorsal gluteal.

25. It is important to aspirate for blood return when administering medications via the IM route to ensure
    A. the airway is patent.
    B. the needle is in a vein.
    C. the needle is in the artery.
    D. the needle is not in a blood vessel.

26. Which of the following is **not** an indication for starting an IV?
    A. replacing fluid and blood
    B. administering a drug
    C. meeting a continuing medical education requirement
    D. obtaining blood samples for lab analysis

27. Which of the following is considered a peripheral vein?
    A. internal jugular
    B. subclavian
    C. femoral
    D. external jugular

28. Which of the following statements is true regarding the use of peripheral veins?
    A. They tend to roll and elude IV placement.
    B. They collapse in hypovolemic patients.
    C. They are often fragile in the elderly.
    D. all of the above

29. The primary role of intravascular proteins is to maintain
    A. hydrostatic pressure.
    B. colloid osmotic pressure.
    C. intracellular pressure.
    D. interstitial pressure.

30. Which of the following solutions is a crystalloid?
    A. plasmanate
    B. dextran

C. hetastarch
D. none of the above

31. Which type of IV solution will remain in the bloodstream initially and not cause a shift in water?
    A. hypotonic
    B. hypertonic
    C. isotonic
    D. hyperlipid

32. Which type of IV solution will rapidly leave the intravascular space?
    A. hypotonic
    B. hypertonic
    C. isotonic
    D. hyperlipid

33. Which type of IV solution will draw water into the vascular space?
    A. hypotonic
    B. hypertonic
    C. isotonic
    D. hyperlipid

34. Lactated Ringer's contains all of the following **except**
    A. proteins.
    B. potassium chloride.
    C. calcium chloride.
    D. sodium lactate.

35. You have infused 2 L of 0.9% sodium chloride into your hypovolemic trauma patient. In one hour, how much will be lost to the intravascular space?
    A. 1 L
    B. 2 L
    C. 660 ml
    D. 1320 ml

36. In a microdrip solution set, _____ drops equal 1 ml.
    A. 10
    B. 15
    C. 30
    D. 60

37. The main difference between normal IV tubing and blood tubing is
    A. the width of the tubing.
    B. the presence of an administration port.
    C. a filter to prevent an embolism.
    D. the absence of a flow clamp.

38. Through which of the following catheters can you deliver the most rapid fluid challenge?
    A. 12 gauge, 4 inch
    B. 12 gauge, 1 inch
    C. 24 gauge, 4 inch
    D. 24 gauge, 1 inch

39. Chills, fever, nausea, and vomiting following IV insertion indicate
    A. an inadvertent arterial puncture.
    B. a pyrogenic reaction.
    C. thrombophlebitis.
    D. an air embolism.

40. In this case (question 39), you should immediately
    A. place the patient head down on his left side.
    B. place warm packs on the IV site.
    C. stop the IV.
    D. clear the IV line of any air.

41. A Huber needle is used with
    A. a venous access device.
    B. an infusion controller.
    C. an infusion pump.
    D. blood tubes.

42. Which of the following IV devices delivers fluids and medications under positive pressure?
    A. the Huber device
    B. an infusion controller
    C. an infusion pump
    D. the Hickman device

Match the following blood tube color tops with their respective anticoagulants:

43. _____ red
44. _____ blue
45. _____ green
46. _____ purple
47. _____ gray

    A. EDTA
    B. none
    C. fluoride
    D. citrate
    E. heparin

48. If you leave the constricting band on your patient's arm too long prior to drawing a venous blood sample, what might be the result?
    A. hemoconcentration
    B. hemolysis
    C. hemophilia
    D. A and B

49. Generally, you will use the intraosseous route for pediatric patients in what age-group?
    A. 3–7
    B. 5–10
    C. newborn–10
    D. newborn–5

50. When inserting an IO needle, you must be careful not to
    A. infuse crystalloids.
    B. damage the epiphyseal plate.
    C. enter the medullary canal.
    D. use the medial tibial plateau.

51. For the adult or geriatric patient, you should insert an IO needle
    A. into the proximal tibia.
    B. into the distal tibia.
    C. superior to the medial malleolus.
    D. B and C

52. When inserting an IO needle, you stop when you
    A. feel an increase in resistance.
    B. feel a "pop."
    C. hear a "whoosh."
    D. see a bone marrow return.

53. Which of the following is a contraindication to IO insertion?
    A. fracture to the tibia
    B. fracture to the ipsilateral femur
    C. osteogenesis imperfecta
    D. all of the above

Make the following conversions:

54. 3 kg   = _____ g

55. 2.5 g   = _____ mg

56. 8 mg   = _____ mcg

57. 3000 ml = _____ L

58. 22 lbs. = _____ kg

Calculate the following drug orders:

DRUG ORDER	PATIENT WEIGHT	ADMINISTER
59. 1 mg/kg	176 lbs.	_____ mg
60. 10 mg/kg	220 lbs.	_____ mg
61. 20 ml/kg	55 lbs.	_____ ml
62. 5 mcg/kg/min	110 lbs.	_____ mcg/min
63. 0.1 mg/kg	22 lbs.	_____ mg

Determine the following drug concentrations:

64. 100 mg/10 ml   _____/ml

65. 50 mg/2 ml   _____/ml

66. 250 mg/20 ml   _____/ml

67. 1 g/10 ml   _____/ml

68. 1 mg/1 ml   _____/ml

Calculate the following drug administrations:

Calculate the following drip rates using microdrip solution sets (60 drops/ml):

DRUG	SOLUTION	MD ORDER	DRIP RATE
69. 1 g	250 ml	3 mg/min	___ drops/min
70. 2 g	500 ml	2 mg/min	___ drops/min
71. 1 mg	250 ml	4 mcg/min	___ drops/min
72. 400 mg	500 ml	5 mcg/kg/min (176 lbs.)	___ drops/min
73. 1 g	500 ml	2 mg/min	___ drops/min

Calculate the following fluid infusion rates:

VOLUME	INFUSION SET	TIME
74. 300 ml	10 gtts/ml	60 min ___ drops/min
75. 200 ml	15 gtts/ml	60 min ___ drops/min

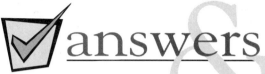

answers & rationales

Following each rationale, you will find a reference to the corresponding objective in the DOT National Standard EMT-Intermediate curriculum. An asterisk denotes material that is supplemental to the DOT curriculum. Page numbers after a rationale indicate where the question topic may be discussed in the Brady text *Intermediate Emergency Care* (Bledsoe, Porter, Cherry).

1.

A. A disinfectant is toxic to human tissue. An antiseptic is not. Therefore, use an antiseptic solution or wipe to cleanse the skin prior to injection. (1-4.11) (IEC p. 275)

2.

D. Nitroglycerin patches, some hypertension medications, and hormones are examples of medications given transdermally. A transdermal medication is absorbed through the skin into the circulatory system. (1-4.21) (IEC p. 277)

Matching (1-4.21) (IEC p. 277)

3.	E	Sublingual
4.	D	Buccal
5.	A	Ocular
6.	C	Aural
7.	B	Nasal

8.

D. Refer to the following Latin abbreviations with regard to the eye drop prescription: (1-4.21) (IEC p. 278)

o.d. (oculus dexter) right eye

o.s. (oculus sinister) left eye

o.u. (oculus uterque) both eyes

9.

B. When setting up a nebulizer—as with Albuterol, for example—set the oxygen source at 5–8 lpm. Any lower setting will not create enough pressure to aerosolize the medication. A setting greater than 8 will create too much pressure and damage the delivery system at its weakest point. (1-4.15) (IEC p. 280)

10.

A. If your patient has a decreased tidal volume, the medication may not reach the lower lungs. In this case, attach the nebulizer to a bag-valve-mask and perform intermittent positive pressure ventilation with the nebulizer running. (1-4.15) (IEC p. 281)

11.

B. In the emergency setting, atropine, lidocaine (Xylocaine), naloxone (Narcan), and epinephrine may be administered safely down the endotracheal tube when vascular access cannot be obtained. (1-4.15) (IEC p. 283)

12.

D. It is very difficult for the untrained person to use a metered dose inhaler effectively because it requires a great deal of coordination and rarely do patients receive proper training. The spacer was invented to help patients use the inhaler. As they simply have to breathe in and out of the device, its operation requires little coordination or training. (1-4.15) (IEC p. 281)

13.

B. When you pour a liquid medication into a medicine cup, it does not form a flat surface. Instead, it clings to the sides at a higher level. Therefore, always measure the liquid at the center, at the lowest point. (1-4.17) (IEC p. 285)

14.

C. A measured teaspoon holds 5 ml of liquid. Since household spoons are notoriously inaccurate, always use a measured spoon or syringe. (1-4.17) (IEC p. 285)

15.

A. After administering an oral medication, you should follow it with at least 4–8 ounces of water or other fluid to help transport it to the stomach. (1-4.17) (IEC p. 286)

16.

A. Because it would alter the slow-release mechanism, you should never administer time-release capsules or enteric-coated tablets through an orogastric tube. (1-4.17) (IEC p. 286)

17.

C. Drugs administered per rectum (PR) are rapidly absorbed through the rich capillary beds of the rectum and do not make a first pass through the liver; thus, hepatic alteration is avoided. (1-4.18) (IEC p. 288)

18.

A. The size of the syringe (the barrel) should be slightly larger than the amount of medication you are going to deliver. Thus, for a 3-cc delivery, select a 5-cc syringe. (1-4.20) (IEC p. 290)

19.

D. A needle's gauge is its diameter. The numbers are in reverse order of their sizes. For example, an 18 gauge is larger than a 27 gauge. (1-4.20) (IEC p. 290)

20.

C. To calculate a drug's concentration, simply divide the amount of drug (250 mg) by the amount of fluid (10 cc). In this case, the concentration is 250 mg/10 ml, or 25/1. (1-4.20) (IEC p. 291)

21.

D. An intradermal injection is administered at a 10–15° angle to the skin. (1-4.20) (IEC p. 298)

22.

A. A subcutaneous injection is administered at a 45° angle to the skin. (1-4.20) (IEC p. 299)

23.

B. An intramuscular injection is administered at a 90° angle to the skin. (1-4.20) (IEC p. 303)

24.

C. You can safely administer 5 ml of medication into the vastus lateralis (lateral thigh), the rectus femoris (anterior thigh), and the dorsal gluteal (buttock). You should administer only up to 2 ml into the deltoid muscle of the lateral shoulder. (1-4.20) (IEC p. 301)

25.

D. It is important to aspirate for blood return when administering medications via the IM (intramuscular) route to ensure that the needle is not in a blood vessel. Administering an IM medication directly into the bloodstream (IV) could be fatal. (1-4.20) (IEC p. 303)

26.

C. There are three reasons for starting an IV: to replace fluid or blood, to administer drugs, and to obtain venous blood samples for laboratory analysis. Initiating an intravenous line is done in order to help manage a patient's condition; starting an IV to meet a continuing medical education requirement is not acceptable. (1-4.20) (IEC p. 305)

27.

D. The external jugular is considered a peripheral vein. The subclavian, internal jugular, and femoral are all considered central veins. (1-4.20) (IEC p. 305)

28.

D. Peripheral veins are the easiest to cannulate during an emergency because of their accessibility. Unfortunately, they often collapse during hypovolemia or circulatory failure or roll and hide during IV placement and can be extremely fragile in elderly patients. (1-4.20) (IEC p. 306)

29.

B. Proteins have numerous responsibilities in the body. One of them is to maintain colloidal osmotic pressure while influencing the amount of water crossing a semipermeable membrane. Since proteins are larger molecules that do not cross membranes easily, they help maintain normal fluid distribution in the body. (1-4.20) (IEC p. 306)

30.

D. Crystalloids contain water and electrolytes but lack the proteins and larger molecules of the colloids. Examples of crystalloids include normal saline, lactated Ringer's, and D_5W. (1-4.20) (IEC p. 306)

31.

C. An isotonic solution has the same concentration (tonicity) on both sides of a semipermeable membrane (the vein). Because of this, there is no gradient (pulling force) created and no resulting water shift initially. (1-4.20) (IEC p. 306)

32.

A. A hypotonic solution has a lower solute concentration on one side of the semipermeable membrane (vein). Because of this, a pulling force (an osmotic gradient) is created, and water is "pulled" from the vein into the interstitial space. Examples include D_5W and 0.45% normal saline (one-half NS). (1-4.20) (IEC p. 307)

33.

B. A hypertonic solution has a higher solute concentration on one side of the semipermeable membrane and creates a gradient that pulls water into the vein. Examples include $D_{50}W$, mannitol, and the colloids. (1-4.20) (IEC p. 307)

34.

A. The isotonic solution named after Sidney Ringer contains sodium chloride, potassium chloride, calcium chloride, sodium lactate, and water. (1-4.20) (IEC p. 307)

35.

D. Two-thirds of an isotonic solution, such as normal saline (0.9% sodium chloride), will leave the intravascular space within 1 hour. (1-4.20) (IEC p. 307)

36.

D. In a microdrip solution set, 60 drops equal 1 ml. (1-4.20) (IEC p. 309)

37.

C. Blood tubing contains a filter to prevent clots or other debris from entering the patient. If a clot or debris enters the bloodstream, it could travel, as an embolus; lodge in a narrowed vessel; and occlude all blood flow distal to the occlusion. (1-4.20) (IEC p. 310)

38.

B. In order to infuse the most fluid the most rapidly, use the largest-diameter cannula with the shortest possible needle length. (1-4.20) (IEC p. 312)

39.

B. A pyrogenic reaction occurs when pyrogens, "foreign particles capable of producing fever," are present in the administration set or intravenous solution. It is characterized by the abrupt onset of fever, chills, backache, headache, nausea, and vomiting. Cardiovascular collapse may also result. (1-4.20) (IEC p. 319)

40.

C. In a case of pyrogenic reaction, terminate the IV immediately and establish another IV in the other arm, using a new administration set and solution. (1-4.20) (IEC p. 319)

41.

A. A Huber needle has an opening on the side of the shaft instead of at the tip. It is used with venous access devices to inject medications or fluid. Every venous access device has its own specialized needle. (1-4.20) (IEC p. 327)

42.

C. An infusion pump is a device that delivers fluids and medications under positive pressure rather than gravity. The major disadvantage of these devices is that you may cause more complications if the vein is infiltrated because of the positive pressure. (1-4.20) (IEC p. 329)

Matching (1-4.22) (IEC p. 331)

43.	B	Red
44.	D	Blue
45.	E	Green
46.	A	Purple
47.	C	Gray

48.

D. If you leave the constricting band on too long prior to drawing a venous blood sample, you run the risk of causing hemoconcentration (elevated numbers of red and white blood cells) and hemolysis (destruction of red blood cells). Both will render the results of the blood sample inaccurate and unusable. (1-4.22) (IEC p. 333)

49.

D. As a rule, you can use the intraosseous (IO) route for rapid venous access in critical patients less than 5 years of age. (1-4.14) (IEC p. 335)

50.

B. At the proximal end of the tibial shaft lies the epiphyseal (or growth) plate. If damaged, it can cause long-term growth complications or abnormalities. Always select an insertion site that is below the tibial tuberosity and on the medial tibial plateau. (1-4.14) (IEC p. 334)

51.

B. For the adult or geriatric patient, you may insert an IO needle into the distal tibia, just superior to the medial malleolus. (1-4.14) (IEC p. 334)

52.

B. When inserting an IO needle with a twisting motion, you should stop pushing when you feel a sudden decrease in resistance, or a "pop." Remember, one pop is good (you are in). Two pops are bad (you have gone through the other side). (1-4.14) (IEC p. 336)

53.

D. Do not attempt an IO line if your patient has a fractured tibia, has a fractured femur on the same side, or has osteogenesis imperfecta, a congenital bone disease that causes fragile bones. (1-4.14) (IEC p. 339)

Math Problems (1-4.3, 1-4.6) (IEC pp. 340–346)

The conversions are based on the following metric system table:

1 g = 1000 mg = 1,000,000 mcg

1000 g = 1 kg

1 kg = 2.2 lbs.

1 L = 1000 ml

54. 1 kg = 1000 g; 3 kg = 3000 g

55. 1 g = 1000 mg; 2.5 g = 2500 mg

56. 1 mg = 1000 mcg; 8 mg = 8000 mcg

57. 1000 ml = 1 L; 3000 ml = 3 L

58. 2.2 lbs. = 1 kg; 22 lbs. = 10 kg

59. 100 mg ÷ 10 ml = 10 mg/ml

60. 50 mg ÷ 2 ml = 25 mg/ml

61. 250 mg ÷ 20 ml = 12.5 mg/ml

62. 1 g (1000 mg) ÷ 10 ml = 100 mg/ml

63. 1 mg ÷ 1 ml = 1 mg/ml

The following calculations are based on the formula:

$$X = \frac{\text{Volume on hand} \times \text{Desired dose (MD order)}}{\text{Drug on hand}}$$

64.

$$X = \frac{5 \text{ ml} \times 75 \text{ mg}}{100 \text{ mg}} \quad X = \frac{375}{100} \quad X = 3.75 \text{ ml}$$

65.

$$X = \frac{1 \text{ ml} \times 0.25 \text{ mg}}{1 \text{ mg}} \quad X = \frac{0.25}{1} \quad X = 0.25 \text{ ml}$$

66.

$$X = \frac{2 \text{ ml} \times 25 \text{ mg}}{50 \text{ mg}} \quad X = \frac{50}{50} \quad X = 1 \text{ ml}$$

67.

$$X = \frac{5 \text{ ml} \times 50 \text{ mg}}{200 \text{ mg}} \quad X = \frac{250}{200} \quad X = 1.25 \text{ ml}$$

68.

$$X = \frac{10 \text{ ml} \times 0.5 \text{ mg}}{1 \text{ mg}} \quad X = \frac{5.0}{1} \quad X = 5.0 \text{ ml}$$

69. Patient weighs 198 lbs. $198 \div 2.2 = 90 \text{ kg}$

MD order is 5 mg/kg $90 \text{ kg} \times 5 \text{ mg} \times 450 \text{ mg}$

$$X = \frac{10 \text{ ml} \times 450 \text{ mg}}{500 \text{ mg}} \quad X = \frac{4500}{500} \quad X = 9 \text{ ml}$$

70. Patient weighs 187 lbs. $187 \div 2.2 = 85 \text{ kg}$

MD order is 1 mg/kg $85 \text{ kg} \times 1 \text{ mg} = 85 \text{ mg}$

$$X = \frac{10 \text{ ml} \times 85 \text{ mg}}{100 \text{ mg}} \quad X = \frac{850}{100} \quad X = 8.5 \text{ ml}$$

71.

$$X = \frac{1 \text{ ml} \times 10 \text{ mg}}{2 \text{ mg}} \quad X = \frac{10}{2} \quad X = 5 \text{ ml}$$

72.

$$X = \frac{10 \text{ ml} \times 120 \text{ mg}}{40 \text{ mg}} \quad X = \frac{1200}{40} \quad X = 30 \text{ ml}$$

73.

$$X = \frac{20 \text{ ml} \times 80 \text{ mg}}{400 \text{ mg}} \quad X = \frac{1600}{400} \quad X = 4 \text{ ml}$$

The following drip rate calculations are based on the formula:

$$\frac{\text{Volume} \times \text{Infusion set}}{\text{Time}}$$

74.

$$\frac{300 \text{ ml} \times 10 \text{ drops/ml}}{60 \text{ min}} = \frac{3000 \text{ drops}}{60 \text{ min}}$$
$$= 50 \text{ drops/min}$$

75.

$$\frac{200 \text{ ml} \times 15 \text{ drops/ml}}{60 \text{ min}} = \frac{3000 \text{ drops}}{60 \text{ min}}$$
$$= 50 \text{ drops/min}$$

Airway Management and Ventilation

unit objectives

Questions in this unit relate to DOT objectives 2-1.1 to 2-1.64. The objectives are listed in the Appendix.

DIRECTIONS

Each of the questions or incomplete statements below is followed by suggested answers or completions. Select the **one answer** that is best in each case.

1. A leaf-shaped cartilage that prevents food from entering the larynx during swallowing is the
   A. arytenoid.
   B. cricoids.
   C. epiglottis.
   D. hyoid.

2. The depression between the epiglottis and the base of the tongue is the
   A. eustachian tube.
   B. vallecula.
   C. hyoid.
   D. pyriform fossa.

3. The narrowest part of the adult upper airway is at the level of the
   A. vocal cords.
   B. cricoid cartilage.
   C. cricothyroid membrane.
   D. hyoid bone.

4. The space between the vocal cords is known as the
   A. eustachian tube.
   B. hyoid process.
   C. cricothyroid membrane.
   D. glottis.

5. The trachea divides into the right- and left-mainstem bronchi at the
   A. hyoid bone.
   B. carina.
   C. vallecula.
   D. parenchyma.

6. A tracheal tube inserted too far will most likely rest in the
   A. right-mainstem bronchus.
   B. left-mainstem bronchus.
   C. lung parenchyma.
   D. carina.

7. The FiO_2 of room air is
   A. 80–100 torr.
   B. .21.
   C. 100%.
   D. 40 torr.

Match the following modified forms of respiration with their respective descriptions:

8. _____ coughing
9. _____ sneezing
10. _____ hiccoughing
11. _____ sighing
12. _____ grunting

   A. prolonged exhalation
   B. respiratory distress sign in infants
   C. protective airway function
   D. caused by nasal irritation
   E. diaphragmatic spasm

13. Minute volume is calculated as
   A. respiratory rate + dead air space.
   B. tidal volume − dead air space.
   C. alveolar volume ÷ dead air space.
   D. tidal volume × respiratory rate.

14. The distensibility of the lungs is known as
    A. capnography.
    B. compliance.
    C. saturation.
    D. atelectasis.

Match the following types of breathing with their respective definitions:

15. _____ eupnea
16. _____ dyspnea
17. _____ tachypnea
18. _____ bradypnea
19. _____ hyperpnea
20. _____ apnea
21. _____ orthopnea

    A. absence of breathing
    B. slow breathing
    C. deep breathing
    D. fast breathing
    E. difficulty breathing
    F. difficulty breathing while lying down
    G. normal breathing

22. Normal SpO_2 should be
    A. under 95%.
    B. 95–99%.
    C. 90–100%.
    D. 80–100%.

23. Which of the following could cause an inaccurate SpO_2 reading?
    A. severe anemia
    B. hypovolemia
    C. CO poisoning
    D. all of the above

24. Immediately following tracheal intubation, you squeeze the esophageal detector device and, once it is applied, you notice that there is a free, effortless return of air after you squeeze the bulb device. This indicates that
    A. you have intubated the esophagus.
    B. you have an obstructed tracheal tube.
    C. you have intubated the trachea.
    D. suction of the trachea is necessary.

25. Your patient is semiconscious with a slight gag reflex. Which of the following airway adjuncts is indicated?
    A. oropharyngeal airway
    B. nasopharyngeal airway
    C. tracheal tube
    D. Esophageal Tracheal CombiTube

26. The major advantage of using a nasopharyngeal airway is that
    A. it isolates the trachea.
    B. it is easy to suction through.
    C. it can be used in the presence of a gag reflex.
    D. none of the above

27. Noncuffed tracheal tubes are typically recommended for children under the age of
    A. 5 years.
    B. 8 years.
    C. 10 years.
    D. 12 years.

28. In which of the following should orotracheal intubation be performed **only** as a last resort of airway management?
    A. a patient without a gag reflex.
    B. anaphylaxis.
    C. respiratory burns.
    D. epiglottitis.

29. Which of the following drugs may **not** be administered down the tracheal tube?

    A. epinephrine

    B. atropine

    C. lidocaine

    D. diazepam

30. Each tracheal intubation attempt should be limited to _____ seconds.

    A. 10

    B. 15

    C. 30

    D. 60

31. Which of the following indicates an esophageal intubation?

    A. continued phonation

    B. absence of breath sounds

    C. gurgling sounds heard over the epigastrium

    D. all of the above

32. The proper position of the head and neck for tracheal intubation in the nontrauma patient is the _____ position.

    A. neutral

    B. hyperextended

    C. sniffing

    D. flexed

33. The curved, or Macintosh, blade is designed to

    A. directly lift the epiglottis.

    B. spread the vocal cords.

    C. fit into the vallecula.

    D. none of the above

34. If your intubated patient has breath sounds only over the right chest, you should

    A. remove the tube immediately and begin BVM ventilation.

    B. secure the tube in place and begin to ventilate.

    C. deflate the cuff, withdraw the tube a few centimeters, and recheck breath sounds.

    D. deflate the cuff, advance the tube a few centimeters, and recheck breath sounds.

35. You have successfully intubated your patient, and your partner has been performing bag-valve-mask ventilation for the past few minutes when he tells you that the bag is becoming harder to squeeze. You notice distended jugular veins and cyanosis. On auscultation, the right chest is silent, and the left has diminished sounds. What do you do immediately?

    A. Insert an oropharyngeal airway as a bite block.

    B. Extubate the patient.

    C. Decompress the right chest with a large-bore catheter.

    D. Perform a cricothyrotomy.

36. Which of the following statements is true regarding pediatric intubation?

    A. The curved blade is the preferred device.

    B. ETT size = (Age in years + 4)/8.

    C. They have greater vagal tone than the adult.

    D. all of the above

37. The Esophageal Tracheal CombiTube (ETC) and the Pharyngo-tracheal Lumen (PtL) airways are similar in that

    A. both are inserted blindly.

    B. both depend on accurate placement assessment.

    C. neither requires maneuvering the head and neck.

    D. all of the above

38. Which of the following is an advantage of using the laryngeal mask airway (LMA)?

    A. It isolates the trachea.

    B. It protects against regurgitation and aspiration.

    C. It can be used in a patient with a gag reflex.

    D. none of the above

39. Which of the following is true regarding suctioning?

    A. Limit the suctioning to 30 seconds.

    B. Apply suction during insertion and during removal.

    C. Hyperoxygenate the patient before and after suctioning.

    D. all of the above

40. When you arrive on the scene of a patient in respiratory arrest, you notice that personnel are performing bag-valve-mask ventilation. You also notice that the patient's abdomen is extremely distended. After you intubate the patient, you notice resistance when you squeeze the bag. Lung sounds are diminished bilaterally, neck veins are normal, and the trachea is midline. What should you do?

    A. Insert a nasogastric tube.

    B. Pull back the tube 2 cm.

    C. Perform a cricothyrotomy.

    D. Decompress both sides of the chest.

41. The nasal cannula delivers oxygen concentrations in the range of

    A. 10–50%.

    B. 50–100%.

    C. 24–44%.

    D. 40–60%.

42. Nasal cannula flow rates should not exceed _____ lpm.

    A. 3

    B. 6

    C. 8

    D. 10

43. The simple face mask delivers oxygen concentrations in the range of

    A. 20–40%.

    B. 40–60%.

    C. 60–80%.

    D. 80–100%.

44. Simple face mask flow rates should never fall below _____ lpm.

    A. 3

    B. 6

    C. 8

    D. 10

45. The nonrebreather mask delivers oxygen concentrations in the range of

    A. 20–40%.

    B. 40–60%.

    C. 60–80%.

    D. 80–95%.

46. To deliver the above oxygen concentration, the nonrebreather mask flow rate should be _____ lpm.

    A. 6

    B. 8

    C. 10

    D. 15

47. The Venturi system delivers oxygen concentrations in the range of
    A. 24–40%.
    B. 40–60%.
    C. 60–80%.
    D. 80–100%.

48. Which of the following statements is true regarding the use of a bag-valve mask?
    A. Always engage the pop-off valve.
    B. Use an oxygen reservoir whenever possible.
    C. Reusable BVMs are acceptable.
    D. Adult BVMs are unacceptable for pediatric patients.

49. Using a pocket mask without supplemental oxygen delivers oxygen in the range of
    A. 16–17%.
    B. 21–22 %.
    C. 20–50%.
    D. 90–100%.

50. A bag-valve-mask device with an oxygen reservoir can deliver up to _____ of oxygen with flow rates at 10–15 lpm.
    A. 50%
    B. 60%
    C. 80%
    D. 95%

51. Using a bag-valve-mask without supplemental oxygen delivers _____ oxygen.
    A. 17%
    B. 21%
    C. 50%
    D. 90%

52. A flow-restricted oxygen-powered ventilation device will deliver up to _____ oxygen at its highest flow rates.
    A. 50%
    B. 60%
    C. 80%
    D. 100%

53. Which of the following complications is associated with use of a flow-restricted oxygen-powered ventilation device?
    A. pneumothorax
    B. subcutaneous emphysema
    C. gastric distention
    D. all of the above

54. Which of the following is true regarding the use of an automatic ventilator?
    A. It delivers higher minute volumes than the bag-valve-mask.
    B. Most units deliver controlled ventilation only.
    C. It can be used safely in all age-groups.
    D. The pop-off valves should be disengaged.

55. In which of the following cases might higher airway pressures be necessary to ventilate the lungs?
    A. cardiogenic pulmonary edema
    B. adult respiratory distress syndrome
    C. bronchospasm
    D. all of the above

56. A function of the epiglottis is to
    A. prevent air from entering the esophagus.
    B. direct food into the thyroid opening.
    C. allow air to enter the esophagus during breathing.
    D. allow air to enter the trachea during inhalation.

57. Which of the following will cause a decrease in the PaO_2 level in the blood?
    A. lactic acidosis
    B. aerobic metabolism
    C. poorly saturated hemoglobin
    D. depressed metabolism

58. An increase in the production of CO_2 may be the result of
    A. diminished respiratory rate.
    B. diminished metabolic rate.
    C. increased respiratory rate.
    D. increased metabolic rate.

59. You arrive on-scene to find a 56-year-old male who is breathing deeply at 32 times a minute. During your assessment, you find no subjective or objective indications of respiratory distress. What would you expect his $PaCO_2$ level to be?
    A. initially increased, then decreased
    B. initially decreased, then increased
    C. most likely lower than normal
    D. most likely higher than normal

60. All of the following statements about the purpose of suctioning are true **except**
    A. it can lower airway resistance during positive pressure ventilation.
    B. it can help remove excess fluid from the alveolar-capillary membrane.
    C. it can promote hypoxia if incorrectly performed.
    D. it can be safely performed on an infant.

61. What is the most effective way of unclogging a partially occluded suction catheter while performing oral suctioning?
    A. Disassemble the tip and clean manually.
    B. Increase the amount of suction applied.

C. Aspirate water through the catheter.
D. Strike the tip against a hard surface.

62. Which statement in regard to the anatomy of the upper airway is most accurate?
    A. The vallecula prevents food from entering the respiratory system while swallowing.
    B. The larynx joins the pharynx with the trachea.
    C. The larynx contains several openings such as the eustachian tube and the posterior nares.
    D. The thyroid cartilage, like the tracheal cartilages, forms a complete circle.

63. Which of the following statements about the vocal cords is true?
    A. The vocal cords are contained within the oropharynx.
    B. The vocal cords are found within the larynx.
    C. The vocal cords are housed within the cricoid cartilage.
    D. The vocal cords represent the opening into the esophagus.

64. Which of the following describes the relationship between the esophagus and the larynx?
    A. The larynx passes food while the esophagus passes water.
    B. The larynx and the esophagus exit at the same point.
    C. The larynx lies anterior to the esophagus.
    D. The larynx and the esophagus are comprised of cartilage.

65. Excess carbon dioxide (CO_2) is removed from the blood by
    A. bradypnea and hypopnea.
    B. urinary excretion.
    C. tachypnea and hyperpnea.
    D. sweating.

66. Suctioning is a priority in emergency care to
    A. prevent fluids from entering the esophagus.
    B. remove excess CO_2 from the respiratory system.
    C. prevent fluids from entering the trachea.
    D. reduce mucus production.

67. Which statement about suctioning is the most accurate?
    A. Suctioning should be limited to 30 seconds.
    B. Apply suction only during the insertion of the catheter.
    C. Oxygenation between suctioning attempts is not necessary.
    D. Suctioning should be limited to 10 seconds in the adult.

68. You are treating an unresponsive nonbreathing 13-year-old male who was involved in a car crash. Tracheal intubation equipment is not available. What is the best alternative for this patient?
    A. a nasal airway and supplemental oxygen
    B. a demand valve
    C. an oral airway and bag-valve-mask with an oxygen reservoir
    D. a nasal pharyngeal airway and a nonrebreather mask

69. You are treating a patient who needs to be intubated. All of the following statements about the tracheal intubation process are true **except**
    A. it is important to place the tracheal tube on the first attempt regardless of how long it takes.
    B. each tracheal intubation attempt should be limited to 30 seconds.
    C. the patient should be hyperoxygenated before each attempt to place the tracheal tube.
    D. during tracheal intubation, hypoxia can result because of operator inexperience.

70. A physician informs you that the 54-year-old male you transported has a PaO_2 of 94 mm Hg on room air. You know that this figure is considered
    A. low.
    B. normal.
    C. high.
    D. extremely high.

71. Which of the following would be considered a normal $PaCO_2$?
    A. 100 mm Hg
    B. 49 mm Hg
    C. 38 mm Hg
    D. 75 mm Hg

72. Which of the following statements would most correctly describe a healthy individual's $PaCO_2$ level and respiratory status during exercise?
    A. hypercarbic, increase in respiratory activity
    B. hypocapnic, increase in respiratory activity
    C. hypocarbic, increase in respiratory activity
    D. hypercapnic, no change in respiratory activity

73. A healthy individual has inhaled a considerable amount of smoke and presents as cyanotic and restless. Which of the following statements would best describe the condition and the expected respiratory rate?

    A. hypoxia, decrease in respirations

    B. hypoxia, increase in respirations

    C. hypercapnia, decrease in respirations

    D. hypoxic drive, decrease in respirations

74. While ventilating a patient who has a tracheal tube in place, you notice that the pilot balloon will not remain inflated. You would suspect

    A. inadequate connection between the bag-valve-mask and the pilot balloon.

    B. the tracheal tube has been misplaced in the esophagus.

    C. increased airway resistance.

    D. a leaking tracheal cuff.

75. The best indicator of proper tracheal tube placement would be

    A. absence of epigastric ventilation sounds.

    B. adequate breath sounds.

    C. ease in bag-valve-mask compliance.

    D. visualization of the tube passing between the vocal cords.

76. Besides preventing inadvertent tube dislodgment, a properly placed tracheal tube should be secured to prevent

    A. the patient from biting down on the tube.

    B. laceration by the metal stylet.

    C. inadvertent cardiovascular stimulation.

    D. rupture of the pilot balloon.

77. The normal range for arterial $PaCO_2$ is

    A. 15–25 mm Hg.

    B. 25–35 mm Hg.

    C. 35–45 mm Hg.

    D. 45–55 mm Hg.

78. What is the effect of hypercapnia on the respiratory rate of a healthy individual?

    A. Respiratory rate and depth are unchanged.

    B. Respiratory rate increases, while the depth is unchanged.

    C. Respiratory rate decreases, while the depth is unchanged.

    D. Respiratory rate and depth increase.

79. What is the effect of hypocapnia on the respiratory rate of a healthy individual?

    A. Respiratory rate and depth are unchanged.

    B. Respiratory rate increases, while the depth is unchanged.

    C. Respiratory rate decreases, while the depth is unchanged.

    D. Respiratory rate and depth increases.

80. Possible causes of increased CO_2 production include

    A. asthma and respiratory depression.

    B. fever and shivering.

    C. head injury and drug overdose.

    D. airway obstruction and paralysis of the respiratory muscles.

81. An oropharyngeal airway is an effective airway adjunct because it prevents the tongue from obstructing the airway and it

    A. isolates the trachea.

    B. allows air to pass around and through the device.

    C. is flexible and fits the airway.

    D. will not stimulate vomiting.

82. Which of the following is a relative contraindication of tracheal intubation?

    A. ingestion of a caustic substance

    B. major facial and neck trauma

    C. esophageal varices

    D. spinal injury

83. Complications associated with suctioning include hypoxia, vagal stimulation, and

    A. improved airway patency.

    B. hyperventilation.

    C. soft-tissue injury.

    D. hyperoxygenation.

84. Which anatomical structure is responsible for regulating the passage of air through the larynx?

    A. vocal cords

    B. epiglottis

    C. arytenoid folds

    D. lesser cornu

85. Which anatomic structure lies directly posterior to the cricoid cartilage?

    A. hyoid bone

    B. esophagus

    C. vallecula

    D. epiglottis

86. Which of the following statements regarding the esophageal opening and its structure is true?

    A. The esophageal opening is surrounded by cartilaginous structures.

    B. The esophageal structure is positioned posterior to the larynx.

    C. The esophageal structure is supported by semicircular cartilage.

    D. The esophageal opening is protected from food by the epiglottis.

87. To visualize the glottic opening when performing direct laryngoscopy, you must first lift which structure?

    A. vocal cords

    B. hyoid bone

    C. vocal fold

    D. epiglottis

88. The most common cause of airway obstruction is

    A. the tongue blocking the airway.

    B. a foreign body obstruction.

    C. aspiration of vomitus or food.

    D. laryngeal spasm constriction.

89. Loss of muscle tone to which muscle may cause the tongue to fall back against the pharynx causing an occluded airway?

    A. rectus femoris muscle

    B. vastus lateralis muscle

    C. submandibular muscle

    D. gastrocnemius muscle

90. Which of the following structures is the primary landmark for insertion of a tracheal tube?

    A. tracheal cartilage

    B. aryepiglottic fold

    C. false vocal cords

    D. true vocal cords

91. All of the following statements about the technique of suctioning are true **except**

    A. the tonsil-tip catheter is used to suction the lower airway.

    B. each suctioning attempt should be limited to 10 seconds.

    C. suction is applied only when withdrawing the catheter.

    D. cardiac dysrhythmias can occur during suctioning.

92. To help prevent viscous secretions from obstructing the suction tubing, you should
    A. reverse the suction action to help expel the thick secretions.
    B. suction water through the tubing between suctioning attempts.
    C. pretreat the tubing before suctioning with a petroleum lubricant.
    D. replace the suction tubing between every suctioning attempt.

93. You are about to suction a patient's mouth and oropharynx using the soft (French) catheter. Which is the proper way to measure the catheter?
    A. Measure from the patient's corner of the mouth to the tip of the ear.
    B. Measure from the tip of the patient's nose to the tip of the ear.
    C. Measure the length of the patient's little finger, then multiply by 2.
    D. Measure from the corner of the patient's mouth to the thyroid cartilage.

94. A limitation of the battery-powered suction unit is
    A. the unit becomes ineffective when the battery runs out.
    B. the unit requires two trained personnel to operate effectively.
    C. the suction created is too strong to use on infants and children.
    D. this suction device is limited to the confines of the ambulance.

95. Which type of suction unit may be more effective when suctioning heavier, tenacious substances?
    A. engine manifold–powered unit
    B. oxygen-powered unit

C. electric-powered unit
D. hand-powered unit

96. All of the following statements about the use of the rigid suction catheter are correct **except**
    A. the rigid suction catheter is used to suction the mouth of unresponsive patients.
    B. the rigid suction catheter is inserted into the mouth only as far as you can see.
    C. the rigid suction catheter is not used to suction the back of the airway of infants.
    D. the rigid suction catheter is used to suction the laryngopharynx and glottic space.

97. Which of the following is **not** a desired feature of the bag-valve mask?
    A. pop-off valve
    B. self-refilling bag
    C. transparent mask
    D. oxygen reservoir

98. Which of the following patients should **not** be intubated by orotracheal intubation?
    A. an unresponsive overdose patient who will not tolerate an oropharyngeal airway
    B. an unresponsive cardiac patient who does not respond to any type of stimulus
    C. a respiratory patient who becomes unresponsive to voice and tactile stimulation
    D. an unresponsive trauma patient who has copious amounts of blood in the airway

99. If after placing the tracheal tube you are unsure if the tube is properly placed, you should
    A. remove the tube and immediately attempt to reintubate the patient.
    B. deflate the cuff and gently withdraw the tube 1–2 cm and recheck.
    C. immediately remove the tube and ventilate using a oropharyngeal airway and a bag-valve-mask.
    D. have your partner reassess if you are unsure if whether the tube is properly placed.

100. All of the following are potential complications of tracheal suctioning **except**
    A. hypoxia may result from a decrease in lung air volume.
    B. cardiac arrhythmias may occur from suctioning the airway.
    C. bronchospasm may occur from insertion past the carina.
    D. stimulating the back of the throat may cause bradycardia.

101. All of the following structures are located in the pharynx **except**
    A. epiglottis.
    B. gag reflex nerves.
    C. vallecula.
    D. vocal cords.

102. Which of the following airway adjuncts completely isolates the trachea, ensuring a patent airway?
    A. oropharyngeal airway
    B. nasopharyngeal airway
    C. tracheal tube
    D. laryngeal mask airway

103. The appropriate equipment for intubating an infant is
    A. a curved laryngoscope blade and cuffed tracheal tube.
    B. a curved laryngoscope blade and uncuffed tracheal tube.
    C. a straight laryngoscope blade and cuffed tracheal tube.
    D. a straight laryngoscope blade and uncuffed tracheal tube.

104. All of the following are alternative airway adjuncts to tracheal intubation for the apneic patient **except** the
    A. nasogastric tube.
    B. laryngeal mask airway (LMA).
    C. Pharyngo-tracheal Lumen (PtL) airway.
    D. Esophageal Tracheal CombiTube (ETC).

105. Select the statement that best describes the relationship between the epiglottis and the larynx.
    A. The larynx is superior to the epiglottis.
    B. The epiglottis is superior to the larynx.
    C. The epiglottis is at the same level as the larynx.
    D. The epiglottis is inferior to the larynx.

106. Select the statement that best describes the relationship between the tongue and the larynx?
    A. The tongue is superior and anterior to the larynx.
    B. The tongue is inferior and anterior to the larynx.
    C. The tongue is inferior and posterior to the larynx.
    D. The tongue is superior and posterior to the larynx.

107. The anterior portion of the larynx that forms a "V" shape is called the
    A. thyroid cartilage.
    B. anterior cartilage.
    C. tracheal cartilage.
    D. cricoid cartilage.

108. What is the relationship between the false vocal cords and the true vocal cords?
    A. The false cords are inferior to the true cords.
    B. The false cords are lateral to the true cords.
    C. The false cords are medial to the true cords.
    D. The false cords are located in the oropharynx.

109. What is the space between the vocal cords called?
    A. septum
    B. vallecula
    C. pyriform fossa
    D. glottis

110. Which statement best describes the relationship of the pharynx to the larynx?
    A. The larynx is anterior to the pharynx.
    B. The larynx is posterior to the pharynx.
    C. The larynx is inferior to the pharynx.
    D. The larynx is superior to the pharynx.

111. What is the most superior region of the pharynx called?
    A. hyperpharynx
    B. oropharynx
    C. nasopharynx
    D. laryngopharynx

112. Which statement best describes a soft suction catheter?
    A. a rigid tube with two openings on the distal end
    B. a part rigid and part flexible tube with two openings on the distal end
    C. a long flexible tube with an open distal end
    D. a rigid tube with three openings on the distal end

113. You are ventilating a patient in respiratory arrest with a bag-valve-mask device. The patient suddenly vomits. What type of suction catheter should you select?
    A. whistle-tip suction catheter
    B. standard-tip suction catheter
    C. tonsil-tip suction catheter
    D. miller-tip suction catheter

114. What type of catheter would you use for tracheal suctioning?
    A. soft suction catheter
    B. standard-tip suction catheter
    C. tonsil-tip suction catheter
    D. miller-tip suction catheter

115. Which of the following is an indication for the use of the Esophageal Tracheal CombiTube airway?
    A. a patient with an intact gag reflex who requires ventilation
    B. a patient with respirations of 4 per minute and significant bleeding in the oropharynx
    C. a patient in respiratory arrest who ingested a caustic substance
    D. an adult trauma patient in whom you are unable to place a tracheal tube

116. All of the following items should be available prior to placing an ETC airway **except**

A. stethoscope.

B. water-soluble lubricant.

C. 35-cc syringe.

D. stylet.

117. Which of the following actions would best prevent deterioration of airway management skills?

A. Constantly read and review your textbook.

B. Watch a videotape reviewing the procedure.

C. Practice the skills on a continual basis.

D. Listen to an audiotape describing the procedures.

118. Tracheal intubation must be accomplished within

A. 30 seconds.

B. 40 seconds.

C. 50 seconds.

D. 60 seconds.

119. A 13-year-old female patient witnessed her pet getting hit and killed by a car. She now presents to you with classic indications of stress-induced hyperventilation syndrome. You would expect her carbon dioxide levels to be

A. diminished because of increased alveolar ventilation.

B. increased because of the extra acid production from breathing so hard.

C. diminished because of the levels of oxygen in her bloodstream rising from the increased ventilation.

D. increased because of the drop in alveolar ventilation.

120. All of the following statements regarding suctioning are correct **except**

A. routine suctioning should not take longer than 5–10 seconds per episode.

B. you should not suction infants because of the inherent danger of hypoxemia.

C. prolonged suctioning may precipitate hypoxemia.

D. application of suction to the suction tip should only occur while the catheter is being removed.

121. All of the following statements regarding the portable suction machine are true **except**

A. the collection bottle should be cleaned and disinfected after use.

B. improper assembly of the equipment may cause the unit to fail the next time it is needed.

C. the unit should be left charging in between calls.

D. the device is not designed to be used with a French-tip catheter.

122. At what level of the airway does occlusion occur when the tongue relaxes and falls against the back of the throat in an unresponsive patient?

A. nasopharynx

B. oropharynx

C. hypopharynx

D. laryngopharynx

123. Which of the following pieces of equipment is not always necessary during tracheal intubation of an adult patient with apnea and no gag reflex?

A. a 10-ml syringe

B. a laryngoscope blade

C. a malleable stylet

D. a laryngoscope handle

124. During the process of intubation, when should the tracheal tube stop being advanced?

A. when the proximal end of the cuff passes through the true vocal cords

B. when the proximal end of the cuff passes alongside the false vocal cords

C. when the distal end of the cuff passes through the true vocal cords

D. when the distal end of the cuff passes alongside the false vocal cords

125. What airway structure houses the vocal cords?

A. pharynx

B. larynx

C. epiglottis

D. carina

126. As you are transporting a patient with severe pulmonary edema, your partner states that the patient's trachea needs suctioned. The most correct statement is

A. tracheal suctioning should not be completed in the prehospital phase.

B. the trachea could be suctioned, but only by an EMT-Paramedic.

C. the trachea could be suctioned, but not for longer than 20 seconds at a time.

D. the trachea could be suctioned, but use lower levels of suction than pharyngeal suctioning.

127. Which one of the following clinical indications would alert you to a possible misplaced tracheal tube?

A. noticeable abdominal distention

B. a decrease in bagging resistance

C. moisture inside the lumen of the tracheal tube

D. high carbon dioxide reading in the end-tidal CO_2 monitor

128. When placing a tracheal tube or Esophageal Tracheal CombiTube in the trachea, the tube must first pass

A. between the esophagus and larynx.

B. through the glottic opening and between the vocal cords.

C. behind the vocal cords and through the larynx.

D. through the cricoid cartilage and between the thyroid cartilage.

129. The esophagus is located

A. inferior to the larynx.

B. anterior to the thryroid cartilage.

C. superior to the aretynoid cartilage.

D. posterior to the glottic opening.

130. A patient begins to choke and gasp for air while drinking a glass of water. Which of the following structures are most likely involved in this event?

A. epiglottis and vocal cords

B. esophagus and cricoid cartilage

C. thyroid cartilage and epiglottis

D. trachea and bronchus

131. You arrive on the scene and find a 26-year-old male patient who is visibly upset because of the breakup with his girlfriend. He is complaining of tingling in his extremities, light-headedness, and a tightness in his chest. His BP is 138/66, HR is 96/min, and respirations are 46/min and deep and full. If an arterial blood gas sample was drawn, what would you expect the PaO_2 level to be?

A. greater than 100 mm Hg

B. 80–90 mm Hg

C. 35–45 mm Hg

D. less than 40 mm Hg

132. You arrive on scene and find a patient who appears to be unresponsive on the floor in the kitchen. The family states the patient began slurring his words and complained of a severe headache followed by unconsciousness. You find the patient supine, with vomitus coming from his mouth and apparently not breathing. Which of the following would be your next immediate action?

   A. Check for a pulse.

   B. Suction the airway and perform a head tilt/chin lift maneuver.

   C. Begin bag-valve-mask ventilation with supplemental oxygen.

   D. Suction the airway and apply a nonrebreather mask at 15 lpm.

133. You are treating a patient with an altered mental status who is not breathing. You have suctioned the oropharynx and have inserted an oropharyngeal airway. The patient has a large amount of vomitus in both nostrils. Which of the following would be your next action?

   A. Begin bag-valve-mask ventilation with supplemental oxygen.

   B. Immediately insert an ETC CombiTube or PTL airway.

   C. Insert a nasopharyngeal airway in the right nasopharynx.

   D. Suction both nasopharyngeal passages with a soft suction catheter.

134. Which of the following is a **disadvantage** of orotracheal intubation?

   A. The tracheal tube can be used as a drug administration route.

   B. Aspiration of oral and nasal secretions cannot occur with a tracheal tube in place.

   C. Oral intubation requires a laryngoscope plus knowledge of the upper airway anatomy, practice, and skill.

   D. The tracheal tube reduces dead-air-space ventilation.

135. You arrive on scene and find a 56-year-old male patient who was involved in a motor vehicle crash. He has a significant amount of facial trauma from striking the windshield. You suction the airway, but the mouth readily fills with blood again. How would you control the airway in this patient?

   A. Continue to suction and insert an oropharyngeal airway.

   B. Insert a nasopharyngeal airway.

   C. Put the patient in a lateral recumbent position and perform a jaw-thrust maneuver.

   D. Insert a tracheal tube.

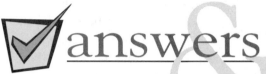
answers & rationales

Following each rationale, you will find a reference to the corresponding objective in the DOT National Standard EMT-Intermediate curriculum. An asterisk denotes material that is supplemental to the DOT curriculum. Page numbers after a rationale indicate where the question topic may be discussed in the Brady Text *Intermediate Emergency Care* (Bledsoe, Porter, Cherry).

1.

C. The epiglottis is a leaf-shaped cartilage that prevents food from entering the respiratory tract during the act of swallowing. (2-1.3) (IEC pp. 145, 202)

2.

B. The depression between the epiglottis and the base of the tongue is known as the vallecula. This landmark is significant because, during intubation, you insert the curved blade into this crevice. (2-1.3) (IEC p. 202)

3.

A. In adults, the narrowest part of the upper airway is at the level of the vocal cords. (2-1.3) (IEC p. 202)

4.

D. The glottis is the slitlike opening between the vocal cords, also known as the glottic opening. (2-1.3) (IEC p. 203)

5.

B. The carina is the point at which the trachea bifurcates into the right- and left-mainstem bronchi. (2-1.3) (IEC p. 204)

6.

A. The right-mainstem bronchus is at a slight angle, while the left-mainstem bronchus angles more acutely to the left. A tracheal tube inserted too far will most likely rest in the right-mainstem bronchus for that reason. (2-1.4) (IEC p. 204)

7.

B. The FiO_2 is a measurement of the concentration of oxygen in the inspired air. The FiO_2 of room air is approximately .21 (21%). (2-1.8) (IEC p. 210)

Matching (2-1.22) (IEC p. 354)

8.	C	coughing
9.	D	sneezing

10.   E hiccoughing
11.   A sighing
12.   B grunting

13.

D. Minute volume is the amount of gas moved in and out of the lungs and respiratory tract in 1 minute. It is measured by multiplying the tidal volume by the respiratory rate. (2-1.6, 2-1.15) (IEC p. 212)

14.

B. Compliance refers to the distensibility of the lung tissue. It is determined by how easily the lungs stretch. Increased compliance indicates the chest or lungs are very easy to inflate and may indicate a loss of some elastic recoil. Decreased compliance—which is often seen in conditions such as emphysema, circumferential chest wall burns, and tension pneumothorax—indicates the chest or lungs are stiff and difficult to inflate. (2-1.31) (IEC p. 356)

Matching (2-1.15) (IEC pp. 211, 354, 412, 424–425)

15.   G eupnea
16.   E dyspnea
17.   D tachypnea
18.   B bradypnea
19.   C hyperpnea
20.   A apnea
21.   F orthopnea

22.

B. Normal SpO_2 should be between 95% and 99%. (2-1.10) (IEC p. 357)

23.

D. Hypovolemia, CO poisoning, severe anemia, high-intensity lighting, certain hemoglobin

abnormalities, and an absent pulse can result in a false SpO_2 reading. Always use pulse oximetry as **one** of your assessment tools. (2-1.10) (IEC pp. 357–358)

24.

C. If there is a free flow of air after you squeeze the bulb device, you are in the wide, uncollapsible trachea. If the bulb does not refill, you are in a collapsed esophagus. (2-1.57) (IEC pp. 358–360)

25.

B. In the semiconscious patient with a gag reflex, the nasopharyngeal airway is an acceptable airway adjunct. (2-1.53) (IEC p. 370)

26.

C. The major advantage of using the nasopharyngeal airway is that it can be used in the presence of the gag reflex. (2-1.53) (IEC p. 370)

27.

B. Noncuffed tracheal tubes are typically recommended for children under the age of 8. In these children, the cricoid cartilage acts as an anatomical cuff since it is the narrowest part of the pediatric airway. (2-1.60) (IEC p. 388)

28.

D. Tracheal intubation should be avoided in patients suspected of having epiglottitis. Any unnecessary agitation of the patient can cause immediate laryngospasm and subsequent airway obstruction. If the patient is rapidly deteriorating or if the patient suffers a complete airway obstruction, orotracheal intubation could be attempted. (2-1.60) (IEC pp. 379, 388, 495, 1224)

29.

D. The following medications can be administered down the tracheal tube: oxygen, naloxone, atropine, epinephrine, and lidocaine. (2-1.55) (IEC pp. 283, 379)

30.

C. Tracheal intubation attempts should be limited to 30 seconds to prevent hypoxia. (2-1.55) (IEC p. 381)

31.

D. Signs of an esophageal intubation include an absence of chest rise and breath sounds with ventilatory support, gurgling sounds heard over the epigastrium, the absence of breath condensation in the tracheal tube, a persistent air leak despite inflation of the distal cuff, cyanosis, progressive worsening of the patient's condition, and phonation. (2-1.57) (IEC p. 381)

32.

C. The proper position of the head and neck for tracheal intubation in the nontrauma patient is the sniffing position. This is accomplished by flexing the neck forward and the head backward or by inserting a rolled towel under the patient's shoulders or the back of the head. (2-1.55) (IEC pp. 382, 384)

33.

C. The curved, or Macintosh, blade is designed to fit into the vallecula and indirectly lift the epiglottis. The vallecula is the space between the base of the tongue and the epiglottis. (2-1.55) (IEC p. 375)

34.

C. If your intubated patient has breath sounds heard only over the right-chest, you should assume a right mainstem bronchus intubation. In this case, deflate the cuff, withdraw the tube a few centimeters, and recheck placement. (2-1.57) (IEC pp. 381–382)

35.

C. The most common cause of tension pneumothorax is positive pressure ventilation. This includes overaggressive bag-valve-mask ventilation. Classic signs include increasing difficulty using the bag, distended jugular veins, absent breath sounds on the affected side, and diminished sounds on the opposite side. Treatment is immediate decompression with a large-bore catheter on the affected side—second intercostal space, midclavicular line. (2-1.55) (IEC p. 382)

36.

C. Intubating an infant or young child is a challenging proposition. The mouth is smaller, the tongue is larger, the larynx is more anterior, and the epiglottis is elongated and floppy. Infants and young children also have greater vagal tone than do adults. (2-1.60) (IEC pp. 386, 388–390)

37.

D. The ETC and the PtL airways are similar in that both are inserted blindly, both depend on the accurate assessment of their placement, and neither requires movement of the head and neck. (2-1.54) (IEC pp. 391–395)

38.

D. The LMA does not isolate the trachea or protect the lung against regurgitation and aspiration. It cannot be used for people with a gag reflex. An advantage of the LMA is that it can be placed rapidly without the need to visualize the airway. (2-1.54) (IEC pp. 395–396)

39.

C. Suctioning should always be limited to 10 seconds. You should hyperoxygenate the patient before and after all suctioning attempts and always apply suction during removal. (2-1.46) (IEC p. 366)

40.

A. Often performing ventilation on an unintubated patient causes gastric distention. The distention puts pressure on the diaphragm, making ventilation more difficult. In these cases, decompress the stomach by inserting a nasogastric tube. (2-1.49) (IEC p. 367)

41.

C. The nasal cannula delivers oxygen concentrations in the range of 24–44%, depending on the liter flow. (2-1.27) (IEC p. 360)

42.

B. Nasal cannula flow rates should not exceed 6 lpm, as this will dry the mucous membrane and cause headaches. (2-1.27) (IEC p. 360)

43.

B. The simple face mask delivers oxygen concentrations in the range of 40–60%. Oxygen is delivered through the bottom of the mask via its oxygen inlet port. (2-1.27) (IEC p. 361)

44.

B. No fewer than 6 lpm should be administered through this device, as expired carbon dioxide can otherwise accumulate in the mask. (2-1.27) (IEC p. 361)

45.

D. The nonrebreather mask consists of oxygen tubing and a face mask with an attached reservoir bag. When the patient inhales, 100% oxygen contained in the reservoir is drawn into the mask and the patient's respiratory passageways. The nonrebreather mask delivers the highest concentration of oxygen. Once applied, a flow rate of 12–15 lpm can deliver an 80–95% oxygen concentration. (2-1.27) (IEC p. 361)

46.

D. In order to deliver an oxygen concentration of 80–95%, the nonrebreather mask flow meter should be set at 15 lpm. (2-1.27) (IEC p. 361)

47.

A. The Venturi system is a high-flow device including oxygen tubing, a face mask, and the Venturi system. As oxygen passes through a jet port in the base of the mask, it entrains room air. Depending on the device used, oxygen concentrations can be delivered in the range of 24–40%. (2-1.27) (IEC p. 361)

48.

B. Proper use of a bag-valve mask (BVM) device includes disengaging the pop-off valve (to prevent underventilation), using disposable devices only, watching for chest rise (to prevent overventilation, especially in the pediatric patient), and always using an oxygen reservoir (to deliver maximum FiO_2). (2-1.31) (IEC p. 363)

49.

A. Using a pocket mask without supplemental oxygen delivers the oxygen in the range of 16–17%—in other words, your own expired percentage of oxygen. (2-1.27) (IEC p. 362)

50.

D. A bag-valve-mask device with an oxygen reservoir can deliver up to 95% of oxygen with flow rates at 15 lpm. (2-1.27) (IEC p. 363)

51.

B. Using a BVM without supplemental oxygen delivers 21% oxygen—in other words, room air. (2-1.27) (IEC pp. 362–363)

52.

D. A flow-restricted oxygen-powered ventilation device will deliver up to 100% oxygen at its highest flow rates. (2-1.27) (IEC p. 364)

53.

D. Using a flow-restricted oxygen-powered ventilation device has its disadvantages. Some of these include creating a pneumothorax, subcutaneous emphysema, or gastric distention. (2-1.31) (IEC pp. 364–365)

54.

A. Automatic ventilators deliver higher minute volumes than the bag-valve mask. (2-1.33) (IEC p. 365)

55.

D. In cases such as cardiogenic pulmonary edema, adult respiratory distress syndrome,

and bronchospasm, higher airway pressures may be necessary to ventilate the lungs. (2-1.31) (IEC p. 356)

56.

D. The epiglottis is a flaplike structure that uncovers the glottic opening during inhalation, thereby allowing inhaled air to gain access to the lungs. It closes over the top of the glottic opening during swallowing so that the material is directed into the esophagus. (2-1.3) (IEC pp. 145, 202)

57.

C. Arterial oxygen saturations decrease when there is a problem with oxygenation of the blood. This results in poorly saturated hemoglobin. Aerobic metabolism is cellular activity in the presence of oxygen, and lactic acidosis is a by-product of anaerobic metabolism. (2-1.10) (IEC p. 210)

58.

D. Heightened metabolic activity is a common cause of elevated CO_2 levels as the cells of the body produce more waste products. A diminished respiratory rate may result in heightened CO_2 levels, but it is a function of diminished elimination and not increased production. Both diminishment of the metabolic rate and elevations in the respiratory activity will lower CO_2 levels. (2-1.11) (IEC p. 210)

59.

C. His $PaCO_2$ would be lower than normal because the arterial level of carbon dioxide is a direct function of alveolar ventilation in the healthy person. An increase in alveolar ventilation will reduce the $PaCO_2$ levels in the bloodstream as it is eliminated at a faster rate through the lungs. (2-1.11) (IEC p. 210)

60.

B. It is impossible to suction fluid from the capillary/alveolar membrane. At this level, the structures are much smaller than even a millimeter! Suctioning a patient removes material from either the pharynx or lower in the trachea if the patient has a tracheal tube placed. (2-1.43) (IEC pp. 365–367)

61.

C. When a suction catheter becomes clogged, try suctioning water through the tip. This will often remove the clog. If that does not work, replace the tip. (2-1.46) (IEC p. 366)

62.

B. The larynx is the structure that joins the pharynx with the trachea. The pharynx, or throat, extends from the back of the soft palate to the esophagus and larynx. The pharynx contains the openings for the eustachian tube and posterior nares. The epiglottis is the structure that prevents food from entering the respiratory tract. The vallecula is just above the epiglottis. The thyroid and tracheal cartilages are open on their posterior surfaces, whereas the cricoid cartilage forms a complete ring. (2-1.3) (IEC pp. 200–203)

63.

B. The vocal cords are found within the larynx. They are actually housed within the thyroid cartilages, which is a part of the larynx. Anatomically, the vocal cords represent the opening into the trachea, not the esophagus. (2-1.3) (IEC p. 203)

64.

C. In terms of location, the larynx is anterior to the esophagus. The larynx and esophagus are separate structures that each serve a different function. The larynx is constructed of cartilage and is a conductor of air, while the esophagus is soft and transports food and water into the stomach. (2-1.3) (IEC p. 203)

65.

C. Tachypnea (fast respirations) and deep breathing (hyperpnea) enhance alveolar ventilation and quickly "blow off" excessive amounts of carbon dioxide. Slow respirations would be ineffective in ventilating the excess CO_2 from the alveoli. Carbon dioxide is not excreted in the urine and sweat. (2-1.11) (IEC p. 210)

66.

C. Securing a patent airway is always the priority in emergency care. Suctioning fluids from the airway is one of many ways to accomplish this task. The fluids are removed, thus preventing them from entering the trachea and ultimately the lungs. Suctioning has little effect on removing CO_2 and does not decrease mucus production. (2-1.43) (IEC p. 365)

67.

D. Suctioning should be limited to 10 seconds in an adult. When possible, the patient should be hyperventilated with 100% oxygen before and between each suctioning attempt. Suction should be applied only after the catheter is properly positioned and during withdrawal. (2-1.46) (IEC p. 366)

68.

C. The oral airway and the bag-valve-mask are the best alternative for the patient in this scenario. The demand valve resuscitator is not recommended in patients under the age of 16. A nasal airway would be acceptable if the patient did not accept an oral airway; however, in a nonbreathing unconscious patient, an oral airway should be attempted. The bag-valve mask is necessary for high-flow oxygen therapy and for assisting ventilations. Both the oral airway and bag-valve-mask come in pediatric sizes. (2-1.50) (IEC pp. 362–364, 372–374)

69.

A. Tracheal intubation requires trained personnel, and intubation efforts should not be a lengthy process. Hypoxia can occur from oxygen delays and operator inexperience. The patient should be hyperventilated before and after each attempt, and each attempt should be limited to 30 seconds. (2-1.55) (IEC p. 381)

70.

B. While the optimal figure for arterial oxygen is 100 mm Hg, the range of 80–100 mm Hg is considered within normal limits. This patient has a PO_2 measured at 94 mm Hg, which falls within the suggested range and is not an immediate concern. (2-1.12) (IEC pp. 357–358)

71.

C. The average range of normal $PaCO_2$ values spans 35–45 mm Hg. 38 mm Hg is within this range and is therefore considered normal. (2-1.13) (IEC p. 209)

72.

A. During exertion, activity at the cellular level increases in an effort to meet the added demand. This heightened cellular activity results in an increase in the by-products of water and CO_2. The $PaCO_2$ would increase and be described as hypercarbic. In an effort to rid itself of the added waste products, the neuroregulatory system increases respiratory activity so as to excrete the CO_2 via pulmonary ventilation. (2-1.11) (IEC p. 210)

73.

B. This individual has experienced a drop in arterial oxygen saturation caused by the toxic inhalation and is therefore hypoxic. In an effort to get more oxygen, the respiratory centers in the brain will increase the respiratory activity. Hypercapnia refers to the retention of CO_2, and the hypoxic drive refers to individuals who have lost their ability to regulate internal CO_2 levels and breath in accordance to their PaO_2, such is as seen with COPD patients. (2-1.10) (IEC p. 211)

74.

D. The pilot balloon serves as a visible indicator of the hidden inflatable tracheal cuff. If the pilot balloon will not remain inflated, the EMT-Intermediate must immediately suspect a problem with the inflatable cuff. In this situation, the tracheal tube should be removed and the patient reintubated with another tube. The bag-valve-mask connects to the 15/22-mm adapter at the proximal end of the tube, not the pilot balloon. (2-1.55) (IEC p. 377)

75.

D. Visualization of the tracheal tube passing between the vocal cords is the greatest assurance of proper tube placement. (2-1.56) (IEC p. 385)

76.

C. An unsecured tracheal tube can slide down inside the trachea, stimulating parasympathetic receptors located near and on the carina. Once activated, these receptors can precipitate bradycardia and hypotension. Securing a tracheal tube does little in terms of preventing a patient from biting down on the tube. A bite block or oropharyngeal airway would better serve to accomplish this task. Also, the metal stylet should be immediately removed once the tube has passed between the vocal cords. Because the pilot balloon is located outside the patient's mouth at the proximal end of the tracheal tube, securing the tube has little to do with the unlikely event of rupture. (2-1.58) (IEC p. 751)

77.

C. The normal range for arterial $PaCO_2$ is 35–45 mm Hg. (2-1.13) (IEC p. 209)

78.

D. Hypercapnia in a healthy individual will cause the respiratory activity to increase. This increase in rate and depth, known as hyperventilation, allows more $PaCO_2$ to be exhaled until it is lowered to normal. (2-1.15) (IEC p. 210)

79.

A. Hypocapnia does not stimulate the central and peripheral chemoreceptors; thus, a decrease in $PaCO_2$ has no immediate effect on the respiratory activity of a healthy individual. The respiratory rate and depth will remain essentially unchanged. The $PaCO_2$ accumulates, gradually returning to normal levels. (2-1.15) (IEC p. 211)

80.

B. Possible causes of increased CO_2 production include any activities that result in increased metabolic activity, like fever and shivering. Asthma, respiratory depression due to drug overdose, head injury, airway obstruction, or paralysis of the respiratory muscles all may contribute to the decreased elimination of CO_2, resulting in respiratory acidosis. (2-1.11) (IEC p. 210)

81.

B. An oropharyngeal airway is an effective airway adjunct because it allows for air passage around and through the device and prevents the tongue from obstructing the airway. However, among its disadvantages are failure to isolate the trachea and inflexibility, and that its insertion may stimulate vomiting. (2-1.52) (IEC p. 372)

82.

B. A relative contraindication for tracheal intubation is major facial and neck trauma that may prevent recognition of landmarks. (2-1.55) (IEC p. 374)

83.

C. Soft-tissue injury is a complication associated with suctioning. Others include hypoxia and vagal stimulation. (2-1.47) (IEC p. 366)

84.

A. The true vocal cords regulate the amount of air that passes through the larynx and produce sound. The epiglottis is a leaf-shaped flap that prevents substances from entering the trachea while swallowing. Arytenoid folds are cupped tissues found posterior to the vocal cords, and the lesser cornu are found superior to the hyoid bone. (2-1.3) (IEC p. 203)

85.

B. The esophagus lies directly behind the cricoid cartilage, which forms a complete cartilaginous ring. The upper portion of the thyroid cartilage is attached to the hyoid bone. The vallecula is located above the epiglottis, and the epiglottis is a leaf-shaped flap that is anterior to the pharynx. (2-1.3) (IEC p. 203)

86.

B. The epiglottis prevents food and drink from being aspirated into the glottis and trachea. The esophagus is positioned posterior to the larynx, and the trachea is anterior to the esophagus and can be felt by palpating the neck. The trachea is supported by cartilage structures, not the esophagus. (2-1.3) (IEC p. 203)

87.

D. The epiglottis must be lifted to visualize the glottic opening. The vocal cords are hidden behind the epiglottis and cannot be visualized until the epiglottis is lifted. The hyoid bone is located below the chin but above the pharynx and is unique in the fact that it is the only bone that does not articulate with another bone; it is suspended by ligaments. The vocal folds are a point of attachment for the arytenoid cartilage and does not affect visualization of the glottic opening. (2-1.56) (IEC p. 375)

88.

A. The most common airway obstruction is the tongue blocking the airway. This occurs when the relaxed tongue falls back against the rear of the pharynx, occluding the airway. (2-1.38) (IEC p. 351)

89.

C. The submandibular (below the mandible or lower jaw) muscle provides direct support of the tongue and indirect support of the epiglottis. Poor muscle tone of this muscle may lead to an obstructed airway. (2-1.38) (IEC p. 351)

90.

D. The true vocal cords, which are pale or pearly white, are the structures in the glottic opening that are easiest to identify. The tracheal cartilage is found in the trachea and gives the trachea its structural form. Aryepiglottic folds are landmarks that help identify the glottic area but do not border the glottis. The false vocal cords lie above the true vocal cords. (2-1.56) (IEC p. 203)

91.

A. Because of its size and structure, the rigid catheter, or tonsil tip, should be used only when suctioning the upper airway. Vigorous insertion can cause lacerations and bleeding. (2-1.44) (IEC pp. 365–366)

92.

B. Suctioning water between each suctioning attempt will clear the tubing as well as lubricate the catheter. The suction cannot be reversed; this would be dangerous, for it would spread secretions. Never use a petroleum lubricant near the airway or rubber tubing. Replacing the tubing would be costly and wasteful but be prepared to replace it if needed. (2-1.46) (IEC p. 366)

93.

A. The correct way to measure the length needed to suction the mouth and oropharynx is from the corner of the mouth to the tip of the ear. When suctioning the nose and nasopharynx, the length is determined by measuring the catheter from the tip of the patient's nose to their ear. (2-1.42) (IEC p. 366)

94.

A. The battery-powered suction unit becomes totally ineffective once the battery runs out. This suction unit can be operated by one rescuer. The suction can and should be reduced when suctioning infants and children and the unit is manufactured as a portable. (2-1.44) (IEC p. 365)

95.

D. The hand-powered unit is the most effective when suctioning thick, tenacious substances. The hand-powered unit also does not require a power source other than that of the EMT-Intermediate. This reduces the maintenance costs and the threat of failure caused by a failed power source. (2-1.55) (IEC p. 365)

96.

D. The rigid suction catheter is not used to suction the laryngopharynx and glottic space. This area of the airway is below the epiglottis and is too far down the airway to effectively suction with the rigid catheter. (2-1.42) (IEC p. 367)

97.

A. A bag-valve mask with a pop-off valve that cannot be disabled may lead to inadequate ventilations in some patients. A self-refilling bag is desired, so there is no need for the oxygen pressure to refill the bag. The transparent mask will permit you to visualize if the patient vomits. The oxygen reservoir will allow you to deliver a high concentration of oxygen rather than the 21% that is found in the air. (2-1.31) (IEC p. 363)

98.

A. An unresponsive patient who will not tolerate an oropharyngeal airway will not tolerate orotracheal intubation. A patient who does not respond to any type of stimulation is a high risk for aspiration and should be intubated. The trauma patient with copious amounts of blood in the airway needs to be suctioned and then intubated to prevent the aspiration of the blood. Do not intubate this patient by hyperextending the head. (2-1.55) (IEC p. 379)

99.

C. If at any time you are unsure that the tube is properly placed, quickly remove the tube and use an alternative method such as an oropharyngeal airway and a bag-valve-mask to ventilate the patient. If the tube is left in the esophagus, the patient will die. The patient must be ventilated with the bag-valve-mask prior to reintubating, or severe hypoxia will result. Remember, if you see the tube pass through the vocal cords, you are in the correct place. (2-1.57) (IEC p. 381)

100.

D. Bradycardia caused by stimulating the back of the throat may occur when suctioning the mouth and oropharynx, not when suctioning down the tracheal tube. (2-1.48) (IEC p. 366)

101.

D. The epiglottis, gag reflex nerves, and vallecula are located in the pharynx. The vocal cords are found in the larynx. (2-1.3) (IEC pp. 202–203)

102.

C. The tracheal tube (also called the endotracheal tube) isolates the trachea, which allows complete control of the airway. It also offers a direct route to the respiratory passages, thereby allowing for easy suctioning and medication administration. (2-1.55) (IEC p. 374)

103.

D. Intubating the pediatric patient requires a straight laryngoscope blade, as the epiglottis is floppy, so it needs to be lifted directly. The narrowest part of the pediatric airway is the cricoid cartilage. When an appropriately sized tracheal tube is inserted, a seal is created at the cricoid level. The cricoid ring serves as a functional cuff. (2-1.60) (IEC p. 388)

104.

A. The laryngeal mask airway, pharyngeal tracheal lumen airway, and Esophageal Tracheal CombiTube airway are acceptable alternative airway adjuncts for the apneic patient. Intubation of the trachea, when possible, is the preferred technique for managing the airway. (2-1.54) (IEC pp. 367, 391–396)

105.

B. The epiglottis is located within the laryngopharynx and is superior to the larynx. (2-1.3) (IEC p. 202)

106.

A. The tongue is located anterior and superior to the larynx. (2-1.3) (IEC pp. 201–202)

107.

A. The anterior portion of the larynx is known as the thyroid cartilage. It is commonly called the Adam's apple. The cricoid cartilage forms the inferior border of the larynx, which makes up the first tracheal ring. (2-1.3) (IEC pp. 202–203)

108.

B. The false vocal cords are located lateral to the true vocal cords. The true vocal cords regulate air entering the larynx. As the muscles of the larynx contract, the vocal cords change shape and vibrate. This change in shape, coupled with the movement of air across the vocal cords, produces sound. Passage of a tracheal tube between the true vocal cords prevents the creation of sound or the production of a cough. (2-1.56)

109.

D. The space between the vocal cords is known as the glottis or the glottic opening. The vallecula is the junction of the tongue and the epiglottis. The pyriform fossa is located on both sides of the epiglottis. (2-1.56) (IEC pp. 202–203)

110.

C. The larynx is located inferior to the pharynx. The lowermost portion of the pharynx is known as the hypopharynx or the laryngopharynx. (2-1.3) (IEC p. 202)

111.

C. The most superior region of the pharynx is called the nasopharynx. The oropharynx and the laryngopharynx are the other functional subdivisions. (2-1.3) (IEC p. 202)

112.

C. The whistle-tip, or soft suction, catheter is a long flexible tube. It is smaller in diameter than the tonsil-tip suction catheter, and for this reason it is not well suited to the removal of large amounts of fluids or blood. The whistle tip is used for deep tracheal suctioning. The tonsil tip is used for the removal of large amounts of blood or secretions in the oropharynx. (2-1.42) (IEC p. 366)

113.

C. For large amounts of fluid or vomit, use a Yankauer, or tonsil-tip, suction catheter. The distal opening is much larger than a whistle-tip suction catheter and better able to handle large volumes and larger particulate matter. (2-1.42) (IEC p. 366)

114.

A. A whistle-tip, or soft suction catheter is thin, flexible, and long enough to provide tracheal suctioning. The whistle-tip catheter may be placed through the external nares, the oropharynx, or an oropharyngeal airway or into a tracheal tube. (2-1.42) (IEC p. 367)

115.

D. If airway patency cannot be achieved with a tracheal tube, an ETC airway is acceptable in the trauma patient. An ETC airway should not be attempted in the patient with an intact gag reflex or excessive bleeding in the oropharynx or if caustic poison has been ingested. (2-1.61) (IEC pp. 392–393)

116.

D. A stylet is used to assist with placement of a tracheal tube. It is not required for ETC airway placement. An assembled esophageal obturator airway complete with mask and tube, suction unit, syringe, lubricant, and stethoscope should also be prepared. (2-1.61)

117.

C. Airway management skills such as tracheal intubation are psychomotor skills. You must practice these skills constantly to maintain your proficiency. Reading, watching, and listening will not take the place of actually performing or practicing the skill. (2-1.2)

118.

A. Tracheal intubation must be accomplished in less than 30 seconds. After 30 seconds, ventilate the patient for 2 minutes prior to attempting the intubation again. Try holding your breath from the time you stop ventilations until you need a breath. If you need a breath, you can be sure the patient does as well. (2-1.55) (IEC p. 381)

119.

A. Carbon dioxide levels in the bloodstream are a direct reflection of alveolar ventilation. As such, any increase in the patient's minute ventilation will cause a lowering of the $PaCO_2$ value. Oxygen levels move opposite of carbon dioxide levels but are not dependent on it. The extra acid produced from the heightened muscular respiratory effort will be buffered by the body's normal mechanisms. (2-1.11) (IEC p. 210)

120.

B. An infant with an airway occlusion needs suctioning just as much as an adult patient, and there are no dangers of inherent hypoxemia as long as the skill is done correctly. You should not suction longer than 5–10 seconds to avoid hypoxemia, and you should suction only while withdrawing the catheter. (2-1.45) (IEC pp. 365–367)

121.

D. Portable suction units can be used with either a tonsil-tip catheter or whistle-tip catheter. Most units will have two levels of suctioning so that you can decrease the suctioning strength with the French tip. Always clean and disinfect all equipment and be sure to assemble it correctly and charge the batteries so it will be functional the next time it is needed. (2-1.44)

122.

B. Directly posterior to the tongue is the oropharynx, and when the unconscious patient becomes supine, gravity causes the tongue to relax backward and block the airway. The nasopharynx is located superior to the oropharynx, and the hypopharynx (also known as laryngopharynx) is located inferior to the oropharynx. (2-1.38) (IEC pp. 201–202, 351)

123.

C. A stylet is an adjunctive piece of equipment needed for intubation when the glottic opening is located anterior or cephalad. The syringe is needed to inflate the tracheal cuff, the blade (#3 or #4 for an adult) is necessary

for visualization, and the laryngoscope handle is necessary and interfaces with the laryngoscope blade. (2-1.55) (IEC pp. 377–378)

124.

A. Insertion of a tracheal tube is very important so that it is not advanced too far. To ensure proper placement, insert the tube until the proximal side of the cuff passes just beyond the true vocal cords, through the glottic opening. (2-1.55) (IEC p. 384)

125.

B. The larynx, comprised of the thyroid, cricoid, and epiglottis cartilage, houses the vocal cords. The pharynx, commonly known as the throat, lies superior to the larynx and is a passageway for both food and air. (2-1.3) (IEC p. 203)

126.

D. When providing tracheal suctioning, use a French catheter and a negative vacuum pressure of 80–120 mm Hg. Pharyngeal or oral suctioning is usually greater than 120 mm Hg. This skill could be completed by the EMT-Intermediate who intubated the patient, but suctioning time should still be limited to 5–15 seconds to avoid undue hypoxemia. (2-1.48)

127.

A. If a tracheal tube becomes misplaced, there will be abdominal distention that may become severe. The presence of moisture in the ET tube is expected, and a decrease in bagging resistance is not characteristic of a misplaced tube; in fact, it should increase if misplaced. Finally, high CO_2 levels are expected with appropriate tube placement. (2-1.57) (IEC pp. 385–386)

128.

B. The tube will first pass through the oropharynx, the hypopharynx, the glottic opening, and then between the vocal cords in the larynx and into the trachea. (2-1.56) (IEC pp. 390, 391)

129.

D. The esophagus is located posterior to the glottic opening in the hypopharynx. Both the glottic opening and the esophagus are located in the hypopharynx. (2-1.3) (IEC p. 203)

130.

A. The larynx begins to spasm, causing the vocal cords to close when water, food, or other substances enter the glottic opening. This protective reflex causes the patient to choke forcefully and perceive a feeling of not being able to catch his breath. (2-1.39) (IEC p. 202)

131.

A. The patient is experiencing hyperventilation syndrome, in which he is breathing fast and deep. His elevated respiratory rate and increased tidal volume will cause him to take in excessive amounts of oxygen and blow off significant amounts of carbon dioxide, resulting in an elevated PaO_2 level exceeding 100 mm Hg and a decreased $PaCO_2$ below 40 mm Hg. (2-1.10, 2-1.11) (IEC p. 210)

132.

B. The priority is to clear the airway with suction then to perform a manual maneuver to open the airway. Once the airway is opened, it is necessary to assess and manage the ventilation before checking the pulse. (2-1.1) (IEC p. 353)

133.

D. It is necessary to suction the nasopharynx. An oropharyngeal airway will not protect the trachea from aspiration of vomitus or other substances. If the nasopharynx is not cleared, the vomitus will likely be aspirated into the trachea with the first few ventilations. (2-1.43)

134.

C. One disadvantage of tracheal intubation is the need for training and skill in performing a laryngoscopy and knowledge of upper-airway anatomy in order to successfully place a tracheal tube. Other devices like the ETC do not require visualization, much skill, or a significant amount of training. (2-1.2) (IEC p. 379)

135.

D. It is necessary to immediately intubate this patient to control the airway and prevent aspiration of blood. An oropharyngeal airway or a nasopharyngeal airway will not prevent aspiration of blood coming from the face or upper airway. The patient cannot be placed in a lateral recumbent position because of the suspicion of a spinal injury and the need to perform manual in-line spinal stabilization. (2-1.55) (IEC p. 386)

1

History Taking

unit objectives

Questions in this unit relate to DOT Objectives 3-1.1 to 3-1.9. The objectives are listed in the Appendix.

DIRECTIONS
Each of the questions or incomplete statements below is followed by suggested answers or completions. Select the **one answer** that is best in each case.

1. Which of the following is an effective method for establishing a positive rapport with your patient when you first meet him?
   A. Stand over him when you introduce yourself.
   B. Avoid eye contact initially.
   C. Introduce yourself.
   D. Use a firm voice to gain control of the situation.

2. You arrive at the nursing home of an elderly woman whose name is Helen Smith. How should you address her until she tells you otherwise?
   A. Honey
   B. Helen
   C. Mrs. Smith
   D. any of the above

3. Which of the following is an open-ended question?
   A. How would you describe your chest pain?
   B. Does your chest hurt?
   C. Are you having any difficulty breathing?
   D. Do you take insulin every day?

4. Your patient tells you about his chest pain. As he relates his story, you maintain sincere eye contact and repeat things like "Mm-hmm" and "Go on." This is an example of
   A. clarification.
   B. reflection.
   C. confrontation.
   D. facilitation.

5. Your patient denies chest pain but keeps rubbing his chest. You say to him, "You say your chest doesn't hurt, but I notice you keep rubbing it." This is an example of
   A. facilitation.
   B. confrontation.
   C. clarification.
   D. reflection.

6. The pain, discomfort, or dysfunction that caused your patient to request help is known as the
   A. primary problem.
   B. nature of the illness.
   C. differential diagnosis.
   D. chief complaint.

Match the following elements of the present illness of the patient who has a chief complaint of chest pain with their respective examples:

7. _____ O
8. _____ P
9. _____ Q
10. _____ R
11. _____ S
12. _____ T
13. _____ AS
14. _____ PN

A. pain is 6 on a scale of 1–10
B. patient also complains of shortness of breath and nausea
C. sudden onset
D. pain began 2 hours ago
E. pain worsens while lying down
F. patient denies dizziness
G. pain goes through to the back
H. pain is heavy and viselike

15. Cardiac chest pain is commonly felt in the jaw and down the left arm. This is known as
    A. sympathetic pain.
    B. tenderness.
    C. referred pain.
    D. associated pain.

16. A person with PND may have orthopnea. You would have elicited this information during which part of your History of Present Illness?
    A. R
    B. AS
    C. P
    D. Q

17. Which of the following is **not** a component of the Past History?
    A. adult diseases
    B. medications
    C. surgeries
    D. accidents

18. Which of the following would **not** be included when eliciting current medications?
    A. illegal substances
    B. prescribed medications
    C. over-the-counter medications
    D. home remedies

19. Your patient has smoked two packs of cigarettes each day for the past 35 years. He is a _____ pack/year smoker.
    A. 35
    B. 70
    C. 730
    D. 25,550

20. The CAGE questionnaire is used as an evaluation tool to assess
    A. alcoholism.
    B. lung disease.
    C. allergies.
    D. pregnancy.

21. Which of the following statements is true regarding the Review of Systems?
    A. The questions asked cover sleep patterns and family history.
    B. You should begin your history with the Review of Systems.
    C. The questions will be determined by your patient's chief complaint, condition, and clinical status.
    D. It is important to use the entire Review of Systems with each patient.

22. The mnemonic GPAL is used to evaluate
    A. alcoholism.
    B. allergies.
    C. pregnancy history.
    D. endocrine dysfunction.

23. Which of the following could be a valid reason why your patient suddenly became silent?
    A. organic brain syndrome
    B. clinical depression
    C. your insensitivity
    D. all of the above

24. A mood disorder characterized by hopelessness and malaise is known as
    A. dementia.
    B. dysmenorrheal.
    C. delirium.
    D. depression.

25. You ask your patient when his headaches began, and he answers, "My head feels like a squirrel." His problem may be due to

A. psychosis.

B. organic disease.

C. head injury.

D. all of the above

Match the following components of the comprehensive history with their respective categories:

26. _____ pertinent negatives

27. _____ current tobacco use

28. _____ current medications

29. _____ HEENT

30. _____ exercise and leisure activities

31. _____ religious beliefs

32. _____ onset

33. _____ allergies

34. _____ adult diseases

35. _____ cardiac

36. _____ diet

37. _____ endocrine

38. _____ provocation

39. _____ prior injuries

40. _____ CAGE

41. _____ family history

42. _____ skin

43. _____ surgeries

44. _____ time

45. _____ region/radiation

46. _____ urinary

47. _____ sleep patterns

48. _____ substance abuse

49. _____ GPAL

50. _____ respiratory

A. History of Present Illness

B. Past History

C. Current Health Status

D. Review of Systems

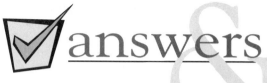

answers & rationales

Following each rationale, you will find a reference to the corresponding objective in the DOT National Standard EMT-Intermediate curriculum. An asterisk denotes material that is supplemental to the DOT curriculum. Page numbers after a rationale indicate where the question topic may be discussed in the Brady text *Intermediate Emergency Care* (Bledsoe, Porter, Cherry).

1.

C. You get only one chance to make a good first impression, and your patient will form an impression of you in the first few moments. A positive, caring, professional impression will put your patient at ease and facilitate your assessment. Make sincere eye contact at eye level, introduce yourself, and offer a handshake or comforting touch. Always remain calm regardless of how your patient presents. (3-1.2) (IEC p. 402)

2.

C. Proper respect for your elders dictates that you use the formal Mrs. Smith until you are told otherwise by your patient. Respect begets respect. (3-1.2) (IEC p. 402)

3.

A. Open-ended questions allow your patient to answer in detail. Closed-ended questions elicit one-word answers, such as "yes" or "no." Used appropriately, both types are effective methods of conducting a patient interview. (3-1.3) (IEC p. 403)

4.

D. Facilitation is a simple method of practicing active listening. You maintain eye contact, listen intently, and follow up his statements with phrases such as "Mm-hmm" or "I'm listening" to let your patient know you are indeed listening. (3-1.5) (IEC p. 404)

5.

B. Sometimes your patients will try to hide the truth. If you suspect they are, you might try confronting them with the discrepancy between what they say and what you see. It may help them open up. (3-1.5)

6.

D. The pain, discomfort, or dysfunction that caused your patient to request help is known as the chief complaint. Elicit the chief complaint with an open-ended question, such as "Why did you call us today?" or "What seems to be the problem?" Document the chief complaint in the patient's own words. (3-1.2) (IEC pp. 406, 512)

Matching (3-1.8) (IEC pp. 406–408, 512)

Note: In the mnemonic OPQRST–ASPN, O = onset, P = provocation/palliation, Q = quality, R = region/radiation, S = severity, T = time, AS = associated symptoms, PN = pertinent negatives. This mnemonic stands for questions that may elicit a description of the patient's pain or other symptoms.

7. C O
8. E P
9. H Q
10. G R
11. A S
12. D T
13. B AS
14. F PN

15.

C. Referred pain is pain that is felt at a location away from its source. For example, cardiac chest pain is referred to the left arm and jaw, gallbladder pain is referred to the right shoulder, and splenic pain is referred to the left shoulder and testicles. (3-1.2) (IEC p. 407)

16.

C. The "P" in the mnemonic OPQRST. ASPN stands for "provocation" (making worse) and "palliation" (making better). PND stands for paroxysmal nocturnal dyspnea, which is sudden shortness of breath while sleeping. It usually indicates orthopnea (difficulty breathing while lying down) from congestive heart failure and is a provocative factor. (3-1.8) (IEC pp. 407, 512)

17.

B. The components of the Past History include general state of health, childhood diseases, adult diseases, psychiatric diseases, accidents or injuries, and surgeries or hospitalizations. (3-1.6) (IEC p. 408)

18.

A. Your patient's current medications include prescriptions, over-the-counter drugs, home remedies, vitamins, and minerals. Always ask your patient to describe any reactions he may have had to any medications. (3-1.8) (IEC p. 510)

19.

B. The number of packs/year is calculated as packs/day times years. Your patient is a 70 pack/year smoker. Anything over 30 packs/year is considered significant. Members of the "Century Club" (100 packs/year) can be expected to exhibit significant lung disease. (3-1.6) (IEC p. 409)

20.

A. The CAGE questionnaire is used to evaluate the presence of alcoholism. The CAGE questionnaire is as follows:

C — Have you ever felt the need to **C**ut down on your drinking?

A — Have you ever felt **A**nnoyed by criticism of your drinking?

G — Have you ever felt **G**uilty about your drinking?

E — Have you ever taken a drink as an **E**ye opener?

Two or more "yes" answers suggest alcoholism and further inquiry. (3-1.6) (IEC p. 409)

21.

C. The Review of Systems is a series of questions designed to identify problems your patient has not already mentioned. The list is categorized by body system and is more comprehensive than the basic history. Your patient's chief complaint, condition, and clinical status will determine how much of the Review of Systems to use. (3-1.6) (IEC pp. 411–413)

22.

C. The mnemonic GPAL is used to evaluate the pregnancy history. It stands for (3-1.6) (IEC p. 412)

Gravida	How many pregnancies?
Para	How many viable births?
Abortions	How many abortions?
Living	How many living children?

23.

D. A patient who becomes silent can be a challenge to even the most experienced EMT-Intermediate. He may have a pathological problem (organic brain disease or dysarthria), he may be upset or scared, or you may have caused the silence by your behavior. If your patient suddenly becomes silent, try to determine why, what is happening, and what you can do about it. (3-1.9) (IEC p. 413)

24.

D. Depression is a mood disorder characterized by hopelessness and malaise. Depression is potentially lethal, so you must recognize its signs and evaluate its severity. (3-1.9) (IEC p. 415)

25.

D. When your patient's answers do not seem to make any sense, it may be due to psychosis (mental illness), organic disease (dementia or delirium), head injury, or a stroke. (3-1.9) (IEC p. 415)

Matching (3-1.6) (IEC pp. 406–413)

26.	A	pertinent negatives
27.	C	current tobacco use
28.	C	current medications
29.	D	HEENT
30.	C	exercise and leisure activities
31.	C	religious beliefs
32.	A	onset
33.	C	allergies
34.	B	adult diseases
35.	D	cardiac
36.	C	diet
37.	D	endocrine
38.	A	provocation
39.	B	prior injuries
40.	C	CAGE
41.	C	family history
42.	D	skin
43.	B	surgeries
44.	A	time
45.	A	region/radiation
46.	D	urinary
47.	C	sleep patterns
48.	C	substance abuse
49.	B	GPAL
50.	D	respiratory

2 Techniques of Physical Examination

unit objectives

Questions in this unit relate to DOT Objectives 3-2.1 to 3-2.48. The objectives are listed in the Appendix.

DIRECTIONS
Each of the questions or incomplete statements below is followed by suggested answers or completions. Select the **one answer** that is best in each case.

1. Which of the following is **not** a physical exam technique?
   A. inspection
   B. palpitation
   C. percussion
   D. auscultation

2. Which of the following should be used to palpate lymph nodes or rib fractures?
   A. the pads of the fingers
   B. the tips of the fingers
   C. the back of the hand
   D. the palm of the hand

3. Which of the following should be used to assess tactile fremitus?
   A. the pads of the fingers
   B. the tips of the fingers
   C. the back of the hand
   D. the palm of the hand

4. Which of the following statements is true regarding abdominal palpation?
   A. Always perform deep palpation first.
   B. Observe your patient's face during the procedure.
   C. Use the heel of one hand to perform deep palpation.
   D. Always palpate the painful area first.

5. A hollow and vibrating resonance heard when percussing the chest indicates the presence of
   A. air.
   B. blood.
   C. pleural fluid.
   D. pus.

6. When reporting and recording lung sounds, you should note the
   A. abnormal sound.
   B. location.
   C. timing during the respiratory cycle.
   D. all of the above

7. You will usually perform auscultation last except in which of the following situations?
   A. acute pulmonary edema
   B. acute abdomen
   C. acute myocardial infarction
   D. arterial bruits

8. A healthy adult's pulse rate at rest should be between _____ and _____ beats per minute.
   A. 50, 90
   B. 60, 120
   C. 50, 100
   D. 60, 100

9. A weak, thready pulse is a common finding in a patient with
   A. circulatory collapse.
   B. high blood pressure.
   C. heat stroke.
   D. increasing intracranial pressure.

Match the following respiratory patterns with their respective definitions:

10. _____ eupnea
11. _____ tachypnea
12. _____ bradypnea
13. _____ apnea
14. _____ hyperpnea
15. _____ Cheyne-Stokes

16. _____ Biot's

17. _____ Kussmaul's

18. _____ apneustic

A. normal rate but deeper

B. prolonged inspiration, shortened expiration

C. normal rate and depth

D. rapid and deep

E. rapid rate

F. increases, decreases, absence

G. slow rate

H. rapid, deep gasps with periods of apnea

I. absence of breathing

19. The amount of air you breathe in and out of your lungs in one breath is known as

A. minute volume.

B. respiratory output.

C. stroke volume.

D. tidal volume.

20. Korotkoff sounds are generated by

A. the heart valves closing.

B. the heart valves opening.

C. blood hitting the arterial walls.

D. blockage in the carotid arteries.

21. A patient with a blood pressure of 150/80 has a pulse pressure of _____ mm Hg.

A. 230

B. 70

C. 100

D. none of the above

22. A widening pulse pressure indicates

A. increasing intracranial pressure

B. pericardial tamponade.

C. tension pneumothorax.

D. decompensated shock.

23. Hypertension in adults is defined as a blood pressure higher than

A. 100/70.

B. 120/80.

C. 130/86.

D. 140/90.

24. You measure the patient's heart rate while he is in a supine position. You then place the patient in a standing position and reassess the heart rate. You note the heart rate has increased by 32 beats per minute while he is in a standing position. You would suspect

A. congestive heart failure.

B. significant blood loss.

C. severe hypertension.

D. coronary artery disease.

25. At which body temperature will brain cells die and seizures become imminent?

A. 102°F

B. 103°F

C. 104°F

D. 105°F

26. The preferred device for measuring temperature in children younger than 6 years old is

A. rectal.

B. oral.

C. tympanic.

D. axillary.

27. You should use the diaphragm of your stethoscope to auscultate
    A. heart sounds.
    B. lung sounds.
    C. bowel sounds.
    D. all of the above

28. Which of the following statements is true regarding stethoscopes?
    A. Thin, flexible tubing transmits sound better.
    B. Longer tubing minimizes distortion.
    C. Angle the earpiece toward the nose.
    D. Use a flexible diaphragm cover.

29. A Broselow tape is used to
    A. calculate infant blood pressure.
    B. measure an infant patient's length.
    C. estimate your patient's weight.
    D. secure an endotracheal tube.

30. If your patient wears shoes that have been altered with slits, holes, or open laces, you might suspect he is suffering from
    A. gout.
    B. bunions.
    C. edema.
    D. all of the above

31. Your patient presents with a bitter almond odor on his breath. This may suggest
    A. hypercarbia.
    B. hypocalcemia.
    C. cyanide poisoning.
    D. methanol overdose.

32. Which is the most reliable location for obtaining an accurate pulse rate on an infant?
    A. apical
    B. carotid
    C. radial
    D. brachial

33. If you are unsuccessful in obtaining a blood pressure, you should wait _____ until trying it again in the same arm.
    A. 15 seconds
    B. 30 seconds
    C. 1 minute
    D. 5 minutes

34. Normal SpO_2 at sea level on room air should be
    A. 80–100%.
    B. 90–120%.
    C. 96–100%.
    D. 90–95%.

35. Your patient is suspected of having carbon monoxide poisoning, yet his SpO_2 is 98%. How is this possible?
    A. The pulse oximeter is inaccurate.
    B. His hemoglobin is saturated with CO.
    C. His hematocrit is below 25%.
    D. He is bleeding out somewhere.

36. The cardiac monitor **does not** provide information about
    A. the cardiac output.
    B. the heart rate.
    C. the cardiac cycle.
    D. dysrhythmias.

37. If your patient's skin color is cyanotic, you should suspect
    A. hypocarbia.
    B. deoxyhemoglobin.
    C. DNA abnormalities.
    D. hypovolemia.

38. Your patient presents with a yellowish tint only to the palms of his hands, the soles of his feet, and his face. He is most likely suffering from
    A. liver failure.
    B. cirrhosis.
    C. carotanemia.
    D. none of the above

Match the following skin conditions with their respective causes:

39. _____ oily skin
40. _____ localized warmth
41. _____ generalized coolness
42. _____ thick skin
43. _____ poor turgor
44. _____ decreased mobility

    A. scleroderma
    B. dehydration
    C. hypothermia
    D. hyperthyroidism
    E. bleeding
    F. eczema

45. Periorbital ecchymosis and mastoid process discoloration are classic signs of
    A. increased intracranial pressure.
    B. basilar skull fracture.
    C. orbital injury.
    D. TMJ dislocation.

46. Placing the tip of your finger into the depression just anterior to the tragus and asking your patient to open his mouth is the procedure for assessing his
    A. gag reflex.
    B. cranial nerve IX.
    C. TMJ.
    D. ability to swallow.

47. You test your patient's pupillary response to light by shining your light directly into one eye and watching its response. When you observe the other eye's reaction, you are testing its _____ response.
    A. indirect
    B. sympathetic
    C. corneal
    D. consensual

Match the following direct pupillary responses to their respective causes:

48. _____ unilateral sluggish pupil
49. _____ bilateral sluggishness
50. _____ constricted pupil
51. _____ fixed and dilated pupil

    A. brain death
    B. opiate poisoning
    C. global hypoxia
    D. increased intracranial pressure

52. The "H" test evaluates
    A. eyelid opening.
    B. peripheral vision.
    C. extraoccular muscles.
    D. the corneal reflex.

53. Which of the following is **not** a chest wall abnormality?
    A. barrel chest
    B. pigeon chest
    C. funnel chest
    D. squirrel chest

54. A hyperresonant percussion sound in the right chest only might indicate
    A. pneumonia.
    B. acute pulmonary edema.

C. pneumothorax.

D. hemothorax.

55. At which point of the respiratory cycle will wheezes typically be heard **first** as a sign of bronchial constriction?

A. beginning of inspiration

B. end of inspiration

C. beginning of exhalation

D. end of exhalation

56. When palpating the carotid arteries, you notice a left-sided thrill or humming. Which procedure should you perform next?

A. auscultate for bruits

B. percuss for dullness

C. carotid sinus massage

D. egophony

57. Which of the following structures is found at the PMI?

A. the upper border of the kidney

B. the apex of the heart

C. the diaphragmatic pouch

D. the carina

58. To make an abdominal exam easier for you and more comfortable for your patient, have him

A. place a pillow under his pelvis.

B. place his hands above his head.

C. empty his bladder prior to the exam.

D. lay laterally recumbent.

59. Cullen's sign and Grey-Turner's sign are classic findings in

A. peritonitis.

B. intraabdominal hemorrhage.

C. appendicitis.

D. hernias in males.

60. A suprapubic bulge suggests a

A. hernia.

B. pregnant uterus.

C. distended bladder.

D. B and C.

61. Which of the following signs suggests an intestinal obstruction?

A. absent bowel sounds

B. decreased bowel sounds

C. increased bowel sounds

D. bruits

62. Rebound tenderness is a classic sign of

A. bowel obstruction.

B. abdominal aortic aneurysm.

C. peritonitis.

D. hernia.

63. The presence of ascites is a classic sign of

A. congestive heart failure.

B. bowel obstruction.

C. paralytic ileus.

D. hernia.

64. You are examining the external genitalia of your female patient and notice a yellow discharge from the urethral opening and a foul-smelling odor. You suspect

A. candidiasis.

B. gonorrhea.

C. a fungal infection.

D. herpes simplex.

65. Your patient complains of nontraumatic left-hand pain and numbness. Following a physical exam, you make a field diagnosis of carpal tunnel syndrome. This involves inflammation of the _____ nerve.

A. radial

B. ulnar

C. median

D. biceps brachii

66. Inflammation of the lateral or medial epicondyles of the elbow suggests

    A. tendonitis.

    B. bursitis.

    C. subluxation.

    D. arthritis.

67. Lateral ankle sprains are more common than medial sprains because the lateral ligaments are smaller and weaker. You should expect severe pain during which range-of-motion movements?

    A. eversion and dorsiflexion

    B. inversion and dorsiflexion

    C. inversion and plantar flexion

    D. eversion and plantar flexion

68. Exaggerated lumbar concavity (swayback) is known as

    A. kyphosis.

    B. scoliosis.

C. lordosis.

D. lumbago.

69. You are reading a patient's chart during your ICU rotation and notice a notation that reads radial pulse 1+. This means that the pulse is

    A. normal.

    B. bounding.

    C. weak and thready.

    D. absent.

70. Your patient has dysarthria. This is best described as a speech defect caused by

    A. vocal cord problems.

    B. damage to the cortex.

    C. motor deficits.

    D. psychotic disorder.

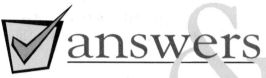
Following each rationale, you will find a reference to the corresponding objective in the DOT National Standard EMT-Intermediate curriculum. An asterisk denotes material that is supplemental to the DOT curriculum. Page numbers after a rationale indicate where the question topic may be discussed in the Brady text *Intermediate Emergency Care* (Bledsoe, Porter, Cherry).

1.

B. The four basic physical exam techniques are inspection, palpation (not "palpitation"), auscultation, and percussion. (3-2.1) (IEC pp. 420–424)

2.

A. The pads of the fingers are more sensitive than the tips for detecting masses, fluid, position, consistency, size, and crepitus. (3-2.2) (IEC p. 421)

3.

D. To detect vibrations, such as fremitus, you should use the palm of your hand because the skin is thinner and more sensitive. (3-2.2) (IEC p. 421)

4.

B. When palpating your patient's abdomen, observe how your patient responds with facial expressions while you palpate tender areas. Even if he is unconscious, he may respond to pain with facial expressions or movement. (3-2.2) (IEC p. 422)

5.

A. Percussion evaluates the surface and the tissue beneath by sending a vibration through it. A hollow and vibrating resonance heard when percussing the chest indicates the presence of air. (3-2.2) (IEC p. 422)

6.

D. When reporting and recording lung sounds, you should note the abnormal sound you hear (crackles, wheezes, rhonchi), the location (bilateral, right lower lobe, bases), and the timing during the respiratory cycle (inspiratory, end-expiratory). (3-2.2) (IEC p. 423)

7.

B. Generally auscultate after you have used other assessment techniques. The only exception to this rule is the abdomen, which you should auscultate before palpating and percussing. (3-2.2) (IEC p. 423)

8.

D. A healthy adult should have a resting heart rate between 60 and 100 beats per minute. (3-2.3) (IEC p. 424)

9.

A. A weak, thready pulse is a common finding in a patient in circulatory collapse, such as in shock. (3-2.3) (IEC p. 424)

Matching (3-2.3) (IEC pp. 424–426)

10.	C	eupnea
11.	E	tachypnea
12.	G	bradypnea
13.	I	apnea
14.	A	hyperpnea
15.	F	cheyne-Stokes
16.	H	biot's
17.	D	kussmaul's
18.	B	apneustic

19.

D. Tidal volume is the amount of air a person breathes in and out of the lungs in one breath. A healthy adult at rest breathes approximately 500 ml of air each breath, just enough to make the chest rise. (3-2.3) (IEC p. 425)

20.

C. Korotkoff sounds are the sounds of blood hitting the arterial walls that you auscultate when you take your patient's blood pressure. (3-2.3) (IEC p. 426)

21.

B. Pulse pressure is the difference between the systolic and diastolic pressures. A patient with a BP of 150/80 has a pulse pressure of 70 mm Hg. (3-2.3) (IEC p. 426)

22.

A. The pulse pressure widens in a patient with increasing intracranial pressure in the body's attempt to perfuse the brain. A narrowing pulse pressure suggests tamponade, tension pneumothorax, or hypovolemic shock. (3-2.3) (IEC p. 426)

23.

D. Blood pressure higher than 140/90 in adults is considered hypertension. (3-2.3) (IEC pp. 426–427)

24.

B. If your supine patient's pulse rate rises more than 10–20 beats per minute when you stand him up, you should suspect a volume loss. This is known as a positive "tilt test," or orthostatic hypotension. When the tilt test provides a heart rate increase by greater than 30 beats per minute, you should suspect significant blood loss. (3-2.3) (IEC p. 427)

25.

D. At temperatures above 105°F (41°C), brain cells die, and seizures may occur. (*) (IEC p. 427)

26.

A. A rectal thermometer is the preferred method for measuring temperature in children younger than 6 years old. (3-2.47) (IEC p. 427)

27.

A. To maximize your ability to auscultate blood pressure, heart sounds, or arterial bruits, use the diaphragm side of your stethoscope. To hear lung or bowel sounds, the bell side is recommended. (3-2.3) (IEC p. 428)

28.

C. To maximize your ability to auscultate sound, use a rigid diaphragm cover and thick, heavy, short tubing; always angle the earpiece toward the nose. (3-2.3) (IEC p. 428)

29.

B. A Broselow tape is a measuring device used to provide you with information regarding airway equipment, drug dosages, and IV calculations based on your patient's height. You simply measure your patient from the feet to the top of the head and use the color-coded information provided. (3-2.47) (IEC pp. 241, 431)

30.

D. Look at your patient's shoes. If they have been altered with slits, holes, or open laces, he may be compensating for a painful foot condition, such as gout, edema, or bunions. (3-2.5) (IEC p. 431)

31.

C. Your patient's breath sometimes can provide important clues that aid you in forming your field diagnosis. The smell of bitter almonds is a classic finding in cyanide poisoning. (3-2.5) (IEC p. 431)

32.

D. When assessing the pulse rate in an infant, use the brachial pulse, located just medial to the biceps tendon. Auscultating the apical pulse provides the sounds of the cardiac valves closing but tells you nothing about the quality of the pulse wave generated. (3-2.47) (IEC p. 433)

33.

B. If you do not obtain a reading, wait 30 seconds to allow the blood pressure to normalize before inflating the cuff again. Failure to wait will render an inaccurate reading. (3-2.3) (IEC p. 433)

34.

C. A pulse oximeter measures the oxygen saturation of the blood. At sea level on room air, your oxygen saturation should be between 96% and 100%. This means that 96–100% of your hemoglobin is saturated, preferably with oxygen. (*) (IEC p. 434)

35.

B. This patient's hemoglobin is saturated with carbon monoxide because the CO molecule binds 200 times more easily with hemoglobin than oxygen does. Therefore, the pulse oximeter reads that 96% of the hemoglobin is indeed saturated and does not distinguish between CO and O_2. (*) (IEC p. 435)

36.

A. Cardiac monitoring is an effective assessment tool for patients requiring advanced life support. It tells you the heart rate, measures the cardiac cycle, and allows you to identify cardiac dysrhythmias. It cannot, however, provide hemodynamic information (i.e., whether the heart is pumping effectively or at all). Always correlate what you see on the monitor with your clinical assessment (taking a pulse and BP). (*) (IEC p. 435)

37.

B. Bright red oxyhemoglobin gives the skin a pink color. As the hemoglobin loses its oxygen to the tissues, it changes color to the darker blue deoxyhemoglobin. Increased deoxyhemoglobin causes cyanosis, a bluish skin color, and signifies decreased oxygen at the tissue level. Cyanosis = hypoxia. (3-2.8) (IEC p. 436)

38.

C. Only your patient's palms, soles, and face appear yellow—he probably has carotanemia, a harmless nutritional condition caused by eating a diet high in carrots and yellow vegetables or fruits. Jaundice, a yellow color that first appears in the sclera and then all over the body, indicates severe liver disease. (3-2.8) (IEC p. 437)

Matching (3-2.8) (IEC p. 437)

39.	D	oily skin
40.	E	localized warmth
41.	C	generalized coolness
42.	F	thick skin
43.	B	poor turgor
44.	A	decreased mobility

45.

B. Periorbital ecchymosis (raccoon eyes) and discoloration at the mastoid process (Battle's sign) are classic signs of a basilar skull fracture. Sinuses in the skull allow blood to pool in the soft tissues around the eyes and behind the ears following a fracture of the base of the skull. (3-2.9) (IEC p. 439)

46.

C. To evaluate your patient's temporomandibular joint (TMJ), place your fingertip into the depression just in front of the tragus and ask him to open his mouth. As he opens his mouth, your finger should drop into the joint space. Palpate it for tenderness, crepitus, swelling, and range of motion. (3-2.10) (IEC p. 439)

47.

D. Shining a light into one eye and observing its reaction to light is checking its direct response. Observing the other eye is checking its consensual response. Both eyes should constrict simultaneously in response to the light. (3-2.12) (IEC p. 439)

Matching (3-2.12) (IEC p. 439)

48.	D	unilateral sluggish pupil
49.	C	bilateral sluggishness
50.	B	constricted pupil
51.	A	fixed and dilated pupil

52.

C. In the "H" test, have your patient follow your finger as you move it in an "H" pattern in front of him. This tests the integrity of the extraoccular muscles and cranial nerves III (occulomotor), IV (trochlear), and VI (abducens). Normal eye movements should be conjugate (together). (3-2.12) (IEC p. 439)

53.

D. Common chest abnormalities include funnel chest (pectus excavatum), pigeon chest (pectus carinatum), and barrel chest. (3-2.26) (IEC pp. 445–446)

54.

C. Hyperresonance suggests an area abnormally filled with air. In a unilateral lung, you would suspect pneumothorax. Bilaterally, you would suspect diseases such as asthma or emphysema, which trap air in the distal alveoli. (3-2.24) (IEC p. 446)

55.

D. Wheezes are caused by bronchiole constriction and mucosal lining inflammation. These tiny airways collapse when the positive pressure exerted on them from the outside is greater than the pressure available on the inside. The first sign of wheezing is typically found at the end of exhalation during your auscultation of the lungs. As the bronchoconstriction and inflammation progress, wheezing may begin to appear earlier in the respiratory cycle. (3-2.25) (IEC p. 448)

56.

A. If, when palpating the carotid arteries, you note a thrill, or humming vibration, immediately auscultate the artery for bruits, the sound of rushing blood around an obstructed artery. Avoid deep manipulative palpation, which could loosen the obstruction (plaque) and cause a cerebral embolism (stroke). (3-2.19) (IEC p. 450)

57.

B. The point of maximum impulse (PMI) signifies the apex of the heart. Here you can find the apical pulse. This point is usually found at the fifth intercostal space, just medial to the midclavicular line. Lateral displacement suggests right-ventricle enlargement from systemic hypertension. (3-2.24) (IEC p. 450)

58.

C. A relaxed patient is the key to an effective abdominal exam. Have him lay supine with a pillow underneath his head and his knees to relax the abdominal muscles. Have him place his arms at his sides and make sure his bladder is empty prior to the exam if possible. (3-2.35) (IEC p. 450)

59.

B. Discoloration over the umbilicus (Cullen's sign) or over the flanks (Grey-Turner's sign) is a classic late sign of intraabdominal hemorrhage. (3-2.36) (IEC p. 450)

60.

D. A bulge just above the pubic bone suggests a pregnant uterus or a distended bladder. A bulge in the inguinal or femoral area suggests a hernia. (3-2.3) (IEC p. 421)

61.

C. Proximal to an intestinal obstruction where the bowels are trying to force debris through the obstruction, you will hear the increased sounds of hyperperistalsis. (3-2.36) (IEC p. 452)

62.

C. An inflamed peritoneum will be very irritable. Even the slightest movement causes severe pain. To test for rebound tenderness, press down gently but firmly on an area away from the patient's complaint and then release your hand quickly. The sudden jarring will cause pain if the peritoneum is irritated. (3-2.36) (IEC p. 452)

63.

A. Ascites is the collection of fluid in the abdominal cavity and flanks caused by congestive heart failure. Test for ascites by causing a fluid wave across your patient's abdomen. (3-2.36) (IEC pp. 450, 452)

64.

B. A yellow, green, or gray genital discharge with a fishy or foul odor suggests a bacterial infection, such as gonorrhea or Gardnarella. If the discharge is white or curdlike and odorless, suspect a fungal infection, such as candidiasis. (3-2.38) (IEC p. 452)

65.

C. Carpal tunnel syndrome is caused by inflammation of the median nerve, which runs through the middle groove at the inside of the wrist. During acute flexion of the wrist, your patient will complain of numbness of the palmar surface of the thumb, the index finger, the middle finger, and part of his ring finger. (3-2.42) (IEC p. 455)

66.

A. Nontraumatic inflammation of the lateral epicondyles (tennis elbow) or medial epicondyles (golfer's elbow) suggests tendonitis at those muscle insertion sites. (3-2.42) (IEC p. 455)

67.

C. Lateral ankle sprains are common. Your patient will present with pain, tenderness, and swelling to the outside of the ankle. During inversion and plantar flexion tests, expect him to complain of severe pain. In these cases, do not continue the exam. (3-2.42) (IEC p. 458)

68.

C. Inspect your patient's spine and note any irregularities. The spine should be straight and plumb from the neck to the buttocks. Abnormal lateral curvature is known as scoliosis. Observe the spine from the side. An exaggerated lumbar concavity is known as lordosis or swayback. An exaggerated thoracic convexity is known as kyphosis or hunchback. (*) (IEC p. 462)

69.

C. Pulse quality is quantified according to the following scale: (3-2.28) (IEC p. 465)

0   Absent

1+ Weak and thready

2+ Normal

3+ Bounding

70.

C. Speech pattern abnormalities can be the result of dysarthria (from a motor deficit), dysphonia (from vocal cord damage), or aphasia (from neurological damage to the brain). (3-2.46) (IEC p. 468)

3

Patient Assessment in the Field

unit objectives

Questions in this unit relate to DOT Objectives 3-3.1 to 3-3.44. The objectives are listed in the Appendix.

DIRECTIONS Each of the questions or incomplete statements below is followed by suggested answers or completions. Select the **one answer** that is best in each case.

1. Which of the following is **not** a component of an assessment conducted on a responsive medical patient?
   A. initial assessment
   B. rapid medical assessment
   C. focused history and physical exam
   D. ongoing assessment

2. Which of the following is **not** a component of the scene size-up?
   A. body substance isolation
   B. mechanism of injury
   C. initial assessment
   D. location of all patients

3. The HEPA mask is designed to protect you from
   A. tuberculosis.
   B. AIDS.
   C. hepatitis.
   D. meningitis.

4. The top priority in any emergency situation is
   A. patient assessment.
   B. bystander cooperation.
   C. customer service.
   D. your personal safety.

5. As you approach a scene, something just does not seem right. It is not anything you can put your finger on, just a sense that something is wrong or is about to happen. What should you do about it?
   A. Wait until law enforcement arrives before entering.
   B. Ignore your feelings and enter the scene.

   C. Enter the scene with something with which to protect yourself.
   D. Call out for the patient to come outside.

6. You are responding to a shooting at a well-known bar. How should you approach the scene?
   A. Stage outside the bar until the police arrive.
   B. Wait for another ambulance or rescue crew before entering.
   C. Just enter the scene.
   D. Stage your ambulance a few blocks away until law enforcement arrives.

7. You arrive on the scene and see that a power line lies close to your pediatric patient. You are fairly sure the line is live and decide to move it with a dry piece of equipment. Which of the following should you use?
   A. a wooden-handled ax
   B. a fallen tree branch
   C. a nylon rope
   D. none of the above

8. When you and your partner arrive at a multiple-patient incident, you should
   A. begin assessing and treating the first patient you encounter.
   B. establish command and begin triage.
   C. provide intensive emergency care to the most critical patient.
   D. start at opposite ends and begin assessing patients.

9. Of the following components of the initial assessment, which should you perform first?

   A. airway assessment
   B. priority determination
   C. circulation assessment
   D. mental status assessment

10. To maintain proper alignment of a child's head and neck, you should place a folded towel under his

    A. head.
    B. neck.
    C. shoulders.
    D. none of the above

11. Your patient presents with his eyes open, and he responds to you when you speak to him. He answers your questions but is obviously disoriented as to time and place. You grade him _____ on the AVPU scale.

    A. A
    B. V
    C. P
    D. U

12. Your patient fails to respond to your shouting commands. When you pinch his fingernails and rub his sternum, he exhibits decorticate posturing. He receives a(n) _____ on the AVPU scale.

    A. A
    B. V
    C. P
    D. U

Match the following upper airway obstruction situations with their respective treatments:

13. _____ snoring
14. _____ gurgling
15. _____ foreign body
16. _____ burns

17. _____ stridor with hives, redness, and itching
18. _____ epiglottitis

    A. vasoconstrictor medications
    B. orotracheal suctioning
    C. blow-by oxygen and a quiet ride
    D. immediate tracheal intubation
    E. abdominal thrusts/Magill forceps
    F. head tilt/chin lift

19. Which of the following is **not** a possible diagnosis for a patient with diffuse expiratory wheezing?

    A. epiglottitis
    B. bronchitis
    C. asthma
    D. bronchiolitis

20. When performing positive pressure ventilation on a nonbreathing patient, provide _____ breaths per minute for adults and _____ breaths per minute for children.

    A. 20, 30
    B. 25, 50
    C. 12, 20
    D. 12, 15

21. You arrive on the scene and find a patient in a supine position on his bed. The patient does not respond to painful stimuli. There is minimal chest wall excursion and you hear sonorous sounds with each breath. Your partner inserts an oropharyngeal airway and the sonorous sounds are eliminated. You should immediately do which of the following?

    A. Intubate the patient with a tracheal tube.
    B. Perform bag-valve-mask ventilation.
    C. Administer 100% oxygen via a nonrebreather mask.
    D. Complete the initial assessment.

22. Your patient presents with warm, pink skin; a radial pulse rate of 80 per minute; and a capillary refill time of less than 2 seconds. From this information, what can you conclude about her circulatory condition?
    A. It is normal.
    B. It shows signs of early circulatory compromise.
    C. It shows signs of severe circulatory collapse.
    D. none of the above

23. Which of the following patients should be prioritized for rapid transport?
    A. cardiac arrest
    B. isolated femur fracture
    C. altered mental status
    D. all of the above

24. Which of the following mechanisms is **not** considered a predictor of serious internal injury for an adult?
    A. fall from 10 feet
    B. ejection from vehicle
    C. vehicle rollover
    D. motorcycle crash

25. You arrive on the scene of a head-on motor vehicle crash and notice that the air bag on the driver's side has been deployed. When you lift the bag, you also notice that the steering wheel is deformed. What is the most likely reason for this finding?
    A. The air bag malfunctioned.
    B. The seat belt was not fastened.
    C. The crash was not of high speed.
    D. The steering wheel was bent before the crash.

26. The rapid trauma assessment is designed to
    A. provide a detailed physical exam.
    B. identify and manage life-threatening injuries.
    C. find and treat minor injuries.
    D. rule out the need for rapid transport.

27. Which of the following is **not** a component of the DCAP-BTLS mnemonic?
    A. lacerations
    B. contusions
    C. deformities
    D. broken bones

28. Your patient presents with a major jugular vein laceration. You must immediately
    A. stop the bleeding with a gauze pressure dressing.
    B. clamp the vessel with a hemostat.
    C. tie the vessel off with a surgical string.
    D. apply an occlusive dressing.

29. Your major trauma patient presents with jugular vein distention while sitting up. Which of the following conditions may be the cause?
    A. pericardial tamponade
    B. massive hemothorax
    C. flail chest
    D. diaphragmatic hernia

30. Your patient's trachea tugs to the left side each time he breathes. The most likely cause for this is
    A. tension pneumothorax.
    B. tracheal tear.
    C. simple pneumothorax on the left.
    D. simple pneumothorax on the right.

31. Infants and small children _____ to maintain back pressure to keep the airways open.
    A. use accessory muscles
    B. use retractions
    C. grunt
    D. flare their nares

32. Which bone fractures more easily and more often than any other in the body?
    A. clavicle
    B. radius
    C. tibia
    D. cranium

33. If your patient presents with fractures of the first three ribs, you should suspect
    A. no major systemic complications.
    B. pericardial tamponade.
    C. major underlying damage.
    D. esophageal damage.

34. Paradoxical chest wall movement is a classic sign of
    A. pneumothorax.
    B. diaphragmatic hernia.
    C. tracheobronchial tear.
    D. flail chest.

35. Your patient presents with jugular vein distention, absent breath sounds on the left side, diminished breath sounds on the right side, tachycardia, and profound hypotension. You should
    A. monitor and transport the patient to the trauma center.
    B. decompress the left chest immediately.
    C. place your patient on his right side.
    D. perform pericardiocentesis.

36. Which of the following is **not** a component of a SAMPLE history?
    A. past medical history
    B. medications
    C. signs
    D. allergies

37. Which of the following do you **not** use to evaluate a basketball player who has twisted his knee?
    A. milking the joint
    B. frawer test
    C. side-to-side test
    D. full range of motion, regardless of the pain

38. The "H" test evaluates the integrity of
    A. the optic nerve.
    B. cranial nerves III, IV, and V.
    C. the extraoccular muscles.
    D. all of the above

39. Your patient complains of chest pain. You should include an examination of the mouth to assess
    A. central oxygenation.
    B. presence of fluids.
    C. buccal pallor.
    D. all of the above

40. Your cardiac patient presents with jugular vein distention while sitting up. This could suggest
    A. right-heart failure.
    B. left-heart failure.
    C. simple pneumothorax.
    D. systemic hypertension.

41. A localized wheeze could be the result of
    A. asthma.
    B. pneumonia.
    C. acute pulmonary edema.
    D. COPD.

42. Your patient presents with unequal femoral pulses and a cool, ashen left leg. This could be the result of a(n)
    A. thoracic aneurysm.
    B. abdominal aneurysm.
    C. pulsus paradoxus.
    D. deep vein thrombosis.

43. Your patient presents with pinpoint pupils, a classic finding in
    A. shock.
    B. anticholinergic poisoning.
    C. brain anoxia.
    D. narcotic overdose.

44. At the far extremes of your "H" test, you note that your patient's eyes begin fine, jerking movements. This is known as
    A. doll's eyes.
    B. nystagmus.
    C. decortication.
    D. hyphema.

45. Which of the following patients should receive a "rapid alternating movements" exam?
    A. acute abdomen
    B. acute myocardial infarction
    C. stroke
    D. arm injury

46. Voluntary abdominal rigidity and guarding suggest
    A. peritoneal irritation.
    B. intraabdominal hemorrhage.
    C. massive infection.
    D. an anxious patient.

47. Which of the following statements best describes the detailed physical exam?
    A. It is only conducted if the patient's condition and time allow.
    B. It is conducted in place of the rapid trauma assessment in significant mechanism of injury.
    C. It is always performed on medical patients with a complaint of chest pain.
    D. It is performed to identify and manage immediate life threats to the patient.

48. The ongoing assessment is designed to
    A. reevaluate the effectiveness of your interventions.
    B. detect trends.
    C. review the ABCs every 5 minutes for critical patients.
    D. all of the above

49. You are transporting a patient with a chest injury following a motor vehicle crash. Your partner has intubated the patient and is performing bag-valve ventilation. He suddenly complains that the bag is becoming increasingly more difficult to squeeze. You reassess your patient and note pronounced JVD, tachycardia, and hypotension. The most likely cause for this sudden change in condition is
    A. pericardial tamponade.
    B. tension pneumothorax.
    C. massive hemothorax.
    D. diaphragmatic hernia.

50. A narrowing pulse pressure, along with JVD and muffled heart sounds, suggests
    A. tension pneumothorax.
    B. cardiac tamponade.
    C. hypovolemic shock.
    D. massive hemothorax.

51. Which of the following activities are done during the scene size-up?
    A. Determine mechanism of injury and identify and treat immediate life threats.
    B. Gather information about present situation, question bystanders, and obtain past medical history.
    C. Complete physical exam, obtain baseline vital signs, and identify treatment priorities.
    D. Identify potential environmental or situational hazards, determine mechanism of injury, secure the scene, and locate patients.

52. You have responded to a call in which the patient was injured during a fight in the parking lot outside a bar. Although police are on-scene, a large hostile crowd gathers as you begin assessing the patient. What should you do to manage this situation?
    A. Leave the patient and return immediately to the ambulance.
    B. Use your body to shield the patient and continue your care.
    C. Move the patient to the ambulance with police assistance.
    D. Continue to provide care while the police deal with the crowd.

53. What is the primary difference in your approach to the assessment of a medical patient versus a trauma patient?
    A. Assessment of the trauma patient focuses on the relationship between the patient's past history and systemic physical findings.
    B. Assessment of the medical patient is directed toward signs of potential problems as suggested by the mechanism of injury.
    C. Assessment of the trauma patient tends to be more interactive with the patient based on detailed questioning of his or her past history.
    D. Assessment of the medical patient is more commonly directed toward gathering a history and performing a physical exam based on the reported symptoms.

54. How is pulmonary ventilation affected by a diaphragmatic injury?
    A. An injury to the diaphragm increases the potential size of the thoracic cavity and thus increases tidal volume with each respiration.
    B. A diaphragmatic injury reduces oxygenation by limiting the amount of expansion of the uninjured lung caused by air in the pleural space.
    C. An injury to the diaphragm impairs its ability to contract normally and reduces the potential size of the thoracic cavity during inhalation.
    D. A diaphragmatic injury compromises ventilation when the accumulation of air in the pleural space and the resulting decrease in pressure maintain lung inflation.

55. An increase in airway resistance may be noticed when ventilating a patient due to all of the following **except**
    A. tension pneumothorax.
    B. occlusion of the airway.
    C. esophageal intubation.
    D. intubation of the right-mainstem bronchus.

56. A deflated reservoir bag observed while using a bag-valve-mask device may indicate all of the following **except**

    A. an empty oxygen cylinder.

    B. an increase in airway resistance.

    C. a leak in the bag-valve-mask device.

    D. a disconnected oxygen supply line.

57. Relative contraindications for oral tracheal intubation include an intact gag reflex, epiglottitis, and

    A. cardiac arrest.

    B. cervical spine injury.

    C. apnea secondary to an acute asthma attack.

    D. hypoxic pulmonary edema patient in respiratory failure.

58. Which of the following statements regarding the use of a tourniquet for hemorrhage control is true?

    A. A sphygmomanometer is an effective tourniquet only if it is inflated to a minimum pressure of 300 mm Hg.

    B. Inadequate tourniquet pressure will only inhibit venous return, thus increasing the rate and volume of blood loss.

    C. Tourniquets provide excellent control of hemorrhage and should be considered as first-line management in most situations.

    D. Once applied, tourniquets should be loosened after 10 minutes to maintain perfusion of uninjured tissue adjacent to the wound.

59. Exposing the trauma patient during the rapid trauma assessment may result in

    A. the development of life-threatening hypothermia.

    B. charges of assault and battery.

    C. quick identification of potentially life-threatening injuries.

    D. exacerbation of unstable cervical or thoracic spine injuries.

60. Of the following statements, which would be an important part of the pertinent past medical history for a 60-year-old male patient complaining of chest pain?

    A. Patient occassionally takes sinus medication.

    B. Patient had a hernia repair 2 years ago.

    C. Patient underwent coronary bypass surgery last year.

    D. Patient's brother died of a heart attack at the age of 78.

61. Which of the following activities would occur during the definitive care phase of the patient care continuum?

    A. administration of medications to control pain en route

    B. placement of a chest tube

    C. transmission of cardiac rhythms to the receiving facility

    D. ventilatory support via bag-valve-mask device

62. Which of the following statements most accurately describes the proper immobilization sequence for a supine patient?

    A. Manually stabilize the head and neck in a neutral position. Logroll the patient onto a long backboard. Strap the torso and legs securely to the board and then secure the patient's head and neck. Secure the backboard to the cot.

    B. Apply a cervical collar to stabilize the head and neck in a neutral position. Roll the patient onto a long backboard. Strap the patient securely to the board and secure the patient's head and neck. Secure the backboard to the cot.

    C. Manually stabilize the head and neck in a neutral position and apply a cervical collar. Logroll the patient onto a long backboard. Strap the torso and legs securely to the board and then secure the patient's head and neck. Secure the backboard to the cot.

    D. Apply a rigid collar to stabilize the head and neck in a neutral position. Logroll the patient onto the cot and strap the patient securely to prevent movement. Secure the patient's head and neck.

63. Which of the following activities should occur as part of your ongoing assessment of a patient while en route to the hospital?

    A. Report patient data to the receiving facility.

    B. Reassess mental status, initial assessment, and vital signs every 5 or 15 minutes and check interventions.

    C. Reassure family members that the patient will be fine.

    D. Document any care provided at the scene on the patient care report.

64. A 73-year-old Alzheimer's patient is found sitting on the steps of a residence at 2:00 A.M. The patient is wet and disoriented and has a decreased mental status. Which of the following would you do immediately following the initial assessment?

    A. Obtain a thorough medical history.

    B. Place the patient in the ambulance.

    C. Ascertain the amount of time the patient has been gone.

    D. Obtain a thorough set of vital signs.

65. Your partner has intubated an unresponsive female with a tracheal tube. After approximately 1 minute of positive pressure ventilation with a bag-valve-mask, she begins to groan loudly. What should your next action be?

    A. Restrain the patient and continue positive pressure ventilation.

    B. Assist the patient in her respiratory efforts.

    C. Leave the endotracheal tube in place without positive pressure ventilation.

    D. Check the tube placement.

66. While assessing a combative 23-year-old male who has been stabbed in the right hemithorax, you note he is dyspneic and cyanotic. Your immediate concern is

    A. determining wound depth.

    B. assessing for a rib fracture.

    C. replacing lost fluid.

    D. managing the hypoxia.

67. You intubate an unresponsive 23-year-old male with a CombiTube airway. The patient has been shot in the back of the mouth and has profuse bleeding. After passing a CombiTube, you note equality in chest rise and fall and breath sounds. How would you continue airway management?

   A. Continue ventilating at a rate of 12–20 ventilations per minute.

   B. Extubate the patient and continue ventilating with a bag-valve-mask.

   C. Continue ventilations with a demand valve resuscitator.

   D. Extubate the patient and reattempt the intubation.

68. A patient has been struck by a car and continues to bleed from an open wound to the deformed right leg. Which of the following, in addition to direct pressure, would control this hemorrhage best?

   A. splinting the right leg

   B. administering oxygen and elevating the extremity

   C. applying an ice pack to the bleeding area

   D. placing the patient in a Trendelenburg position

69. An individual's mental status can be easily determined during the initial assessment by which of the following?

   A. directly observing whether the patient is talking

   B. a description as to whether the patient is semiconscious or coherent

   C. a minineurological exam using the AVPU method

   D. the level of consciousness is not ascertained during the initial assessment

70. Which of the following best describes the Glasgow Coma Scale?

   A. a scale related to eye, verbal, and sensory function

   B. a quantification as to exact patient injury

   C. a numerical system to identify trends in the neurologic status of the patient

   D. a system that dictates what interventions the EMT-Intermediate must initiate

71. You are immobilizing a 32-year-old female onto a backboard. The patient has fallen down a flight of stairs and has suffered a large laceration to the frontal region of her head. The patient is on the backboard, and manual spinal stabilization is being held. What is the **best** order to apply the backboard straps?

   A. legs, torso, head

   B. torso, legs, head

   C. head, torso, legs

   D. torso, legs, no strap for the head because of the laceration

72. An elderly female who refused your treatment after falling and striking her head has died from a cerebral hemorrhage. Your best protection in this situation is

   A. the witness testimony of your partner.

   B. the verbal report you gave your supervisor following the refusal.

   C. a written narrative attached to a standard refusal form.

   D. none—the standard refusal form is adequate.

73. You are called to a factory to treat three unconscious employees who were overcome by fumes. They are still in the building. How should you proceed at the scene?

   A. Immediately enter the building and retrieve the patients.

   B. Park the ambulance upwind from the factory and wait for the fire department.

   C. Park the ambulance downwind from the factory and enter the building with oxygen on.

   D. Prevent escape of additional fumes by closing all windows.

74. You are called to the scene of a shooting. The patient has been shot in the abdomen. You see the assailant as you approach the scene. You should

   A. immediately approach the injured person for treatment.

   B. confront the person with the gun so you can begin treatment of the patient.

   C. keep your ambulance at a safe distance and wait while your dispatcher calls for police assistance.

   D. park the ambulance between the patient and the assailant and approach the patient.

75. You arrive on the scene of multiple-system trauma patient who is unresponsive. Paramedic backup is en route to the scene. You should:

   A. wait for the paramedic backup prior to performing any treatment of the patient.

   B. immediately perform an initial assessment followed by a rapid trauma assessment and begin treatment of the patient.

   C. immediately begin transport of the patient and rendevous with the paramedic unit.

   D. immediately initiate an intravenous line, attempt tracheal intubation, and load the patient for rapid transport.

76. A patient has been struck in the anterior neck with a baseball. The patient is dyspneic and unable to speak. You would suspect an injury to what structure?

   A. oropharynx

   B. esophagus

   C. larynx

   D. the temporal lobe

77. Steam burns with secondary edema would be most concerning if they involved what structure?

   A. hands

   B. oropharynx

   C. chest

   D. arms

78. You are called to the scene of a car/pedestrian crash. The pedestrian was thrown to the side of the road. What airway maneuver would be most appropriate for this patient?

   A. tracheal intubation

   B. head tilt/chin lift

   C. jaw thrust

   D. a manual airway maneuver is not needed

79. While ventilating a 73-year-old cardiac arrest patient, you are having difficulty maintaining the seal between the patient's face and the mask of the bag-valve-mask. You should

   A. insert an oropharyngeal airway.

   B. remove the patient's dentures.

   C. change to a pocket mask.

   D. secure the mask to the face with tape.

80. As you are ventilating your patient with a bag-valve-mask, you note minimal bag resistance and rapid emptying. This would be associated with

    A. an airway obstruction.

    B. normal ventilations.

    C. a mask leak.

    D. a hole in the bag.

81. You are ventilating an intubated patient with a bag-valve-mask, with supplemental oxygen connected to a reservoir. All of the following are signs of effective ventilation **except**

    A. equal chest rise and fall.

    B. bilateral breath sounds.

    C. abdominal distension.

    D. decrease in cyanosis.

82. You are treating a patient from a car crash. You suspect he is suffering from decreased perfusion. The patient's skin most likely will be

    A. warm and dry.

    B. cool and pale.

    C. warm and pale.

    D. red and hot.

83. You are attending to an elderly male who lacerated his right forearm with an ax. He informs you that the accident occurred 2 hours ago and that he immediately applied a tourniquet. The distal extremity is now deeply discolored, and all bleeding has stopped. You would

    A. remove the tourniquet to restore distal circulation.

    B. loosen the tourniquet slightly to restore distal circulation and replace after 5 minutes.

    C. gradually loosen the tourniquet so as to gradually restore distal circulation.

    D. leave the tourniquet in place and transport.

84. During the middle of winter, you respond to a call where a 60-year-old female has been hit by a car. The patient is unresponsive. How should you proceed with your treatment?

    A. Perform the initial assessment, expose the patient, and do the rapid trauma assessment on-scene.

    B. Establish responsiveness, perform the initial assessment, expose the patient, and continue with the rapid trauma assessment on-scene.

    C. Perform the initial assessment and immobilization on-scene. Expose the patient and continue the rapid trauma assessment in the ambulance.

    D. Perform the initial assessment and rapid trauma assessment. Exposing the patient is not necessary.

85. You are transporting a 65-year-old female who has fractured her right hip in a fall. During your reassessment of the patient, what information would be most important?

    A. allergies the patient may have

    B. complaint of nausea

    C. the severity of the pain

    D. presence or absence of a distal pulse

86. You are treating an elderly male patient who fell and has a possible hip fracture. The patient tells you he was dizzy before he fell. How should you prepare this patient for transport?

    A. Packaging includes immobilization only.

    B. Packaging is complete once you finish the initial assessment.

    C. Packaging should include fracture stabilization and transport.

    D. Packaging should include complete spinal immobilization and fracture stabilization.

87. Which statement is most accurate about securing a patient to the cot?

    A. The patient needs to be secured to the cot only when the ambulance is moving.

    B. There should be a minimum of four straps holding the patient to the cot.

    C. If the patient is secured to the backboard, it is not necessary to secure the patient to the cot.

    D. The patient should be secured to the cot before transfer to the ambulance.

88. You are treating a 60-year-old male complaining of chest discomfort. The family wants the patient transported to a hospital in the next town, which is 12 miles away. While en route, the patient's condition starts to deteriorate and his mental status decreases. What should be your next decision?

    A. Continue transport to the facility of family choice.

    B. Call the family for permission to take the patient to a closer hospital.

    C. Transport the patient to the closest hospital for stabilization.

    D. Speed up your transportation to the facility in the next town.

89. The primary purpose of performing an initial assessment is

    A. to determine if rapid transport is necessary.

    B. to determine if a BLS unit can transport this patient without tying up an Intermediate Life Support unit.

    C. to manage life threats and establish priorities of care.

    D. to determine vital signs.

90. Which of the following hazards are you most likely to encounter at a medical emergency?

    A. broken glass

    B. infectious pathogens

    C. risk of fire

    D. confined spaces

91. You are dispatched to a motor vehicle crash that requires using extrication tools to free the patient. In addition to ensuring your safety, you should

    A. park your vehicle downwind to avoid any hazardous materials.

    B. provide protection for your patient with a blanket or similar device.

    C. ask the tool operator to stay away from the patient's side of the vehicle.

    D. notify medical control that there may be additional injuries from the extrication.

92. All of the following are elements of the initial assessment **except**

    A. checking carotid and radial pulses.

    B. assessing the skin color, temperature, and condition.

    C. assessing the volume of inspired breaths.

    D. checking the patient's vital signs.

93. Which of the following would be most likely to cause an airway obstruction?

    A. pulmonary edema

    B. epiglottitis

    C. laryngitis

    D. acute bronchitis

94. Hypoxia caused by something other than a direct ventilation disturbance occurs in which of the following?

    A. epiglottitis

    B. pneumonia

    C. pneumothorax

    D. pulmonary embolism

95. Which of the following is a sign of inadequate ventilation?

    A. The heart rate begins to decrease.

    B. Gastric distention develops.

C. The SpO$_2$ reading increases.

D. The skin color becomes less cyanotic.

96. Which of the following would be appropriate when suctioning?

    A. Use only a rigid tonsil-tip catheter to suction.

    B. Apply suction while slowly removing the catheter.

    C. Set the suction at no more than −60 mm Hg.

    D. Apply suction while slowly inserting the catheter for 15 seconds.

97. A minineurological exam can be conducted using the following mnemonic:

    A. SAMPLE

    B. PQRST-A

    C. AVPU

    D. APGAR

98. You have been dispatched to the home of a 17-year-old female who was injured while playing soccer. She is complaining of leg pain. Her father states that sometime during the game he saw her get hit in the shin by another player's foot. Which of the following would **not** be part of the initial assessment?

    A. asking her name and how old she is

    B. checking her radial pulses

    C. evaluating her skin condition, color, and temperature

    D. exposing and palpating the lower extremity

99. All of the following are benefits of drawing a blood sample for the hospital prior to initiating an IV line **except**

    A. obtaining blood glucose levels.

    B. typing and cross-matching.

    C. determining baseline chemistries.

    D. determining the proteinuria levels.

100. You are called to the scene of a motor vehicle crash. On arrival, you find a 30-year-old male who was the unrestrained driver. Your initial assessment reveals that he is unresponsive; radial pulse is absent, carotid pulse is rapid and weak, and respirations are about 42 per minute and shallow. You note a contusion on the chest that approximates the steering wheel. Your priorities for managing this patient include

    A. take in-line spinal stabilization, insert an oropharyngeal airway, and begin positive pressure ventilation.

    B. take in-line spinal stabilization and apply a nonrebreather mask at 15 lpm.

    C. insert an oropharyngeal airway, begin bag-valve-mask ventilation, and apply the PASG.

    D. take in-line spinal stabilization, begin bag-valve-mask ventilation, and start two large-bore IVs of normal saline.

101. You have responded to the scene of a motorcycle-versus-car crash. Your patient was the motorcycle rider, who was thrown 30 feet from the bike. His injuries include an open skull fracture with brain matter exposed, oral trauma with blood and broken teeth in the mouth, chest trauma resulting in a left-thoracic flail segment, and bilateral femur fractures. His vitals are BP 92/60, HR 128, and RR 40 and shallow. After taking in-line spinal stabilization, your next treatment priority is to

    A. perform a head tilt/chin lift and begin bag-valve-mask ventilation.

    B. suction the mouth and begin positive pressure ventilation with O$_2$

    C. suction the oropharynx and apply a nonrebreather mask at 15 lpm.

    D. stabilize the flail segment.

102. Of the following assessments or interventions, which one would be performed last during the rapid trauma assessment of an unresponsive patient with severe head, face, and neck trauma?

    A. auscultation of breath sounds

    B. palpation of the head

    C. palpation of the thorax

    D. application of the cervical spinal immobilization collar

103. You arrive on the scene of a tractor-trailer rollover that has pinned the male driver under the rig. As you approach the driver, you notice a placard on the trailer denoting its contents as flammable. You should immediately

    A. continue to the patient's side and begin your assessment.

    B. quickly scan the trailer for leaks and, if none are noted, proceed.

    C. stop and call for the fire department.

    D. retreat and leave the scene.

104. During extrication of a patient trapped in an automobile, the fire department prepares to cut off the roof. Which of the following will provide the best protection to the patient during the procedure?

    A. stay outside the auto and instruct the patient to lie still

    B. stay inside the auto and place a thick blanket over both of you

    C. stay outside the auto and place a flame-retardant blanket over the patient

    D. stay inside the auto and place protective eyewear on the patient

105. In an unresponsive patient, the tongue may fall posteriorly and occlude the airway at what anatomic site?

    A. oropharynx

    B. carina

    C. nasopharynx

    D. laryngopharynx

106. You have just placed an oropharyngeal airway in an unresponsive patient. In order to ensure a patent airway, you must also

    A. perform the head tilt/chin lift maneuver.

    B. insert a gastric levine tube to decompress the stomach.

    C. use the two-hand BVM technique.

    D. apply oxygen tubing to the pocket mask.

107. What is the major pathophysiologic change that occurs with a simple pneumothorax?

    A. loss of perfusion around the alveoli

    B. loss of negative pressure in the pleural space

    C. loss of diaphragmatic function

    D. loss of phrenic nerve innervation

108. Which of the following properly describes how to secure a pocket mask to the face when performing mouth-to-mask ventilations?

    A. Place one hand around the top portion of the mask and apply pressure downward to ensure an adequate seal.

    B. Encircle both hands around the top portion of the mask and apply pressure downward to ensure an adequate seal.

    C. Place your thumbs along each side of the mask using your palms to push downward while lifting the mandible with your fingers to help ensure a good seal.

    D. Place your thumbs under the mandible and lift while holding the mask in place with your fingers and use your palms to ensure a good seal.

109. Which of the following would indicate the need for immediate positive pressure ventilation?
   A. a pulse oximeter (SpO$_2$) reading of 89%
   B. a respiratory rate of 30 with adequate chest rise and fall
   C. peripheral cyanosis
   D. a respiratory rate of 24 with shallow depth

110. You are treating a patient with an open upper-right-leg fracture with spurting blood. Which anatomic structure is probably responsible for the bleeding?
   A. femoral artery
   B. tibial artery
   C. iliac artery
   D. femoral vein

111. Of the following, which would be found through the process of inspection during the assessment?
   A. crepitus to the left hemithorax
   B. bilateral wheezing
   C. hyperresonance to right hemithorax
   D. paradoxical movement to right thorax

112. You are treating a patient who fell 30 feet off a scaffold. The patient is responsive but is complaining of severe pain to his back and neck. The patient also has a puncture wound to the abdomen. His arms are cool and moist while his legs are warm and dry, capillary refill is delayed, pupils are reactive to light, and abdomen is soft to palpation. His vitals are BP 86/50, HR is 60, and RR is 18. The patient is most likely suffering from
   A. vasogenic shock.
   B. ruptured aortic artery.
   C. myocardial contusion.
   D. hypovolemic shock.

113. Of the following interventions, which should be delayed until you are en route to the hospital when treating a trauma victim?
   A. applying a nonrebreather at 15 lpm
   B. dressing and bandaging all wounds
   C. applying a cervical spinal immobilization collar
   D. applying a traction splint

114. Which of the following is performed last when immobilizing a patient to a backboard?
   A. assess pulse, motor, and sensory function
   B. apply cervical spinal immobilization collar
   C. secure the legs to the board
   D. apply a head immobilization device

115. You are reassessing a patient while en route to the hospital. During this phase of patient assessment, which one of the following injuries should already have been managed?
   A. puncture wound to the left thigh
   B. foreign body in the eye
   C. right humerus protruding through skin
   D. open wound to the posterior thorax

116. List the following in order according to priority care performed on the patient.
   1. control bleeding from a small laceration
   2. initiate bag-valve-mechanical ventilation
   3. assess the carotid pulse
   4. perform a jaw thrust
   A. 1, 2, 3, 4
   B. 4, 2, 1, 3
   C. 4, 2, 3, 1
   D. 2, 4, 3, 1

117. Which of the following hazards would you be least concerned with during the scene size-up?

    A. blood spurting from an open soft-tissue injury

    B. an extremely cold home in the winter

    C. a hostile crowd at an accident scene

    D. extremely hot pavement

118. Which of the following would be **incorrect** regarding scene size-up?

    A. Consider all power lines to be energized at a crash scene.

    B. Delay entry to a hostile scene until arrival of an additional EMS unit.

    C. Do not enter water to perform a rescue unless specially trained to do so.

    D. Assume that confined spaces contain toxic substances or are low-oxygen areas.

119. Which technique listed below is most effective in controlling the crowd at the scene of an emergency?

    A. Assign two EMT-Intermediates to provide crowd control.

    B. Have the patient's family members stand around the patient.

    C. Contact the police to control the scene.

    D. Involve crowd members for crowd control.

120. Additional resources that are commonly required to assess emergency scenes include all of the following **except**

    A. law enforcement.

    B. fire/rescuer resources.

    C. electric utility.

    D. coroner's investigation.

121. The following list pairs common classifications of emergencies with a description. Which items are **incorrectly** paired?

    A. medical—illness

    B. behavioral—abnormal behavior

    C. gynecology—childbirth

    D. trauma—injury

122. The first step in the initial assessment is to assess the

    A. breathing rate and depth.

    B. airway patency.

    C. presence of a pulse.

    D. general impression.

123. Which statement most correctly describes the purpose of performing the initial assessment?

    A. Identify all injuries and treat them as found.

    B. Identify all potential threats to life first, then manage them according to priority.

    C. Evaluate clinical findings and vital signs

    D. Identify immediate life threats and manage them as they are found.

124. Which airway management method is **incorrectly** paired with description?

    A. head tilt/chin lift—displaces the jaw forward and extends the head

    B. chin lift—pulls the chin forward displacing the tongue.

    C. jaw thrust—extends the head and moves the mandible forward.

    D. airway adjunct—displaces the tongue away from the posterior oropharynx

125. You are dispatched to a local restaurant. You arrive on-scene and observe a 40-year-old patient clutching his throat and coughing forcefully. You should immediately
   A. deliver repeated abdominal thrusts until the obstruction is removed.
   B. encourage the patient to continue to cough.
   C. insert a laryngoscope and remove the object with Magill forceps.
   D. perform a tongue-jaw lift and attempt to ventilate.

126. The preferred method to maintain an airway in the suspected spine injured patient is the
   A. head tilt/chin lift.
   B. chin lift.
   C. jaw thrust.
   D. nasopharyngeal airway.

127. What is typically the **earliest** detectable clinical sign of decreased blood volume?
   A. increased heart rate
   B. increased cardiac stroke volume
   C. peripheral vasoconstriction
   D. diaphoresis

128. If the radial pulse is absent because of poor perfusion, which of the following other pulses would you suspect would also be absent?
   A. carotid pulse
   B. femoral pulse
   C. apical pulse
   D. dorsalis pedis pulse

129. After intubating the patient with a tracheal tube, to check for proper placement you must
   A. ventilate the patient for one minute before auscultating breath sounds.
   B. attach the pulse oximeter and check the reading.
   C. ventilate the patient and auscultate over the epigastrium and then each hemithorax.
   D. check for condensation in the ET tube with each ventilation.

130. Which of the following is true regarding tracheal suctioning?
   A. To determine the catheter length, measure from the lips to the ear lobe.
   B. Insert the catheter down the endotracheal tube with suction applied.
   C. Advance the catheter to the level of the carina.
   D. Apply suction for at least 20 seconds.

131. Hypoperfusion or shock is described as inadequate
   A. fraction of inspired oxygen.
   B. removal of carbon dioxide from the alveolar tissue.
   C. levels of hemoglobin that prevent the movement of oxygen from the blood plasma.
   D. delivery of oxygen to and elimination of carbon dioxide from cells.

132. Physiologically unstable patients should be reassessed every
   A. 5 minutes.
   B. 10 minutes.
   C. 15 minutes.
   D. 20 minutes.

133. You are dispatched to a patient who has been stabbed in the neck. You observe a responsive patient in obvious respiratory distress. His neck appears to be swollen, and you feel crepitation on palpation. This finding is described as
    A. pericardial tamponade.
    B. subcutaneous emphysema.
    C. tension pneumothorax.
    D. hematoma.

134. The parameters evaluated in the revised trauma score are
    A. respiratory effort, diastolic blood pressure, and Glasgow Coma Score.
    B. respiratory rate, diastolic blood pressure, and Glasgow Coma Score.
    C. respiratory effort, systolic blood pressure, and Glasgow Coma Score.
    D. respiratory rate, systolic blood pressure, and Glasgow Coma Score.

135. Which of the following is least important when initially taking a patient history?
    A. the patient's last oral intake
    B. the patient's allergies
    C. the patient's father's medical history
    D. radiation of pain to another body region

136. Which of the following is **not** a laboratory test routinely performed by the hospital on prehospital blood samples?
    A. human immunodeficiency virus
    B. blood glucose
    C. complete blood count
    D. type and cross-match

137. Which of the following is true regarding reassessment of the patient?
    A. It is performed to detect changes in the patient's condition, assess other complaints, and guide continued care.
    B. It is a complete head-to-toe physical exam repeated every 5 or 15 minutes.
    C. Reassessment of patients during transport should be conducted only if time or the patient's condition permits it.
    D. It is an assessment of the airway, breathing, and circulation that is performed every 30 minutes.

138. The most important factor to consider when determining the appropriate medical facility to transport the patient to is the
    A. patient's choice.
    B. closeness in distance.
    C. patient's condition.
    D. patient's physician.

139. Which statement best describes the potential results from using lights and siren while transporting a patient?
    A. Patient care is improved dramatically by the use of lights and siren.
    B. Patient care is distracted from by the use of lights and siren.
    C. Patients typically request lights and sirens and are calmed by their use.
    D. Accidents occur less frequently when using lights and siren.

140. An order you receive from medical direction appears to be improper. Select the statement that best describes the action to be taken.

A. Follow the order without question.

B. Follow the order and then document it carefully.

C. Repeat the orders, as given, back to medical direction.

D. Follow the order and consult with medical direction once at the hospital.

141. The ongoing assessment should always include reassessment of which of the following items?

A. initial assessment

B. focused physical exam

C. detailed history

D. detailed physical exam

142. Scene safety begins

A. with the call received from the dispatch center.

B. once you approach the scene at that location.

C. after exiting the vehicle.

D. while visualizing the scene by walking the perimeter.

143. Your unit is the first on-scene of a serious vehicle crash. You notice that wires are lying across the roof of the vehicle. You should

A. stage outside the scene and call for specially trained personnel.

B. carefully approach the vehicle by shuffling your feet and quickly gain entry through a window.

C. cut the wire closest to the pole.

D. cautiously remove the wires by using a wooden or fiberglass pole.

144. You are at the scene of a fight when a group of bystanders suddenly become hostile and threatening. You should

A. try to reason with the group so that you can continue to provide treatment.

B. quietly call for police, continue care, and protect the patient.

C. immediately leave the scene until it is secured.

D. clear the crowd by using necessary force.

145. While approaching a vehicle crash site, you are unsure what level of body substance isolation (BSI) precautions you will need. You should at least

A. apply gloves, protective eyewear, and a HEPA mask.

B. assess the scene further and then decide what is needed.

C. use gloves and return to your vehicle if other BSI is necessary.

D. use gloves and eye protection.

146. You are treating a patient in a busy department store. Which of the following is the best way to protect the patient from the gaze of the public?

A. Ask the bystanders to leave the scene, or you will be forced to have them removed.

B. Have your partner hold a blanket up with outstretched arms to block their view.

C. Have the bystanders turn their backs to the patient while holding an unfolded sheet.

D. Shield the patient from the curious bystanders by placing the stretcher between them.

147. You arrive on a scene of a multiple vehicle crash and find eight critically injured patients. Only three ambulances are immediately available. Your next immediate action should be to
    A. divide the critically injured patients and transport immediately.
    B. initiate the multiple casualty incident plan.
    C. quickly treat all immediate life threats first, then move to other injuries.
    D. immediately transport the most critical patient.

148. You find your patient standing on the roof of a vehicle that is partially submerged in fast-moving water. You should immediately
    A. call for personnel who are specially trained in water rescue.
    B. form a human chain with bystanders and assist the patient to shore.
    C. throw the patient a rope and ask him or her to hold on, then pull the patient to safety.
    D. tie a rescue rope to yourself and make an attempt to reach the patient.

149. You are dispatched to a female patient complaining of respiratory difficulty. The scene size-up does not reveal any unusual situations or hazards. A bystander states that the patient has had this problem before. From this information, you would initially categorize the patient's problem as
    A. trauma.
    B. behavioral.
    C. medical.
    D. obstetric.

150. Stridor is caused by
    A. presence of fluids in the upper airway.
    B. constriction of the bronchioles.

C. tracheal obstruction.
    D. laryngeal edema.

151. The Magill forceps may be used in conjunction with _____ to remove an airway obstruction.
    A. four back blows
    B. direct laryngoscopy
    C. index finger sweeps
    D. oropharyngeal airway

152. After you have inserted an oropharyngeal airway, the patient begins to gag. You should
    A. turn the patient on his or her side.
    B. prepare to suction the airway.
    C. quickly remove the airway.
    D. immediately coach the patient to relax.

153. You are preparing to insert a nasopharyngeal airway. You should
    A. lubricate it with a water-soluble lubricant and insert it at a 45-degree lateral angle to the septum.
    B. lubricate it with a petroleum jelly and insert the airway into the more patent nostril.
    C. lubricate it with a water-soluble lubricant and insert it with the bevel toward the septum.
    D. lubricate it with a petroleum lubricant and insert it in the right nostril only.

154. You are treating an unresponsive adult patient involved in a vehicle crash. As you perform the initial assessment, you hear sonorous sounds. You should immediately
    A. do a head tilt/chin lift and hold in-line stabilization.
    B. suction and continue with the assessment.

C. apply Sellick's maneuver and begin bag-valve mask ventilation.

D. do a jaw thrust and insert an oropharyngeal airway.

155. Which of the following is **not** an initial sign of suspected spine injury?

A. pale, cool, clammy skin below the site of injury

B. diaphragmatic breathing

C. priaprism

D. loss of sensation in lower extremities

156. All of the statements regarding the bag-valve mask are true **except**

A. tidal volumes delivered by bag-valve mask are less than those delivered by pocket mask.

B. two rescuers are recommended when using the bag-valve mask.

C. the bag-valve mask is the recommended device to use when only one person is available to ventilate.

D. nearly 100% oxygen concentration can be delivered by bag-valve mask when using a reservoir.

157. Which of the following may indicate inadequate ventilation?

A. Heart rate decreases from 124 to 100 per minute.

B. Chest rises with each ventilation.

C. Patient's skin is warm, dry, and pink.

D. Pop-off valve releases air with each ventilation.

158. All of the following may result from decreased perfusion **except**

A. cells will begin to move from aerobic to anaerobic metabolism.

B. glucose metabolism will produce lactic acid.

C. cell death may result from the accumulation of acids.

D. pyruvic acid breaks down into carbon dioxide and water.

159. Which of the following is the leading cause of cardiac arrest and sudden death?

A. coronary artery disease

B. acid-base imbalance

C. cerebrovascular accident

D. pulmonary embolism

160. Which of the following is the most reliable indicator of poor perfusion in the adult patient?

A. pale, cool, clammy skin

B. capillary refill that is less than 2 seconds

C. skin that is cool to the touch

D. constricted pupils that are brisk to respond to light

161. You arrive on the scene and find a 23-year-old male patient who was stabbed in the chest. On your assessment, you find blood in the mouth and a respiratory rate of 42 and shallow. You should immediately

A. assess the radial and carotid pulse.

B. obtain a set of baseline vital signs.

C. administer oxygen by nonrebreather at 15 lpm.

D. suction the mouth and begin bag-valve-mask ventilation.

162. You have responded to the scene of a serious motor vehicle crash. While performing the rapid trauma assessment, you should

A. remove all jewelry.

B. manage non–life-threatening bleeding.

C. dress all wounds.

D. expose the patient.

163. In which circumstance should you **not** expose the patient to perform an assessment?

  A. in an environment that may lead to hypothermia

  B. a motor vehicle crash in which the patient was ejected

  C. if a crowd has gathered at the scene

  D. if your partner is treating another patient

164. The most reliable component of the ongoing assessment to reassess in the head-injured patient to identify deterioration or improvement in the patient's condition is

  A. the blood pressure.

  B. pupil reactivity to light.

  C. the skin.

  D. the mental status.

165. Which assessment or management technique is **not** a part of the detailed physical exam?

  A. application of a cervical spinal immobilization collar

  B. palpating for abdominal masses and rigidity

  C. inspecting the sclera for icterus

  D. auscultation of breath sounds

166. Your patient has fallen approximately 20 feet onto a concrete floor. While palpating the chest, you feel a crackling sensation at the upper chest and base of the neck. You can best describe this as

  A. a flail segment.

  B. subcutaneous emphysema.

  C. paradoxical motion.

  D. suprasternal notch reaction.

167. The GCS evaluates all of the following parameters **except**

  A. eye opening.

  B. respiratory rate per minute.

  C. best verbal response.

  D. best motor response.

168. In which of the following would emergency care **not** be conducted **until after** the removal of the patient from a vehicle?

  A. The patient is not oriented and not cooperating.

  B. There will be a delay in extrication.

  C. The vehicle is on its side and unstable.

  D. The patient complains of cervical pain.

169. During transport, the patient begins to complain of abdominal pain. You should

  A. increase the oxygen flow.

  B. perform a complete detailed physical exam.

  C. administer nitro to the patient.

  D. perform a focused assessment of the area of the complaint.

170. Which physical findings would cause you to categorize the patient as a priority?

  A. BP 100/60 mmHg, pulse 82 BPM, R13 per minute and adequate

  B. side impact in a motor vehicle collision with intrusion into the passenger compartment of 6 inches

  C. Glasgow Coma Score less than 9

  D. open humerus fracture with no major bleeding

171. The purpose of providing a brief, concise, relevant oral report to the hospital staff when transferring care is

  A. that it is a requirement of the hospital staff to receive a report from EMS.

  B. to provide the hospital staff the legal right to treat the patient.

C. to ensure a continuation of care.

D. to avoid being charged with negligence.

172. Which statement regarding the prehospital care report is **not** true?

A. The report will prevent you from being sued.

B. You should use a standardized format.

C. Reports become a permanent part of the patient's medical records.

D. Your report becomes your best legal defense in a court of law.

173. You arrive on the scene and find a 23-year-old male patient who was involved in a fight. On your initial assessment, you find blood in the mouth and tachypnea that is shallow and labored. The skin is extremely pale, cyanotic, and diaphoretic. Your next immediate actions are to

A. suction the mouth and apply a nonrebreather at 15 lpm.

B. take in-line immobilization, suction, and begin positive pressure ventilation.

C. expose the patient and inspect for open wounds to the thorax.

D. check the radial pulse and capillary refill, then apply a nonrebreather mask at 15 lpm.

174. You arrive on the scene of a patient complaining of severe crushing substernal chest pain. As you approach the patient, he states, "I am having a difficult time breathing." Your next immediate action is to

A. perform a head tilt/chin lift and assess the tidal volume.

B. assess breath sound and begin bag-valve mask ventilation.

C. assess the radial pulse and apply a nonrebreather mask.

D. take a set of vitals and gather a SAMPLE history.

175. You open the airway of an unresponsive medical patient using a jaw thrust. The patient continues to produce sonorous sounds. You should immediately

A. begin bag-valve-mask ventilation.

B. reposition the mandible using the jaw thrust.

C. insert an endotracheal tube.

D. assess the respiratory status.

176. You arrive on the scene and find a male patient in his 30s lying supine on the street. There are no bystanders at the scene. He is not alert and appears grossly cyanotic. Your first immediate action is to

A. open the airway and begin bag-valve-mask ventilation.

B. call for additional resources.

C. take in-line immobilization and perform a jaw thrust.

D. quickly scan the scene for any hazards.

177. Which of the following would not be discovered during the initial assessment of the patient?

A. decreased minute ventilation

B. tachycardia

C. poor skin turgor

D. hypotension

178. During the spinal immobilzation process, you should ensure that

A. the feet are strapped to the board.

B. a cervical collar is applied after the logroll.

C. the head is secured after strapping the torso.

D. backboard straps are applied to the abdomen and across the lower legs.

179. You arrive on the scene to find an alert 46-year-old female patient complaining of severe abdominal pain. You place the patient on a nonrebreather mask and assess the radial pulse and skin color, temperature, and condition. Your next immediate actions are to

A. obtain a SAMPLE history, conduct a focused physical exam, and get a set of baseline vital signs.

B. start an IV of normal saline and obtain a set of vital signs.

C. perform a detailed physical exam and obtain a SAMPLE history.

D. prepare the patient for transport and conduct an initial assessment en route to the medical facility.

180. You are at the residence of a patient who is complaining of abdominal pain. The patient is stable at this time. Which of the following would guide your continued care?

A. orders from the patient's son who is a physician

B. your local protocol

C. orders from the family physician

D. the advice from your partner

181. You arrive on the scene and find an unresponsive elderly male patient in his bed. As you approach the patient, you note snoring-type respirations. You should immediately

A. insert an oropharyngeal airway.

B. insert a nasopharyngeal airway.

C. perform a head tilt/chin lift.

D. begin bag-valve-mask ventilation.

182. Adequate ventilation, when using a tracheal tube, is best confirmed by

A. an absence of gastric insufflation.

B. absence of cyanosis.

C. equal bilateral breath sounds in all lung fields.

D. absence of end-tidal CO_2 production.

183. Which of the following conditions would cause an obstructive type of shock?

A. congestive heart failure

B. hemorrhage

C. allergic reaction

D. pericardial tamponade

184. The following are true regarding the prehospital care report **except**

A. it can be admissible as evidence in a court of law.

B. it may be used for quality assurance monitoring.

C. it is used by some EMS systems for billing purposes.

D. it does not become a part of the permanent patient record.

185. In which of the following patient presentations would obtaining a venous blood sample be most important?

A. altered mental status with bizarre behavior

B. acute onset of respiratory distress

C. abdominal pain with specks of blood in the vomitus

D. severe headache that is chronic in nature

186. You have a patient who is entrapped in a car whose fuel tank has ruptured and is burning. As efforts are expended to free the victim, what would best protect the patient from being harmed by the heat and flames?

A. Place the patient in firefighter's turnout gear.

B. Shield the patient with a short spine board.

C. Cover the patient with a flame-retardant blanket.

D. Nothing can be done at this point for the patient.

187. A flail segment impairs adequate ventilation by

A. decreasing the effectiveness of thoracic movement.

B. causing an upper-airway obstruction.

C. paralyzing the diaphragm.

D. allowing air to collect in the pleural space.

188. During the management of a patient in cardiac arrest, the major purpose for providing CPR is to

A. treat the underlying cause of cardiac arrest.

B. provide artificial ventilation and circulation so that defibrillation and drug therapy can be provided.

C. give the family hope that all that can be done is being done.

D. restore normal cardiac activity.

189. A 17-year-old vehicle crash victim sustained the following injuries. Which one of these would be treated during the detailed physical exam?

A. an abdominal evisceration

B. lacerations to the dorsum of the hand

C. an open femur fracture

D. knife wound to the posterior thorax

190. A patient cut her hand while peeling an apple with a paring knife. Which of the following would be most appropriate to control the bleeding?

A. tourniquet applied to the forearm

B. digital pressure on the radial artery

C. digital pressure on the ulnar artery

D. direct pressure to the site of injury

191. You are summoned to a fast-food restaurant where someone is reportedly choking on chicken nuggets. Initial attempts to clear the airway by providing subdiaphragmatic thrusts have failed. As an EMT-Intermediate, you should now

A. initiate transport to the hospital.

B. wait for the patient to go into cardiac arrest and then treat the patient as a cardiac arrest victim.

C. perform a visual laryngoscopy and retrieve the foreign object.

D. lay the patient on the ground and deliver sharp back blows.

192. What would be considered as appropriate body substance isolation when preparing to intubate?

A. gown, gloves

B. mask, gloves, eye protection

C. gloves only

D. gown, gloves, eye protection, mask

193. Disentangling a person from a car or removing him from an awkward location in a home is generally known as patient _____

A. extraction.

B. extrication.

C. removal.

D. interaction.

194. A person who is successfully intubated with a tracheal tube cannot speak because

A. the vocal cords cannot vibrate.

B. the BVM mask covers the face.

C. the delivery of PPV precludes the contraction of vocal cord muscles.

D. air is not passing over the cords during inspiration.

195. You are called for a patient who is complaining of chest pain and severe shortness of breath. Your first action on arrival at the scene is to
    A. open the airway and assess the breathing status.
    B. apply a nonrebreather at 15 lpm.
    C. begin bag-valve mask ventilation and check for a pulse.
    D. assess the scene for safety hazards.

196. You are called to the scene of a possible shooting. When you arrive, the wife of the patient meets you at the curb and states that the patient is bleeding profusely from a wound to the chest. You should immediately
    A. determine if the scene is safe to enter.
    B. stop the bleeding with direct pressure.
    C. apply your gloved hand over the wound.
    D. begin bag-valve-mask ventilation with supplemental oxygen.

197. You are called to the scene for a patient who is complaining of feeling ill for the past week. He has a fever, a cough with blood-tinged sputum, and shortness of breath. Before entering the scene, you should
    A. call for a backup in case it is a cardiac arrest.
    B. put on gloves, eye protection, and a HEPA respirator.
    C. contact medical direction for orders to treat the patient.
    D. put on gloves and eye protection.

198. You are treating a patient at the scene of an auto crash at a busy intersection. A crowd gathers to see what is going on. As you conduct your physical assessment of the patient, it is necessary to
    A. disperse the crowd immediately.
    B. move the ambulance between the crowd and the patient.
    C. cover the patient with a sheet as you expose the body to conduct the exam.
    D. have the crowd form a human barrier to protect you from oncoming traffic.

199. You arrive on the scene for a patient who is complaining of shortness of breath. As you enter, you note a large male patient weighing approximately 400 pounds sitting in a recliner. He is cyanotic and is on a nasal cannula at 2 lpm. You should immediately
    A. increase the oxygen flow to 6 lpm on the nasal cannula.
    B. call for a backup crew to assist with lifting and moving the patient when ready to leave the scene.
    C. place the patient on the floor and begin chest compressions.
    D. ask the patient if he is able to walk down to the ambulance cot.

200. You are treating a patient who was struck in the head by a piece of machinery at a factory. Your partner tells you that the patient's airway is clear and that he has a respiratory rate of 16 per minute. You should immediately
    A. check for a radial pulse.
    B. begin hyperventilating the patient by bag-valve mask.

C. look at the chest for rise and fall and listen for air movement.

D. apply a nonrebreather at 15 lpm.

201. Your partner asks you to apply pressure to the anterior surface of the neck while he is ventilating in an attempt to reduce the risk of regurgitation and gastric distention. You will apply pressure to what anatomic structure?

   A. glottic opening

   B. epiglottis

   C. thyroid cartilage

   D. cricoid cartilage

202. Which of the following statements about using an oropharyngeal airway is **true**?

   A. It should never be removed once it is inserted.

   B. It cannot be used while performing mouth-to-mask ventilation.

   C. A head tilt/chin lift or jaw-thrust maneuver must be maintained even with the airway in place.

   D. A longer oropharyngeal airway can be used in cases of laryngeal swelling to facilitate airflow past the larynx.

203. You arrive on the scene of a construction site where you find a 26-year-old male patient who fell off a scaffold from about 25 feet. He is unresponsive, has blood in his mouth, and is breathing shallow at a rate of 24 per minute. You should immediately

   A. check for a radial and carotid pulse.

   B. establish in-line spinal stabilization, suction the airway, and begin bag-valve-mask ventilation.

   C. expose the patient and inspect for any open wounds to the chest.

   D. establish in-line spinal stabilization, suction the airway, and apply a nonrebreather mask at 15 lpm.

204. The major complication associated with flail segment is

   A. pain on deep inhalation.

   B. hypoxia associated with an underlying pulmonary contusion.

   C. decreased breath sounds and tracheal deviation.

   D. stomach contents herniating into the chest cavity and impeding ventilation.

205. What should the pressure be set at when suctioning the oropharynx of an adult patient?

   A. less than -120 mm Hg

   B. -120 mm Hg

   C. greater than -120 mm Hg

   D. -80 to -100 mm Hg

206. You are applying direct pressure to a large wound on the left forearm. The wound continues to bleed profusely even with the direct pressure. You should consider

   A. applying a tourniquet.

   B. elevating the arm and applying pressure to the brachial artery.

   C. lowering the arm and applying cold packs to the wound.

   D. applying additional dressings and compressing the femoral artery.

207. Fractures not associated with major bleeding should be identified and managed during the
    A. initial assessment.
    B. resuscitation phase.
    C. detailed physical exam.
    D. ongoing assessment.

208. Which of the following signs or symptoms would be an indication of an esophageal rupture?
    A. bowel sounds in the chest cavity
    B. jugular venous distention
    C. subcutaneous emphysema
    D. hemoptysis

209. Which of the following would **not** be considered a part of the history of the present illness (chief complaint)?
    A. medications
    B. onset
    C. severity
    D. duration

210. You are treating a 21-year-old female who was thrown from her horse. She is responding to painful stimuli with flexion of her arms. Her BP is 100/82 mm Hg, heart rate is 126 per minute, and respirations are 34 per minute and shallow. She has an obvious deformity and fracture to her left humerus. Prior to transport, you should
    A. apply a nonrebreather mask, immobilize the humerus with a vacuum splint, and cover her with a blanket.
    B. begin bag-valve-mask ventilation, immobilize her to a backboard, and immobilize the humerus to the backboard.
    C. immobilize her to a backboard, apply a nonrebreather mask, and splint the humerus with long boards and cravats.
    D. apply a cervical collar, apply a nonrebreather mask, and splint the humerus with wire ladder splints.

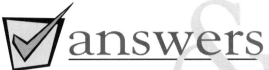

answers & rationales

Following each rationale, you will find a reference to the corresponding objective in the DOT National Standard EMT-Intermediate curriculum. An asterisk denotes material that is supplemental to the DOT curriculum. Page numbers after a rationale indicate where the question topic may be discussed in the Brady text *Intermediate Emergency Care* (Bledsoe, Porter, Cherry).

1.

B. For the responsive patient who can answer your questions, you conduct an initial assessment, a focused history and physical exam, and an ongoing assessment en route to the hospital. (3-3.27) (IEC pp. 511–517)

2.

C. Scene size-up is the essential first step at any emergency. A proper scene size-up includes body substance isolation, scene safety, location of patients, mechanism of injury, and nature of illness. (3-3.4, 3-3.7, 3-3.8) (IEC pp. 481–491)

3.

A. The high-efficiency particulate air (HEPA) mask is designed to filter out the tuberculosis bacillus. Always wear the mask when performing high-risk procedures, such as endotracheal intubation, or suctioning on patients suspected of having tuberculosis. (3-3.5) (IEC p. 483)

4.

D. Never forget this! Your personal safety is jeopardized every time you answer an alarm. The safety of you and your crew is the top priority at any emergency scene. (3-3.5) (IEC p. 484)

5.

A. Your instincts are the subconscious sum of your experiences. Listen to them. They are probably correct. (3-3.3) (IEC p. 484)

6.

D. Entering an unstable or dangerous environment without law enforcement is the foolish behavior of inexperienced emergency personnel. Better to stage your ambulance a few blocks away from the scene so as not to rile the bystanders and wait for the police to secure the scene. (3-3.5) (IEC p. 485)

7.

D. Another example of foolish behavior by inexperienced emergency personnel is to try to move a live wire with **any** piece of equipment. No matter how dry you believe the wooden handles are, they contain moisture and will conduct electricity. Leave it for the professionals with equipment tested to do the job safely. A foolish hero is not a hero. (3-3.5) (IEC p. 486)

8.

B. The first crew on the scene of a multiple-patient incident must avoid the urge to begin treating patients. It is more important to establish a command center, assess your needs, call for help, and begin triage. These steps are patient care. (3-3.9) (IEC p. 484)

9.

D. The initial assessment consists of the following steps: forming a general impression, stabilizing the cervical spine as needed, assessing a baseline mental status, assessing the airway, assessing breathing, assessing circulation, and determining priority. (3-3.12–3-3.24) (IEC p. 491)

10.

C. A child's occiput is very large. To compensate for this, place a folded towel under his shoulders to maintain proper alignment of his head and neck. (3-3.14) (IEC pp. 492–493)

11.

A. An awake patient, as evidenced by open eyes, is classified as alert even though he is disoriented. (3-3.13) (IEC p. 494)

12.

C. If your patient responds to your painful stimulus by abnormal posturing, he receives a P on the AVPU scale. (3-3.13) (IEC p. 494)

Matching (3-3.14) (IEC pp. 494–496)

13.	F	snoring
14.	B	gurgling
15.	E	foreign body
16.	D	burns
17.	A	stridor with hives, itching, and redness
18.	C	epiglottitis

19.

A. Expiratory wheezing is usually the result of lower-airway spasm or obstruction. This can be the result of diseases such as asthma, bronchiolitis, emphysema, and bronchitis. Epiglottitis is an upper-airway problem that causes stridor. (3-3.14) (IEC p. 495)

20.

C. According to the American Heart Association, when performing positive pressure ventilation on a nonbreathing patient, provide 12 breaths per minute for adults and 20 breaths per minute for children. (3-3.17) (IEC p. 496)

21.

D. If your patient presents as unresponsive, without a gag reflex, and with a decreased minute volume, you should first perform bag-valve-mask ventilation. Once you begin ventilating the patient, supplemental oxygen will be provided through the bag-valve mask. Since inadequate breathing is considered an immediate life threat, you must intervene prior to continuing with your assessment. Tracheal intubation can be considered following completion of the initial assessment. (3-3.17) (IEC p. 496)

22.

A. Normal circulatory status in the healthy adult is evidenced by warm, dry skin; the presence of a radial pulse at a rate of 60–100 per minute; and a capillary refill time of less than 2 seconds. (3-3.20) (IEC p. 497)

23.

C. Top priority and rapid transport are reserved for patients with significant airway, breathing, or circulation problems and those with an uncorrectable altered mental status. Cardiac arrest patients can be managed effectively and more efficiently on the scene. (3-3.24) (IEC p. 500)

24.

A. Predictors of serious internal injury for an adult patient include ejection from the vehicle, fall from higher than 20 feet, vehicle rollover, high-speed collision, motorcycle crash, and penetration of the trunk or head. (3-3.24) (IEC p. 501)

25.

B. Within seconds after inflation, an air bag deflates so as not to suffocate the patient. Unfortunately, if your patient does not have his seat belt fastened, he could be propelled into the steering wheel and sustain life-threatening injuries. (3-3.6) (IEC p. 502)

26.

B. The rapid trauma assessment is conducted on trauma patients with a significant mechanism of injury or an altered mental status. It is designed to identify and manage life-threatening injuries. (3-3.29) (IEC p. 503)

27.

D. When performing a rapid trauma assessment, use the mnemonic DCAP–BTLS. It stands for **D**eformities, **C**ontusions, **A**brasions, **P**enetrations, **B**urns, **T**enderness, **L**acerations, and **S**welling. (3-3.31) (IEC p. 503)

28.

D. Aside from major blood loss, consider the possibility of an air embolism because of the negative pressure generated each time your patient inhales. The negative pressure in the chest may draw air into an exposed jugular vein. An occlusive dressing will prevent this. (3-3.19) (IEC p. 505)

29.

A. Jugular vein distention following chest trauma is usually caused by either pericardial tamponade or tension pneumothorax, in which blood is inhibited from returning to the heart. To differentiate, listen for lung sounds. They will be clear bilaterally in pericardial tamponade and absent in tension pneumothorax. (3-3.31) (IEC p. 505)

30.

C. If the trachea tugs to one side during inspiration, the probable cause is a simple pneumothorax on that side. (3-3.31) (IEC p. 505)

31.

C. Grunting is a sign of serious respiratory distress in infants and children. They grunt to create back pressure to keep their lower airways open in such diseases as asthma and bronchiolitis. If your patient is grunting, it is serious. (3-3.26) (IEC p. 505)

32.

A. The clavicles, being so thin and so unprotected and vulnerable, fracture more easily and more often than any other bones in the body. (3-3.31) (IEC p. 505)

33.

C. The first three ribs are well supported and well protected. It takes a tremendous force to cause a fracture. Thus, you should expect major damage to organs lying underneath these ribs, especially vascular structures. (3-3.31) (IEC pp. 505–506)

34.

D. A flail chest is defined as two or more rib fractures in two or more places, causing a floating segment. The floating segment moves in opposition to the rest of the chest wall in a paradoxical fashion. (3-3.31) (IEC p. 507)

35.

B. Jugular vein distention, absent breath sounds on one side and diminished breath sounds on the other, tachycardia, and hypotension paint the classic picture of a left-sided tension pneumothorax. You would immediately decompress the left chest with a large-bore angiocatheter. (3-3.31) (IEC p. 507)

36.

C. The SAMPLE history is comprised of the following components: **S**ymptoms, **A**llergies, **M**edications, **P**ast history, **L**ast eaten, and **E**vents preceding the incident. It is used to elicit a quick history from a trauma patient. Signs are indications you observe; they are not obtained during the history. (*) (IEC p. 510)

37.

D. For a person with an isolated injury, such as a twisted knee, you inspect and palpate the joint for any irregularities, which includes "milking the joint" for a fluid wave. You then conduct the side-to-side test to evaluate the stability of the medial and lateral collateral ligaments. You use the drawer test to assess the stability of the anterior and posterior cruciate ligaments. Finally, you put the knee through its passive range of motion unless this causes pain. (3-3.31) (IEC pp. 510, 524)

38.

C. Anyone with an eye injury should receive a full eye exam. This includes inspection and palpation of the external eye for discoloration, deformity, tenderness, and hyphema; a visual acuity test; direct and consensual response to light; the near–far reflex; accommodation; and the "H" test. The "H" test evaluates the integrity of the cranial nerves and the extraoccular muscles they innervate: CN-III (occulomotor) superior rectus, inferior rectus, inferior oblique; CN-IV (trochlear) superior oblique; and CN-VI (abducens) lateral rectus. An easy way to remember this is SO4–LR6–AR3. In other words, **S**uperior **O**blique is CN-IV, **L**ateral **R**ectus is CN-VI, and **A**ll the **R**est are CN-III. (3-3.31) (IEC p. 522)

39.

D. Examining the mouth of a chest pain patient may reveal important clues as to the seriousness of his condition. Examine the buccal mucosa for signs of central hypoxemia (cyanosis) and circulatory collapse (pallor). Also observe for any fluids, such as pink frothy sputum, which could indicate acute pulmonary edema. (3-3.26) (IEC p. 513)

40.

A. Jugular vein distention (JVD) indicates that blood return to the heart is inhibited. Some common causes for JVD include tension pneumothorax, cardiac tamponade, massive pulmonary embolism, and right-heart failure. (3-3.26) (IEC p. 513)

41.

B. Localized wheezing is the result of a lower airway obstruction in one area of the lung from conditions such as an infection (pneumonia), a pulmonary embolism, or foreign body aspiration. Diffuse, or global, wheezing is the result of conditions that affect the entire lung, such as asthma, COPD, and acute pulmonary edema. (3-3.26) (IEC p. 514)

42.

B. An abdominal aneurysm usually blocks the blood flow path to one or the other leg. This results in a weaker femoral pulse on the affected side, absent pulses in the foot, and cool, ashen skin. (3-3.26) (IEC p. 514)

43.

D. Pinpoint pupils, along with unconsciousness and depressed respirations, are a classic sign of narcotic drug overdose. They also can suggest a pontine (from the pons) hemorrhage. (3-3.26) (IEC p. 515)

44.

B. A nystagmus is a fine, jerking movement of the eyes during an extraoccular muscle exam. If it occurs at the far extremes of the test, it is normal. If it occurs during the entire range of motion, it is considered pathological. (3-3.31) (IEC p. 515)

45.

C. The "rapid alternating movements" test is used to evaluate the integrity of the cerebellum and the pyramidal system. Any patient with neurological deficits should receive a complete cerebellar exam, which also includes point-to-point and heel-to-shin tests. (3-3.31) (IEC p. 515)

46.

D. If you detect abdominal rigidity or guarding, you must determine whether it is voluntary, because your patient is anxious or resisting your exam, or involuntary, suggesting peritoneal irritation. (3-3.31) (IEC p. 515)

47.

A. The detailed physical is a thorough head-to-toe exam that is designed to identify all other injuries or signs associated with the patient's injury or condition. It is only performed if the patient's condition allows it and if there is adequate time to perform it without jeopardizing the patient's condition or delaying rapid transport when necessary. The detailed physical exam is performed after the focused history and physical exam, which includes the rapid trauma or medical exam. (3-3.40) (IEC p. 519)

48.

D. The ongoing assessment is designed to reevaluate the ABCs to detect trends in vital signs and to record the effectiveness of your interventions. (3-3.42, 3-3.43) (IEC p. 525)

49.

B. A bag that becomes increasingly more difficult to squeeze is cause for great concern because something is inhibiting lung inflation. This is a classic description of a tension pneumothorax. If you assess lung sounds, you will note absence on the affected side and diminished on the other side. In this case, immediately decompress the chest with a large-bore catheter on the affected side. (3-3.31) (IEC p. 527)

50.

B. Cardiac tamponade is characterized by a narrowing pulse pressure, JVD, and muffled heart sounds—known as Beck's triad. (3-3.31) (IEC p. 527)

51.

D. In the scene size-up, you identify potential environmental or situational hazards, secure the scene, determine MOI, locate patients, determine the number of patients, and assess the need for additional resources. (3-3.1, 3-3.5–3-3.8) (IEC pp. 481–491)

52.

C. Using police assistance, if necessary, you should move the patient to your ambulance. The best way to deal with an environment that has become hostile is to get out of it. (3-3.5) (IEC pp. 484–486)

53.

D. The assessment of a medical patient is more commonly directed toward history gathering and a physical exam that tends to support the reported symptoms. Assessment of the trauma patient is directed toward identifying signs of injury. (*) (IEC p. 511)

54.

C. An injury to the diaphragm can impair its ability to contract normally. This reduces the size of the thoracic cavity, reducing ventilation. Some diaphragmatic injuries can result in the protrusion of abdominal contents into the thoracic cavity. (3-3.31) (IEC p. 805)

55.

C. Esophageal intubation may be recognized by the absence of any resistance to ventilation, gastric distention, or the presence of breath sounds over the epigastrium. Increased airway resistance may be due to tension pneumothorax, occlusion of the airway, or intubation of the right-mainstem bronchus. (3-3.31) (IEC p. 381)

56.

B. An increase in airway pressure would increase resistance to ventilation, making it more difficult to deflate the reservoir. Deflated reservoir bags may indicate an empty oxygen cylinder, a leak in the system, or a disconnected oxygen supply line. (3-3.31)

57.

B. Cervical spine injury, an intact gag reflex, and epiglottitis are relative contraindications to oral intubation. (3-3.31)

58.

B. Inadequate tourniquet pressure will only inhibit venous return and will not affect arterial flow, thus increasing the rate and volume of blood loss. Tourniquets should be used only as a last resort for hemorrhage control and, once applied, should not be released. A sphygmomanometer can be an effective tourniquet if it is inflated to 20–30 mm Hg above the patient's systolic blood pressure. (3-3.31) (IEC p. 646)

59.

C. It is important to fully expose your trauma patient during the assessment. Only through visualization, auscultation, palpation, and inspection can you identify potentially life-threatening injuries. (3-3.31) (IEC p. 421)

60.

C. For a 60-year-old male patient complaining of chest pain, it would be important to include information about his coronary bypass surgery last year. Pertinent past medical history should include information about preexisting medical problems, recent surgeries, medications, allergies, and the name of the patient's personal physician. (3-3.26) (IEC pp. 408, 512)

61.

B. The definitive care phase of the patient care continuum includes the patient's admission to an appropriate receiving facility for surgical evaluation of traumatic injuries or management of an acute medical problem. (*)

62.

C. Manually stabilize the head and neck in a neutral position and apply the cervical collar. Then maintain cervical spine stabilization while logrolling the patient onto a long backboard. Strap the torso and legs securely to the board, then secure the patient's head and neck. Secure the backboard to the cot. Immobilizing in this order improves control over the spine and reduces extraneous movement. (3-3.15) (IEC pp. 760–766)

63.

B. Continued evaluation, including serial measurement of vital signs, will provide important information about a patient's condition. Vitals should be reassessed every 5 minutes in an unstable patient and every 15 minutes in a stable patient. During the ongoing assessment, you should also reassess the mental status, airway, ventilation, and circulatory status. Also, check all interventions and further assess any patient complaints. (3-3.42) (IEC pp. 525–528)

64.

B. Following an initial assessment, putting the patient in the ambulance is a priority based on the possibility of hypothermia. Since it is 2:00 A.M. and the patient is wet, the EMT-Intermediate must be alert to the likelihood of hypothermia and its potential effects on the patient. Removing the patient from the cold environment is a critical concern. (3-3.26) (IEC p. 1295)

65.

D. If the patient is groaning loudly, one must assume that the endotracheal tube has been misplaced in the esophagus. The vocal cords lie in the larynx and function to produce sound as passing air vibrates the cords. If an endotracheal tube is properly placed, air should not be vibrating the cords. In this case, one must deduce that the patient is able to produce sound because of the misplaced tube, so the tube placement must be checked immediately. (3-3.26, 3-3.31) (IEC pp. 385–386)

66.

D. This patient appears to be suffering from an open pneumothorax that is compromising ventilatory status and creating a hypoxic state. Therefore, your primary concern involves correcting this poor oxygenation state. An EMT-Intermediate should never open a chest wound to determine depth. Rather, the chest wound should be covered with an occlusive dressing to prevent the worsening of a pneumothorax. (3-3.31) (IEC pp. 505–507)

individual patient assessment/treatment process.(3-3.12) (IEC pp. 1015–1016)

67.

A. You would continue to ventilate at a rate of 12–20 per minute. (3-3.31) (IEC p. 393)

68.

A. Splinting this extremity would be the best way to control and prevent further hemorrhage. Splinting prevents the movement of sharp bone fragments that could lacerate other vessels and promulgate any bleeding. Also, the bones themselves contain vessels that must be stabilized so as to allow proper clotting mechanisms to take effect. The administration of oxygen is always indicated but does little for direct hemorrhage control. (3-3.31) (IEC pp. 657–658)

69.

C. A minineurological examination utilizing the mnemonic AVPU is a simple, objective way of quickly determining and conveying a patient's mental status. A = **A**lert, responds appropriately; V = responds to **V**erbal stimuli; P = responds to **P**ainful stimuli; and U = **U**nresponsive. (3-3.12) (IEC pp. 493–494)

70.

C. The Glasgow Coma Scale is a useful scoring system that can assist with monitoring neurologic status. Repeated values of the GCS can provide trends in mental status over a period of time. The parameters used for evaluation include eye, verbal, and motor response, not sensory. A number should not dictate the interventions an EMT-Intermediate must provide. Patient care is based on

---

71.

B. Any time the EMT-Intermediate immobilizes an individual to a long board, the straps must be secured in the order of torso first and head last. Straps are secured in this order to avoid further manipulation of the cervical spine as might happen if the head was secured initially and the torso moved during strapping. It is easiest to secure the legs after the torso. (*) (IEC pp. 760–766)

72.

C. Complete, accurate, and thorough documentation written at the time of patient refusal is always your best protection. "If it wasn't written down, it wasn't done" applies to every aspect of EMS from ambulance checklists to patient assessment and refusals. It is often hard to prove that verbal discussions took place, and the present testimony of your partner may not accurately reflect the events that took place some time ago. Also, a standard refusal form without a written narrative is incomplete in that there is nothing to prove that any assessment was ever completed. (*) (IEC pp. 576–577)

73.

B. Your safety should be the first consideration. You should never enter a building that is not safe. When dealing with gas fumes or leaks, you should park your ambulance on the same level or above and upwind from the hazardous material site. Hazardous materials experts will need to deal with the toxic substance and will be responsible for extricating the patients from the building. (3-3.5) (IEC pp. 484–486)

74.

C. You should keep your ambulance at a safe distance until the scene is safe. An injured EMT-Intermediate cannot render aid to the patient. Explain the situation to your dispatcher and have him or her notify the police for assistance. Take cover from the person with the weapon. (3-3.5) (IEC p. 485)

75.

B. A multi-system unresponsive trauma patient requires immediate transport; however, an initial assessment and rapid trauma assessment must be performed to identify and manage life threats. Once these are complete, consideration may be given to rendezvous with the paramedic unit if it is not on scene. (3-3.9) (IEC pp. 500–501)

76.

C. Since the vocal cords are responsible for the production of sound and the larynx contains the vocal cords, an injury to this structure could cause voice and airway dysfunction. Sounds could still be produced with injuries to the other structures listed. (3-3.7) (IEC pp. 145, 202–203)

77.

B. Edema from any cause to the oropharynx is critical. The oropharynx serves to conduct air from both the nose and the mouth into the larynx. An occlusion at any level of the upper airway may compromise ventilation and oxygenation. (3-3.31) (IEC pp. 689–690)

78.

C. The jaw thrust is the appropriate airway maneuver for the trauma patient because it allows neutral alignment of the cervical spine. The head tilt/chin lift requires hyperextension of the head, which is inappropriate for the trauma patient; a finger sweep and an attempt to ventilate, in that order, are appropriate. (3-3.14) (IEC pp. 368–369)

79.

C. When using a pocket mask, both hands can be utilized to maintain proper head tilt and a tight seal to the face while blowing through the protruding tube with your mouth. The bag-valve-mask requires one hand on the bag and the other on the mask, thus making it difficult to maintain a mask seal. Utilizing a second person would improve the dilemma but was not an option in this scenario. Inserting an oropharyngeal airway serves only to secure the tongue and does nothing for the seal. Removal of the patient's dentures could worsen the situation by creating a void if the bag-valve-mask has difficulty fitting. Finally, taping the mask is inappropriate. (3-3.17) (IEC pp. 362–363)

80.

C. Minimal bag resistance and rapid emptying is associated with a mask leak. During normal ventilations, there should be moderate resistance. An airway obstruction creates significant resistance, and a bag-valve-mask would not function correctly with a hole in the bag. (3-3.17) (IEC p. 363)

81.

C. Abdominal distention can be a sign of too much pressure while ventilating, which causes air to be forced into the stomach. Abdominal distention can decrease the effectiveness of ventilations. Chest rise and fall, bilateral breath sounds, and decreased cyanosis are all signs of effective ventilation. (3-3.17) (IEC p. 363)

82.

B. The patient would present as pale, cool, and clammy because of the body's compensatory mechanisms. The body shunts blood to the core organs in an effort to preserve them. (3-3.20, 3-3.21) (IEC p. 497)

83.

D. Leave the tourniquet in place and transport. Because the tourniquet was applied 2 hours ago, the EMT-Intermediate can assume that clots and acid have accumulated in the stagnant circulation. Any loosening or removal of the tourniquet could dislodge such clots and send the acidic blood into the systemic circulation. (3-3.24) (IEC p. 788)

84.

C. Exposing the trauma patient is necessary to find life-threatening injuries. This should be limited only when the environment, bystanders, or the situation hinders exposure. Because of the weather, this patient should be exposed in the back of the ambulance. Make sure the patient is kept warm. (3-3.9) (IEC p. 1295)

85.

D. Priority would be given to the reassessment of the patient's distal pulse. When reassessing the patient, one must repeat the initial assessment, check vital signs, and conduct a focused assessment of the patient's complaint and a check of all interventions. (3-3.31) (IEC pp. 525–528, 772)

86.

D. Packaging includes all the actions necessary to prepare the patient for transportation. This includes emergency care procedures such as initiating airway control, ventilations, IVs, fracture stabilization, bandaging, and immobilization. (3-3.16) (IEC pp. 756–766, 780)

87.

D. All patients should be secured to the cot before transfer to the ambulance. Many of the transport devices today have only three straps to secure the patient to the device. Patients who are secured to a backboard must also be secured to the cot. (*)

88.

C. Family wishes should be considered; however, the patient's condition can dictate which facility is most appropriate. When a patient's condition deteriorates, such as in this scenario, he or she should be transported to the closest appropriate facility for stabilization. Once stable, the patient can always be transferred to another hospital if the family wishes. (3-3.24) (IEC p. 22)

89.

C. An assessment of the patient is necessary to identify and manage life threats and establish priorities of care. Transport decisions are made based on the assessment, but that is not the sole purpose of the assessment. Vital signs are only one component of the physical assessment and not its purpose. (3-3.11–3-3.24) (IEC p. 491)

90.

B. Biological agents or germ-infested materials are some of the environmental dangers that an EMT-Intermediate would most likely face at the scene of a medical emergency. (3-3.32) (IEC p. 484)

91.

B. Once you have ensured your safety, you have the responsibility to protect the patient from further injury using whatever protective equipment is necessary. (3-3.5) (IEC p. 486)

92.

D. Vital signs are a part of the secondary assessment or focused history and physical exam. The initial assessment includes AVPU, airway, breathing, and circulation. (3-3.12–3.22) (IEC p. 491)

93.

B. In laryngitis, the vocal cords become inflamed, but this does not impede airflow to the lungs. There can be both congenital and peripheral causes for decreased ventilation. Some of the peripheral causes include trauma, drowning, foreign bodies, burns, anaphylaxis, laryngospasm, hematomas, and bilateral vocal cord paralysis. Epiglottitis can lead to airway obstruction caused by laryngospasm. (3-3.26) (IEC pp. 495, 1222–1224)

94.

D. All the choices can affect oxygen concentrations in the blood. However, pulmonary embolism decreases a portion of pulmonary circulation because of a clot, reducing blood flow to the alveoli and available oxygen in the blood. (3-3.26) (IEC pp. 830–832)

95.

B. Gastric distention is an indicator of improper positioning of the head or overinflation of the lungs. If a patient is being ventilated adequately, which is every 5 seconds for an adult or every 3 seconds for the pediatric patient, the chest should rise and fall with each ventilation, skin color will improve, the heart rate will return to normal, and the pulse oximeter (SPO_2) reading will increase. Ventilations that are delivered too quickly will cause gastric distention. The adult ventilation should be delivered over a 1.5- to 2-second period and an infant and child over a 1- to 1.5-second period. (3-3.17) (IEC p. 367)

96.

B. Suction should be applied only while slowly removing the catheter. Suctioning can be accomplished by using either a rigid, tonsil-tip catheter only as far as one can visualize or using a flexible, soft suction catheter. Additionally, the soft suction catheter can be inserted into the endotracheal tube. Suction is usually set at greater than 120 mm Hg for oral suctioning or less than 120 mm Hg for endotracheal suction. (3-3.14) (IEC pp. 365–367)

97.

C. The AVPU scale is the acronym used for evaluating a patient's mental status in the initial assessment. AVPU stands for A—Alert, V—responds to **V**erbal stimuli, P—responds to **P**ainful stimuli, and U—Unresponsive. (3-3.12) (IEC p. 493)

98.

D. It is important to expose areas of the body that are pertinent to the patient's complaint or situation. In this instance, her leg should be exposed for evaluation and treatment but not as part of the initial assessment. This will be conducted as part of the focused history and physical exam.(3-3.11–3.24) (IEC p. 491)

99.

D. Proteinuria is related to the amount of protein excreted in the urine. This is checked by analyzing the urine and not the blood. (*) (IEC pp. 330–333)

100.

A. At the conclusion of your initial assessment, you should have ascertained that this patient is in need of immediate ventilatory support. Do not delay transport to initiate IV therapy or apply a cardiac monitor. These procedures can be done en route to the closest appropriate trauma facility. (3-3.17, 3-3.31) (IEC pp. 396–397)

101.

B. The primary concern for this trauma patient is airway management. While the other injuries may also be considered life threats, failure to establish and maintain an airway will doom any other resuscitative interventions. Therefore, suction the oral cavity and begin ventilation because of the high respiratory rate and poor tidal volume. (3-3.14, 3-3.31) (IEC pp. 494–497)

102.

A. Auscultation of breath sounds would be performed after application of the cervical collar and palpation of the head and chest. (3-3.31) (IEC pp. 503–509)

103.

C. Scene safety is a primary concern on any call. Failure to actively notice hazards places you, your partner, the patient, and bystanders at risk. On identification of a hazard, you must immediately notify the proper services to handle the emergency prior to entering the scene. In this instance, notifying the fire department is the best course of action to prevent possible injuries to yourself and others. (3-3.5) (IEC pp. 494–496)

104.

B. During patient extrication, care must be taken to minimize the chance of additional injury. This typically includes covering the patient with a protective medium while the fire department removes the body panels. It is also beneficial to have an EMT-Intermediate in the auto with the patient to explain what is going on since extrication can be a frightening experience. (3-3.5) (IEC p. 486)

105.

A. Of particular concern in an unresponsive patient is airway patency. Unresponsive patients are often unable to keep their airway open and clear of secretions. In unresponsive patients, the tongue may become displaced posteriorly from hypotonicity of the mandibular muscles and occlude the airway at the level of the oropharynx. The nasopharynx is superior to the oropharynx, while the laryngopharynx (also called the hypopharynx) is inferior to the oropharynx and contains the epiglottis.(3-3.14) (IEC p. 494)

106.

A. The oropharyngeal airway is an adjunct to establishing a patent airway. Manual maneuvers must be maintained to ensure the airway is open and clear. (3-3.14) (IEC pp. 495–496)

107.

B. A simple closed pneumothorax occurs when air enters the pleural space between the visceral and parietal pleura. This causes a loss of negative intrapleural pressure, causing the lung to partially collapse. (3-3.31) (IEC p. 805)

108.

C. Trying to maintain an adequate seal of the mask while performing mouth-to-mask ventilations is one of the most common causes of difficulty. To perform this skill effectively, the EMT-Intermediate should be positioned behind the patient with his or her thumbs along each side of the mask; using the palms to push downward helps ensure a good seal. The index, middle, and ring fingers should then be placed on the mandible to lift and displace the mandible anteriorly. (*)

109.

D. Positive pressure ventilation is indicated whenever there is inadequate tidal volume or inadequate rate. While the normal minute volume is a function of respiratory rate and depth, if the depth is inadequate, it does not matter what the rate is. While both a low SpO_2 reading and cyanosis indicate poor oxygenation, they do not directly reflect respiratory tidal volume or rate and would warrant further evaluation. (3-3.17) (IEC p. 496)

110.

A. The femoral artery, by nature of carrying a large amount of blood under high pressure, is responsible for the profuse and spurting hemorrhage. Veins bleed continuously with a steady flow. The tibial and iliac arteries are not located in the upper thigh. (3-3.31) (IEC p. 644)

111.

D. Paradoxical movement of the right thorax would be found during inspection. Inspection allows the EMT-Intermediate to identify external signs of trauma/illness. Auscultation is necessary to discern bilateral wheezing, hyperresonance is a function of percussion, and crepitus is found during palpation. (3-3.31) (IEC p. 507)

112.

A. Hypotension with bradycardia, differences in skin temperature and moisture, and a bounding pulse are characteristic of vasogenic shock secondary to spinal cord injury. The injury causes an interruption in the sympathetic nerve transmission; therefore, there is not a reflexive increase in the heart rate from the hypotension, and the interruption also results in compensatory changes above the level of injury and none below. Hypovolemic shock presents with hypotension, tachycardia, and diaphoresis. (3-3.31)

113.

B. Management of non–life-threatening injuries is completed while en route to the hospital. Any life-threatening injury should be managed during the initial assessment and rapid trauma assessment. (3-3.24) (IEC p. 500)

114.

A. After fully immobilizing a patient to a long backboard, the motor, sensory, and perfusion (MSP) status should be assessed in each extremity. (*) (IEC pp. 761–762)

115.

D. An open wound to the thorax is considered an immediate life-threatening injury that must be managed during the initial assessment or rapid trauma assessment. (3-3.31) (IEC pp. 505–507)

116.

C. The sequence is based on potential "threats to life." The airway is managed first, followed by breathing, then circulation. (3-3.14–3-3.22) (IEC p. 491)

117.

B. A cold home is not a hazard that you are concerned with because of your short on-scene exposure. However, the cold home could provide important scene size-up clues as to the potential for hypothermia. (3-3.3) (IEC pp. 484–486)

118.

B. Delay entry into a hostile scene until the arrival of law enforcement personnel. While an additional EMS unit may be needed, law enforcement is responsible for controlling a hostile scene. Numerous hazards can result in injury or death to the EMT-Intermediate. Think before taking a particular action and always assume the worst. Additional sources of hazards to the EMT-Intermediate include unstable surfaces, ice, and crowds. (3-3.5) (IEC pp. 484–486)

119.

C. Crowd control is primarily a law enforcement function. However, sometimes this may be provided by EMS until arrival of law enforcement. The use of EMT-Intermediates is acceptable only if enough resources are available. (3-3.5) (IEC pp. 484–486)

120.

D. The three common resources requested at emergency scenes include law enforcement, fire and rescue services, and electric utilities. The coroner's investigator may be frequently called, but he or she should not be needed to enter the scene or begin patient care. (3-3.10) (IEC pp. 484–486)

121.

C. All items are correctly paired. The best answer is the incomplete answer. Obstetrics refers to pregnancy or childbirth. Gynecology is anything having to do with the female reproductive system. (3-3.31) (IEC pp. 489–491, 581–1153)

122.

D. The first item to evaluate in the initial assessment is the general impression. During the general impression, you look for major life threats and determine the age and gender of the patient. (3-3.22) (IEC pp. 491–493)

123.

D. The purpose of the initial assessment is to quickly determine immediate life threats that may be present. Once discovered, these threats to life need to be managed immediately. (3-3.11–3-3.24) (IEC p. 491)

124.

C. The use of the jaw-thrust maneuver maintains the head in a neutral position while moving the jaw forward. This displaces the tongue off the posterior oropharynx and opens the airway. Because the head is maintained in a neutral position, it is the airway method of choice for a trauma patient with a suspected spinal injury. (3-3.14) (IEC pp. 368–369)

125.

B. The patient has a partial airway obstruction. He is moving enough air to produce a cough, so he should be encouraged to continue to cough. Watch the patient carefully for signs of inadequate breathing, such as a weak, ineffective cough; high-pitched wheezing during inhalation; increased difficulty in breathing; or the development of cyanosis. If any of these are present, treat this patient as if he had a complete airway obstruction. Deliver repeated abdominal thrusts until the patient loses consciousness or the obstruction is removed. If you are able to intubate, perform a laryngoscopy and remove the obstruction with the Magill forceps. (3-3.14) (IEC pp. 816–817)

126.

C. The jaw thrust is the only procedure listed that maintains the head in a neutral position. In the suspected spine-injured patient, the spine must not be flexed, extended, or moved laterally. (3-3.14) (IEC pp. 368–369)

127.

A. The earliest detectable change that occurs with diminished blood volume is an increased heart rate. Increased cardiac stroke volume is difficult to detect clinically. Peripheral vasoconstriction will occur causing the skin to become pale, cool, and clammy. (3-3.25) (IEC p. 427)

128.

D. If the radial pulse is absent because of poor perfusion, it is likely that the donsalis pedis and posterior tibial pulses would also be absent. The carotid and brachial arteries may still be perfused. It takes less blood pressure to perfuse the carotid, femoral, and brachial pulses as compared to a greater pressure to perfuse the posterior tibial and dorsalis pedis arteries. The apical pulse will be felt with any contraction of the heart. (3-3.25) (IEC pp. 427, 655)

129.

C. After tube placement, auscultate over the epigastric region and then over the right and left apex of the lungs. No gurgling sounds should be heard while auscultating over the stomach during ventilation. Note the equality of right and left breath sounds and watch for the chest to rise and fall. Air escaping from the nose and mouth is a sign of improper inflation or a leak in the cuff. The pulse oximeter is not used to check for proper tube placement because the reading may not be available in the patient and is delayed in many. (3-3.17) (IEC p. 390)

130.

C. The suction catheter must initially be inserted into the endotracheal tube without suction applied. Measuring from the lips, then to the ear, and then to the nipple line places the suction catheter at about the level of the carina. Suction is applied, and the catheter is removed with a twisting motion. Suction should not exceed 15 seconds. (3-3.14) (IEC pp. 366–367)

131.

D. The statement that best describes shock is inadequate delivery of oxygen to cells and inadequate elimination of CO_2 and other waste by-products. (*) (IEC p. 195)

132.

A. The unstable patient should be reassessed every 5 minutes. The stable patient should be reassessed every 15 minutes. (3-3.42) (IEC p. 525)

133.

B. Subcutaneous emphysema is a collection of air trapped under the skin. It is a sign of trauma to the airway, respiratory tract, lungs, or esophagus. Observe the patient closely for signs of a developing pneumothorax, tension pneumothorax, or hemothorax. A pericardial tamponade is a collection of fluid in the pericardium. A tension pneumothorax is a condition resulting from collection of air in the pleural space. A hematoma is a collection of blood under the skin. (3-3.31) (IEC p. 505)

134.

D. The revised trauma score evaluates the respiratory rate, systolic blood pressure, and Glasgow Coma Scale score. The respiratory rate and systolic blood pressure are assigned a numerical value based on preestablished criteria. The Glasgow Coma Scale is performed and assigned a point value based on a fixed scale. These two values are then added together to determine the patient's total trauma score. The trauma score is valuable to receiving hospitals for categorization and reassessment purposes. (3-3.31) (IEC p. 747)

135.

C. Determining the patient's father's medical history is not considered a necessity during initial history taking. A SAMPLE history should be obtained and includes S = **S**igns and symptoms, A = **A**llergies, M = **M**edications, P = **P**ast medical history, L = **L**ast oral intake, and E = **E**vents prior to

illness. Radiation of pain is an important component of the history of the present illness. (*) (IEC pp. 510, 745–746)

136.

A. HIV testing is not a routine reason for the prehospital collection of blood samples. Blood glucose, CBC, and type and cross-match are common lab tests performed. (*)

137.

A. The ongoing assessment is performed to detect changes in patient condition, assess additional patient complaints, and evaluate the treatment provided. The reassessment of patients should be performed every 5 minutes in the unstable patient and every 15 minutes in the stable patient. An ongoing assessment must be performed on a routine basis on all patients regardless of time or patient condition. (3-3.42) (IEC p. 525)

138.

C. The most important factor to determine the destination medical facility depends primarily on which facility is best able to manage the patient. The transport of patients to specialized care centers will improve patient outcomes. Thus, the patient condition is a primary consideration. For the stable patient, the decision should be a joint determination reached between the patient and the EMT-Intermediate. (3-3.24) (IEC pp. 22–23)

139.

B. Patient care is frequently compromised when using the lights and siren. Additional stress is placed on the patient, the EMT-Intermediate, and the driver. Higher accident rates are associated with the use of lights and siren, not lower rates. Drive professionally and use lights and siren only when necessary. (*)

140.

C. Question the order by "echoing" the orders back to the medical direction physician. Medical direction may have misunderstood your description of the patient condition or history. Echoing the orders allows the physician to hear and correct a potentially inappropriate order. (*)

141.

A. During the ongoing assessment, the initial assessment of mental status, airway, breathing, and circulation is always repeated. The vital signs are also reassessed, and a focused physical exam is performed if there are additional complaints. (3-3.41) (IEC p. 525)

142.

A. The process of ensuring scene safety begins well before you arrive on the scene. Dispatch information may alert you to many hazards, such as fallen wires, chemical hazards, potentially harmful diseases, and violent settings. (3-3.3) (IEC pp. 735–736)

143.

A. It is best to stage your vehicle and not approach the vehicle to avoid scene hazards. Wait for personnel that are specially trained to manage downed wires. Never attempt to remove any wires unless you have been specially trained. (3-3.5) (IEC pp. 484–486)

144.

C. If for any reason the scene turns hazardous, immediately remove yourself from the scene and return only when you are sure that it is safe. Always protect yourself and your partner first. Usually you cannot reason with a hostile crowd. Furthermore, asserting authority on a hostile scene will usually only exacerbate the situation. (3-3.5) (IEC pp. 484–485)

145.

D. There will be little time to go back to the vehicle for protective gear. You should have eye protection and gloves on before you exit your vehicle. An exposure can happen quickly. If you wait until you are at the patient's side before you have body substance isolation (BSI), the public may perceive this as not being prepared or not wanting to touch the patient. In addition, it delays patient care. (*) (IEC pp. 482–483)

146.

C. You accomplish two objectives by having the onlookers hold the unfolded sheet. You protect the patient's dignity while giving the bystanders a task to do. (*)

147.

B. If you determine that the number of patients exceeds your available resources, first get more help on the way by implementing the multiple-casualty plan. The number of critically injured is not as important as requesting additional resources. Quickly treating life threats will come in the triage phase of the multiple-casualty incident plan. Finally, making patient contact prior to calling for additional resources will cause you to become focused on the patient's needs and not the needs of the entire situation. (3-3.10) (IEC pp. 481, 488–489)

148.

A. If you are not trained for this special situation, you should immediately call for a specially trained swift-water rescue team. You are taking an unnecessary risk by trying to rescue the patient without the proper training in swift-water rescue. The bystanders may be swept downriver and require rescuing. Even the strongest person cannot hold on to a rope for very long in a swift current. (3-3.10) (IEC pp. 484–486)

149.

C. Your first impression is based on several things. The dispatcher's information, scene size-up, and bystander's remarks should lead you to categorize this patient as medical. As you gather more information and complete an assessment, you may need to recategorize the patient. (3-3.6) (IEC p. 491)

150.

D. Stridor is associated with a life-threatening upper-airway obstruction and can be caused by a foreign body, severe swelling, or a metabolic process. Presence of fluids in the upper airway will present with gurgling sounds. Constriction of the bronchioles present with wheezing. (3-3.26, 3-3.31) (IEC p. 448)

151.

B. Direct laryngoscopy is the visualization of the vocal cords and glottic opening using a laryngoscope. The Magill forceps can be used for foreign body removal but only in conjunction with direct visualization. Back blows should not be performed on an adult. This may cause further obstruction of the airway. Finger sweeps are not performed in conjunction with the Magill forceps. The oropharyngeal airway may push the obstruction farther into the airway. (3-3.14) (IEC p. 378)

152.

C. If the patient begins to cough or gag, you must quickly remove the oropharyngeal airway, or the patient may vomit and aspirate. Turning the patient to the side will not prevent the patient from vomiting; however, this position may decrease the chance of aspiration. Be prepared to use suction but remove the airway first. Reassuring the patient will not reduce the gag reflex and stimulations that may cause vomiting and aspiration. (3-3.14) (IEC p. 372)

153.

C. Use only water-soluble lubricants with the airway. Petroleum products may cause further injury to the nasal mucosa and tissue, and damage the nasopharyngeal airway. Insert the airway with the bevel toward the septum, then straight back into the nasopharynx. The airway is measured from the tip of the nose to the tip of the earlobe. (3-3.14) (IEC p. 371)

154.

D. The jaw-thrust maneuver is used to open the airway in patients with suspected spine trauma. Sonorous sounds indicate that the tongue is partially occluding the airway. Thus, using the jaw thrust and an oropharyngeal airway, the airway should be opened adequately. This technique does not require hyperextension of the head to open the airway. The Sellick's maneuver describes the pressure applied to the cricoid cartilage to close off the esophagus and improve the view of the vocal cords during intubation. (3-3.14) (IEC pp. 368–369)

155.

A. The skin above the site of spine injury becomes pale, cool, and clammy, whereas the skin below the site becomes warm and dry. (*)

156.

C. The bag-valve-mask is more difficult to use than a pocket mask; therefore, one-person ventilation is achieved better with the pocket mask. Two EMTs are recommended to maintain a good mask seal and deliver a greater tidal volume. The pocket mask can deliver a greater tidal volume than the bag-valve-mask. Nearly 100% concentration of oxygen can be delivered by the bag-valve-mask when used with supplemental high-flow oxygen as well as a reservoir bag or tubing. (3-3.17) (IEC p. 363)

157.

D. A pop-off valve that continues to vent air may not allow sufficient volumes to be delivered. A heart rate that returns to normal is a sign of adequate ventilations. Good chest rise indicates an adequate tidal volume, which indicates adequate ventilation. Dry, warm, and pink skin are good indications of adequate ventilation. (3-3.17) (IEC p. 363)

158.

D. When sufficient oxygen is present (aerobic metabolism) and perfusion is adequate, pyruvic acid breaks down into carbon dioxide, water, and energy. This is known as the Kreb's cycle. The others may result from decreased perfusion and lead to cellular death, which may lead to death of the organism. (*)

159.

A. Coronary artery disease is the leading cause of cardiac arrest and sudden death (death that occurs within 1 hour of the onset of symptoms). The other answers are all causes of cardiac arrest; however, they do not occur more frequently than death from coronary artery disease. (*) (IEC p. 838)

160.

A. Delayed capillary refill is not a reliable indicator of inadequate perfusion in the adult patient. Environmental factors, gender, and medications can alter capillary refill in the adult. Capillary refill is a quick method to check peripheral perfusion in young children. Cool skin does not alone indicate poor perfusion. The pupil will dilate and respond sluggishly to light in poor perfusion states. (3-3.26, 3-3.31) (IEC p. 497)

161.

D. The next immediate action in this patient is to establish an airway followed by management of the inadequate ventilation status. A pulse will be assessed after establishing a patent airway and adequate ventilations. Vitals will be assessed after the initial assessment and during the rapid trauma assessment. (3-3.14, 3-3.17) (IEC pp. 494–496)

162.

D. To properly assess a trauma patient, you must completely expose the body. Non–life-threatening injuries are treated after the rapid trauma assessment is complete. (*)

163.

A. When the patient is in a cold environment, it may be dangerous to expose the patient until transfer to the ambulance. If a crowd is present, protect the dignity of the patient by covering him or her with a sheet. (*)

answers & rationales

164.

D. The most reliable indicator of a head injury is deteriorating mental status. (3-3.43) (IEC p. 525)

165.

A. Application of a cervical spinal immobilization collar is not done during the detailed physical exam. It is applied during the rapid trauma assessment. (3-3.36) (IEC pp. 519–524)

166.

B. Subcutaneous emphysema is air trapped under the skin. It is a good indicator of a significant chest injury. The air that is trapped may come from a leak in the trachea, bronchus, lungs, or esophagus. A flail segment may cause the paradoxical movement and is a serious chest injury. Suprasternal notch retraction is a serious sign that the patient is having a difficult time breathing and needs immediate management. (3-3.31) (IEC p. 507)

167.

B. The respiratory rate is not evaluated when using the Glasgow Coma Score. The GCS is a system used to monitor neurologic status. The trauma score incorporates the evaluation of the respiratory rate and effort in addition to perfusion status. (3-3.32) (IEC p. 1016)

168.

C. The primary concern at the scene is safety. An unstable vehicle should not be entered until it is made safe. (3-3.5) (IEC pp. 484–486)

169.

D. You should perform a focused assessment of the complaint. Oxygen or nitroglycerin will not relieve the pain. Performing a detailed physical exam is unnecessary. (3-3.40) (IEC p. 527)

170.

C. A Glasgow Coma Score of less than 9 indicates a significant neurologic deficit. A humerus fracture with no major bleeding is not a great concern. The frontal collision is a mechanism that needs to be correlated with clinical signs and symptoms to determine the priority status of a patient. (3-3.24) (IEC pp. 500, 1016)

171.

C. When you provide a complete report, care can be continued without interruption. Medical care consists of events that require consistency to enhance patient care. (*) (IEC pp. 548–549)

172.

A. Your written report will not prevent you from being sued in court; however, a well-written report is your best defense in a court of law. You should use a standardized format. All run reports do become a permanent part of the patient's medical record. Many physicians, nurses, and other health care providers rely on the run report to convey the complete picture of the event. (*) (IEC p. 561)

173.

B. Assessment and treatment priorities of the initial assessment, threats to the airway, breathing, and circulation are treated immediately on identification. It is necessary to take in-line spinal immobilization, clear the airway, and then manage the insufficient ventilating status. (3-3.14–3-3.17) (IEC p. 491)

174.

C. The patient is alert and talking; therefore, the airway is patent and the breathing adequate. Your next immediate action is to administer oxygen and assess circulation. (3-3.14–3-3.22) (IEC pp. 494–497)

175.

B. Managing the airway on an unresponsive patient may be challenging, especially if the gag reflex is still intact. If a manual technique fails in the patient, reposition the airway again before going to a mechanical airway. (3-3.14) (IEC p. 370)

176.

D. Scene safety is the first priority on any call. It takes precedence over all other assessments or interventions. (3-3.5) (IEC p. 484)

177.

D. The initial assessment is performed to identify and manage life threats to the airway, breathing, and circulation. Hypotension will be identified by a blood pressure, which is not taken until the rapid assessment or focused physical exam. (3-3.11–3-3.24) (IEC p. 491)

178.

C. During the process of immobilization, you must be careful to not aggravate any existing injuries. Once on the backboard, immobilize the torso of the body first and then head. Strapping in this order allows the rescuer to protect the head and neck from pivoting. (*) (IEC p. 765)

179.

A. In the responsive medical patient, the most reliable information is gained from the patient in the history. The physical exam is then guided by the complaint of the patient. Therefore, you obtain a SAMPLE history followed by a focused physical exam and then obtain a set of baseline vital signs. (*) (IEC pp. 511–513)

180.

B. The EMT-Intermediate should provide treatment based on his or her protocol given the patient's chief complaint. The wishes of others on-scene (physicians, family, bystanders, or partners) may be considered, but if it causes deviation from your protocol, you must first contact medical control to get approval. (*) (IEC pp. 532–534)

181.

C. During the management of a patient with a partially occluded airway, the EMT-Intermediate should progress in a systematic fashion, employing those techniques that are most likely to work first and the most quickly. As such, if the patient displays sonorous respirations, the EMT-Intermediate should first use manual airway techniques, followed by simple and then advanced mechanical techniques to open the airway. (3-3.14) (IEC p. 495)

182.

C. Adequate ventilations are best confirmed by equal breath sounds in all lung fields. Although the EMT-Intermediate should note diminishing cyanosis as the patient is oxygenated, this will take longer to become apparent. The absence of gastric sounds indicates only that the ET tube is not in the esophagus. Adequate ventilation should produce CO_2 that can be detected by an end-tidal CO_2 monitor. (3-3.14) (IEC p. 385)

183.

D. Whenever the body is not meeting the metabolic demands, shock (or hypoperfusion) will result. Obstructive shock results from a tension pneumothorax, pulmonary embolism, and pericardial tamponade. (3-3.26)

184.

D. A run report is the most important document you will complete following any emergency call. It can be used for quality improvement purposes, it can become a part of billing, it may be reviewed for legal concerns, and it is needed to ensure that appropriate treatment is rendered after delivering the patient to the emergency department. The prehospital care report becomes a part of the patient's permanent record. (*) (IEC p. 561)

185.

A. Generally, you should obtain a venous blood sample whenever an IV is initiated in the prehospital environment. You should always consider drawing blood on a patient suspected of being hypoglycemic, especially prior to the administration of 50% dextrose. A patient with an altered mental status and bizarre behavior may potentially be hypoglycemic. (*) (IEC pp. 330, 516)

186.

C. There is no best way around this situation. A car on fire is not a safe scene by any means. Until it is possible to attempt extrication, you need to offer some type of protection. Since trying to outfit the patient in turnout gear would be nearly impossible, attempt to cover him or her with some flame-retardant material, such as a blanket. (3-3.5) (IEC p. 486)

187.

A. A flail segment diminishes the bellows action of the chest. This does not allow that portion of the underlying lung to expand with the rest of the thorax. This diminishes the tidal volume and will result in hypoxemia and hypercapnia. A flail segment does not impact the airway or guarantee that a hemo- or pneumothorax is present. Diaphragm paralysis is not a result of fractured ribs. (3-3.31) (IEC p. 507)

188.

B. Realistically, the provision of cardiopulmonary resuscitation (CPR) is to prolong the viability of the patient until defibrillation and advanced life support providers can provide additional drug therapy and airway skills. CPR alone does not treat the underlying cause of arrest and rarely (if ever) restores normal cardiac activity. (*) (IEC p. 939)

189.

B. The purpose of the detailed physical exam is to identify and treat non–life-threatening injuries. Evisceration, open femur fracture, and the knife wound are all considered life-threatening injuries that should be detected and treated in the initial assessment phase. (3-3.36) (IEC p. 519)

190.

D. In the management of a patient with an active hemorrhage, the progression of management should be direct pressure, elevation, application of cold, pressure point, and tourniquet. (3-3.19) (IEC pp. 497, 646)

191.

C. After manual techniques have failed to remove a foreign body airway obstruction, the next best thing is to perform a laryngoscopy and retrieve the obstruction with Magill forceps. Initiating transport will do nothing for the airway obstruction, and waiting until the patient arrests only makes the situation worse. Finally, back blows are not recommended as appropriate treatment for adults. (3-3.14) (IEC p. 817)

192.

B. During intubation, it is important that you take appropriate BSI precautions to protect yourself from splashes or droplets. Since it is not uncommon for the patient to gag or cough during the skill, the bare minimum protection you would want is gloves for your hands, eye protection, and a mask for your mouth. A gown is usually not warranted unless there is a large amount of blood or other body fluids that may be splashed on you. (3-3.5) (IEC pp. 482–483)

193.

B. The appropriate term to use when removing a patient from their initial location is known as extrication. Since using appropriate terminology is imperative when interfacing with other health care providers and rescue personnel, you should use the correct term whenever possible. The other terms may be similar or understandable, but they still do not represent the most correct term. (*) (IEC p. 764)

194.

A. When a person is intubated, the vocal cords are spread by the endotracheal tube. This means that no air will pass over the cords during exhalation, and, as such, no sound can be produced. A face mask is irrelevant because one is not used once the patient is successfully intubated. Finally, PPV has no bearing on whether the vocal cords contract. (*)

195.

D. Your first priority at any scene is to establish scene safety. If the scene is not safe, you must either make it safe or retreat until another agency, such as law enforcement or the fire service, can make it safe for you. (3-3.1) (IEC p. 484)

196.

A. Your first priority is to determine that the scene is safe. If the scene is not safe, you should, if possible, make it safe or retreat until the scene becomes safe or the patient is brought to you. (3-3.1) (IEC p. 485)

197.

B. Body substance isolation is considered a priority in your scene size-up. A patient who is ill, has a fever, and is coughing up blood-tinged sputum may have tuberculosis or another respiratory illness. It is necessary to use gloves, eye protection, and a high-efficiency particulate air (HEPA) respirator to protect you from the potential transmission of the TB bacteria or other infectious material. (3-3.5) (IEC pp. 492–493)

198.

C. Even when the scene is very hectic and uncontrolled, it is necessary to always protect the patient's modesty. Once you have exposed the trauma patient and inspected for injuries, cover the patient with a sheet or blanket to protect him or her. This may be enough to drastically reduce the patient's anxiety. (*)

199.

B. During your scene size-up, you are also looking for personal hazards that may cause injury to you or your partner. When you note an extremely large patient whom you feel you and your partner cannot safely lift or move, you should immediately call for assistance. By calling for a backup during the scene size-up, you may reduce the time you are on the scene by having extra personnel available as soon as the patient is ready to be moved. (3-3.10) (IEC p. 481)

200.

C. In order to ensure that the breathing is adequate, you must assess both rate and tidal volume. In this scenario, the rate was assessed; however, the quality of breathing was not. The patient could be breathing 16 per minute with a minimal tidal volume in which the patient would need to be ventilated. A respiratory rate alone does not establish adequate or inadequate breathing. (3-3.17) (IEC p. 496)

201.

D. The cricoid cartilage is the circumferential ring that is compressed while performing cricoid pressure, also known as Sellick's maneuver. The cricoid ring is the big bulky cartilage immediately inferior (below) the thyroid cartilage (Adam's apple). Between the cricoid and thyroid cartilage is the cricothyroid membrane. (3-3.14) (IEC p. 369)

202.

C. Oropharyngeal or nasopharyngeal airways are considered airway adjuncts. Even with either of these airways in place, you must still maintain a manual maneuver, such as a head tilt/chin lift or jaw thrust. (3-3.14) (IEC pp. 468–474)

203.

B. According to your priority of care, you should establish in-line spinal stabilization, suction the airway, and begin bag-valve-mask ventilation. The patient's breathing is shallow, indicating the need to ventilate. Once you have cleared the airway and begun ventilation, you then move on to check the pulse and skin. (3-3.14, 3-3.16, 3-3.17) (IEC p. 491)

204.

B. The major problems associated with a flail segment are the underlying lung injury (pulmonary contusion) and the hypoxia associated with it. You can easily correct the pressure disturbance caused by an ineffective bellow action of the chest by simply ventilating the patient. However, it is the disturbance in gas exchange and oxygenation at the alveolar level from tissue destruction and bleeding in the lung tissue that is not easily corrected. (3-3.31) (IEC p. 507)

205.

C. When suctioning the oropharynx of an adult patient, set the suction to exceed 120 mm Hg of pressure. When performing endotracheal suctioning, the pressure is set at 80–120 mm Hg. (3-3.14)

206.

B. If direct pressure fails to control the bleeding, your next method for bleeding control is pressure points. In this scenario, the brachial artery will be compressed to reduce the blood flow to the lower forearm while direct pressure is maintained. The tourniquet is a last resort if all other bleeding control measures fail. (3-3.19) (IEC pp. 646–647)

207.

C. Fracture management is done during the detailed physical exam. Fractures are not considered life-threatening injuries unless they are associated with major bleeding. One exception is a femur fracture because a patient can lose up to 2 liters of blood around each femur. (3-3.36) (IEC p. 524)

208.

C. Subcutaneous emphysema, or air trapped under the skin, is a sign of an air leak in the thorax or neck. Air may come from the trachea, bronchi, bronchioles, alveoli, or esophagus. (3-3.26, 3-3.31) (IEC pp. 505, 721)

209.

A. Medications are not considered part of the history of the present illness. The OPQRST mnemonic is used to gather information about the chief complaint. Medications are part of the SAMPLE history. (*) (IEC p. 512)

210.

B. You would perform bag-valve-mask ventilation because of the inadequate volume of respiration, immobilize the patient to the backboard because of suspicion of a spinal injury related to the mechanism of injury, and simply strap the humerus to the backboard as a method of immobilization. This patient is considered a priority patient. Taking the time to immobilize the humerus fracture at the scene is not appropriate unless it will not lengthen the scene time. The backboard will serve as a splint until further immobilization can be performed en route. (3-3.15, 3-3.17, 3-3.24) (IEC p. 491)

UNIT

4 Clinical Decision Making

unit objectives

Questions in this unit relate to DOT Objectives 3-4.1 to 3-4.8. The objectives are listed in the Appendix.

DIRECTIONS
Each of the questions or incomplete statements below is followed by suggested answers or completions. Select the **one answer** that is best in each case.

1. Another word that describes your patient's severity is
   A. nulliparity.
   B. acuity.
   C. tonicity.
   D. accommodation.

2. Which patient acuity level poses the greatest challenge to the EMT-Intermediate?
   A. obvious critical life threat
   B. potential life threat
   C. non–life threatening
   D. none of the above

3. A schematic flowchart that outlines patient care procedures is known as a(n)
   A. protocol.
   B. standing order.
   C. algorithm.
   D. advance directive.

4. You are authorized to administer an albuterol treatment to patients with diffuse wheezing. This is an example of a(n)
   A. protocol.
   B. algorithm.
   C. mandate.
   D. standing order.

5. The major disadvantage to using protocols is that they
   A. apply only to atypical patients.
   B. apply only to patients with vague presentations.
   C. do not allow the EMT-Intermediate the flexibility to adapt to an atypical patient with an unusual presentation.
   D. all of the above

6. The style that requires you to focus on the most important aspect of a critical situation is known as
   A. anticipatory.
   B. reflective.
   C. divergent.
   D. convergent.

7. The style that requires you to respond instinctively to a situation rather than thinking about it is known as
   A. impulsive.
   B. reflective.
   C. divergent.
   D. anticipatory.

8. To raise your skill level to the pseudoinstinctive level means to be able to
   A. describe each step in detail.
   B. do it without thinking about it.
   C. consider all the possibilities before attempting a skill.
   D. perform the skill while blocking out all other thoughts.

9. Place the following steps of the decision-making process in chronological order:
   A. maintain control
   B. stop and think
   C. reevaluate
   D. scan the situation
   E. decide and act

10. Which of the following is **not** a part of the critical decision process?
   A. forming a concept
   B. evaluating
   C. reflecting
   D. researching

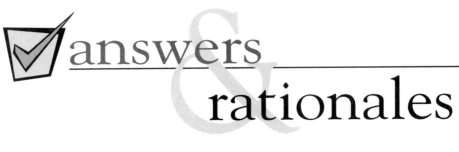

answers & rationales

Following each rationale, you will find a reference to the corresponding objective in the DOT National Standard EMT-Intermediate curriculum. An asterisk denotes material that is supplemental to the DOT curriculum. Page numbers after a rationale indicate where the question topic may be discussed in the Brady text *Intermediate Emergency Care* (Bledsoe, Porter, Cherry).

1.

B. Acuity is a term that describes the severity or acuteness of your patient's condition. There are three general classes of patient acuity: obvious critical life threats, potential life threats, and non–life-threatening presentations. (3-4.2) (IEC p. 532)

2.

B. Patients who fall between minor and life threatening on the acuity scale pose the greatest challenge to the EMT-Intermediate because, while stable, they may become unstable at any time. These patients require extreme vigilance and ongoing assessments. (3-4.2) (IEC p. 532)

3.

C. An algorithm is a schematic outline of patient care procedures for specific signs and symptoms. An example is the algorithm recommended by the American Heart Association for managing a patient in recurrent ventricular fibrillation. (3-4.3) (IEC pp. 532–533)

4.

D. Standing orders are treatments you can perform before contacting the medical direction physician for permission. (3-4.3) (IEC p. 532)

5.

C. Protocols are standard guidelines for managing certain patient conditions. Unfortunately, they address only typical patients with classic presentations and rarely allow the EMT-Intermediate to adapt to the atypical patient with an unusual presentation or with multiple symptoms. (3-4.3) (IEC p. 532)

6.

D. The convergent approach to decision making requires you to focus on the most important aspect of your patient's situation and not be distracted by other stimuli. (3-4.4) (IEC p. 536)

7.

A. There is a time to think and a time to act. When confronted with a patient with a sucking chest wound, an uncontrollable hemorrhage, or a complete airway obstruction, EMT-Intermediates need to react impulsively and fix the situation (seal the wound, stop the bleeding, perform the Heimlich). (3-4.4) (IEC p. 536)

8.

B. As an EMT-Intermediate, you must raise your technical skill level to the pseudoinstinctive level. This means that you have developed such muscle memory that you can perform the skill while you think about something else, such as managing the scene and carrying out the treatment plan. You should be able to start an IV the same way you tie your shoes—without thinking about each step. (3-4.5) (IEC p. 537)

9.

D, B, E, A, C. First, scan the situation (take a look around), stop and think (don't just jump in), decide and act (do something; even a bad plan is better than no plan), maintain control (control yourself first, then others), and finally reevaluate (if things are going badly, change your plan). (3-4.8) (IEC pp. 537–538)

10.

D. The critical decision process includes forming a concept (field diagnosis), interpreting the data (patient assessment), applying the principles (treatment plan), evaluating (ongoing assessment), and reflecting (postcall critique). (3-4.8) (IEC pp. 538–540)

5 Communications

unit objectives

Questions in this unit relate to DOT Objectives 3-5.1 to 3-5.25. The objectives are listed in the Appendix.

DIRECTIONS
Each of the questions or incomplete statements below is followed by suggested answers or completions. Select the **one answer** that is best in each case.

1. Responsibilities of the emergency medical dispatcher include all of the following **except**
   A. acting as the initial contact with the public.
   B. allocating the appropriate resources for the emergency response.
   C. diagnosing the medical problem of the patient.
   D. alerting EMS personnel and directing them to the scene.

2. In order to ensure that radio transmission is clear, all of the following guidelines should be followed **except**
   A. press the transmit button for 1 second before speaking.
   B. speak slowly and clearly into or across a microphone that is at close range.
   C. speak in a normal pitch and know what information you are going to relay before transmitting.
   D. communicate to the hospital using codes when possible.

3. A device that receives a transmission from a low-power source on one frequency and retransmits it at a higher power on another frequency is a(n)
   A. mobile transmitter.
   B. repeater.
   C. encoder.
   D. decoder.

4. A group of radio frequencies that are close together is called a
   A. band.
   B. spectrum.

C. multiplex.
D. UHF configuration.

5. Which of the following radio bands is best suited for cities?
   A. VHF lo
   B. VHF hi
   C. UHF
   D. AM

6. Which of the following radio bands is best suited for large rural areas?
   A. VHF lo
   B. VHF hi
   C. UHF
   D. FM

7. Of the following, which is the **least** important for the EMS dispatcher to get at the time of the call?
   A. the location of the call
   B. the closest cross street to the call
   C. the callback number
   D. the nature of the call

8. Which of the following is **not** a feature of an enhanced 911 system?
   A. caller telephone number
   B. caller location
   C. instant callback
   D. best route of travel

9. A typical EMS event is said to consist of several components. These can include event detection and notification of EMS, response of EMS, treatment, transport, and delivery to the hospital. All of these components are linked by
    A. medical direction.
    B. medical protocols.
    C. medical personnel.
    D. communications.

10. Which of the following is a component of a priority dispatch system?
    A. medically approved caller interrogation
    B. predetermined response configurations
    C. prearrival instructions
    D. all of the above

11. At a minimum, which one of the following must be obtained by the EMS call taker prior to dispatching the ambulance?
    A. phone number from which the caller is calling
    B. existing hazards on the scene
    C. patient's level of consciousness
    D. age of the patient

12. In which type of communications system do transmission and reception occur on the same frequency?
    A. simplex
    B. duplex
    C. multiplex
    D. biotelemetry

13. In which type of communications system can transmission and reception occur simultaneously?
    A. simplex
    B. duplex
    C. multiplex
    D. biotelemetry

14. All of the following are proper radio transmission techniques **except**
    A. use codes whenever possible.
    B. press the button for 1 second before talking.
    C. speak slowly and clearly and avoid difficult words.
    D. use the "echo" system when receiving directions.

15. In which type of communications system can biotelemetry information be transmitted during conversation on the same frequency?
    A. simplex
    B. duplex
    C. multiplex
    D. biotelemetry

16. All of the following are acceptable and pertinent information to relay to a receiving hospital by radio **except**
    A. patient's name.
    B. patient's age.
    C. patient's complaint.
    D. patient's weight.

17. Trunking is a communications term that describes
    A. computerized frequency allocation.
    B. hardwiring for ambulance radios.
    C. base station radio procedures.
    D. multiple-antenna installation.

18. The **first** link in the EMS communication chain is
    A. communication between the EMT-Intermediate and medical control.
    B. completion of a written report.
    C. dispatch of EMS unit.
    D. notification of EMS dispatch.

19. Which of the following statements is true regarding digital technology?
    A. It is much faster and more accurate than analog.
    B. It causes frequency overcrowding.
    C. Digital communications are monitored by scanners.
    D. none of the above

20. Which of the following is an advantage of using cellular communications?
    A. Twelve-lead EKGs can be transmitted.
    B. Fax and computer messages can be transmitted.
    C. Dedicated EMT-Intermediate lines can be established.
    D. all of the above

21. Place the following information into the proper order for a radio report for a medical patient:
    A. SAMPLE
    B. ETA
    C. unit and provider ID
    D. patient age, sex, weight
    E. treatment prior to calling
    F. OPQRST
    G. scene description
    H. chief complaint
    I. request for orders
    J. physical exam

22. The echo procedure refers to
    A. repeating a transmission for clarification.
    B. writing down the address as dispatched.
    C. using the siren as you pass underneath a bridge.
    D. pushing the microphone button and waiting for a few seconds before speaking.

23. All of the following statements about the written EMS run report are true **except**
    A. the documentation allows for personal opinions about the patient.
    B. it provides a record of the patient's initial condition and care.
    C. it documents a patient's refusal of care and transport.
    D. it becomes a legal record of the prehospital care.

24. The government agency that regulates all radio communications is the
    A. Department of Transportation.
    B. Department of Communications.
    C. Federal Communications Commission.
    D. National Association of Broadcasting.

25. The Federal Communications Commission controls and regulates radio communications through the allocation of frequencies and
    A. establishing technical standards for radio equipment.
    B. licensing every EMS provider who communicates by radio.
    C. reviewing patient care reports for completeness and accuracy.
    D. conducting training programs for radio repair personnel.

26. Which one of the following responsibilities related to prehospital radio use does **not** belong to the Federal Communications Commission?
    A. assigns radio frequencies
    B. requires the use of special codes for EMS communication
    C. monitors frequencies for appropriate use
    D. grants site licenses for EMS base station transmitters

27. During a radio report to the hospital, you tell the receiving physician that you have defibrillated the patient at 200 joules and 300 joules. This information is useful to him for

    A. proper billing purposes.
    B. ensuring that the patient is receiving optimal care.
    C. allowing him or her the opportunity to adequately prepare for your arrival.
    D. all of the above

28. Which of the following is **not** an example of one of the phases of communication in an EMS event?

    A. You contact your backup crew to advise them of the situation and what equipment to bring into the scene.
    B. The crew is paged and notified of the nature and location of the call.
    C. The dispatcher contacts the police to respond to the scene.
    D. The EMT-Intermediate at the scene notifies the family of the patient of the seriousness of the illness.

29. The first person who can assist the patient is the

    A. EMT-Intermediate.
    B. First Responder.
    C. Emergency Medical Dispatcher.
    D. EMT-Intermediate.

30. The written EMS report following a call should

    A. be discarded because of patient confidentiality issues.
    B. be filed with the hospital emergency department to ensure a continuum of care.
    C. not be used for billing purposes.
    D. not be used for collection of data because of the differences in patient care reporting among EMS personnel.

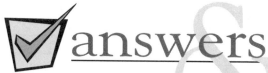

answers & rationales

Following each rationale, you will find a reference to the corresponding objective in the DOT National Standard EMT-Intermediate curriculum. An asterisk denotes material that is supplemental to the DOT curriculum. Page numbers after a rationale indicate where the question topic may be discussed in the Brady text *Intermediate Emergency Care* (Bledsoe, Porter, Cherry).

1.

C. Although some EMS systems have the knowledge and capacity to provide medically approved prearrival instructions, the emergency medical dispatcher is not capable of diagnosing a patient's medical problem. Emergency medical dispatch is the nerve center of the EMS system. The emergency medical dispatcher is the initial—and perhaps the only—contact with the public. The emergency medical dispatcher must be knowledgeable about all resources available in the system and how to access them. (3-5.18) (IEC p. 547)

2.

D. When communicating medical information to the hospital, codes can be confusing unless understood by everyone. Using plain English is the best way to reduce the likelihood of misinterpreted information. (3-5.22) (IEC p. 543)

3.

B. A repeater is a device that receives a transmission from a low-power portable or a mobile radio on one frequency and retransmits it at a higher power on another frequency. Repeaters are important in large geographical areas because portable and mobile radios may not have enough range to communicate with each other, with medical control, or with the dispatcher. (*) (IEC p. 544)

4.

A. A group of radio frequencies that are close together on the electromagnetic spectrum is called a band. Some examples of radio bands are AM, FM, citizen band, shortwave, UHF, and VHF. (*) (IEC p. 544)

5.

C. Ultrahigh frequency (UHF; 300–3000 MHz) penetrates concrete and steel well and is less susceptible to interference, making it an excellent radio band for cities. (*) (IEC p. 544)

6.

A. Very high frequency (VHF) lo (150–170 MHz) follows the curvature of the earth and is best suited for large areas with varied geographical terrain. (*) (IEC p. 544)

7.

B. While all the mentioned bits of information are important, the cross streets for the call, while helpful, are not absolutely necessary. It is vital that the dispatcher have the location, nature, and callback number prior to dispatching the ambulance and any other necessary resources (police, fire, etc.). Ultimately, it is the EMT-Intermediate's responsibility to be familiar with the territory he or she responds to. (3-5.19) (IEC p. 547)

8.

D. With an enhanced 911 system, you receive the caller's location and telephone number and instant callback capability. (*) (IEC p. 546)

9.

D. Communications play a vital role in linking the typical components of an EMS event. Medical direction aids in the connection of transport and delivery but does not apply to notification by the layperson. The same can be said of medical personnel in that they are not required to link occurrence and actual detection. Finally, medical protocols are specific to patient care and cannot be said to link all of the components. (3-5.1) (IEC p. 546)

10.

D. A priority dispatch system includes medically approved caller interrogation, predetermined response configurations, and prearrival instructions. This system, developed by Dr. Jeff Clawson for the Salt Lake City Fire Department, is used throughout the country. (3-5.21) (IEC p. 547)

11.

A. One of the items that must be obtained by the EMS call taker prior to dispatching the initial ambulance is the callback number so that they can be recontacted should they be disconnected. Other items that must be obtained include the location and the nature of the event. The remaining answers provide information about the patient that is useful after the ambulance is already en route. (3-5.19) (IEC p. 546)

12.

A. In a simplex system, transmission and reception cannot occur at the same time because both occur on the same frequency. A person must transmit a message, release the button, and wait for a response. (3-5.15) (IEC p. 550)

13.

B. In a duplex system, two frequencies are used much like telephone communications. This means that transmission and reception can occur at the same time. (3-5.15) (IEC p. 551)

14.

A. Codes can be difficult to use in medical communications. If privacy is necessary, use the phone. Never use the patient's name over the radio. Pressing the button for 1 second before speaking will permit the repeater to function. Speaking slowly and clearly reduces confusion. By immediately repeating the directions, accurate confirmation will be accomplished. (*) (IEC p. 555)

15.

C. In a multiplex system, radio communications and other data, such as EKG, can be transmitted simultaneously, using multiple frequencies. (3-5.15) (IEC p. 551)

16.

A. Transmitting the patient's name over the radio may cause a breach in patient confidentiality by permitting the name to be picked up on scanners and other radios. (3-5.22) (IEC p. 555)

17.

A. In a trunked system, all frequencies are pooled. A computer routes a radio transmission to the first available frequency. All subsequent transmissions are routed in the same manner. This eliminates the need to search for unused frequencies. (3-5.15) (IEC p. 551)

18.

D. This is the first of the five communication "phases" of a typical EMS event: (1) notification from the caller by 911 to EMS dispatch, (2) notification of appropriate EMS unit, (3) communications between EMT-Intermediate and medical control, (4) direct face-to-face communications with emergency department personnel, and (5) notification of dispatch that the unit is back in service. (3-5.24) (IEC p. 546)

19.

A. Digital technology is the wave of the present and is here to stay. It translates sound into

digital code for transmission. It is much faster, more accurate, and more secure than analog communications. You cannot monitor digital transmissions without a decoder, and this technology eases the overcrowding of emergency frequencies. (*) (IEC p. 552)

20.

D. Many EMS systems are using cellular communications. Advantages include the ability to transmit 12-lead EKGs as well as fax and computer messages and the ability to establish dedicated EMT-Intermediate lines into the base station hospital. (*) (IEC p. 552)

21.

C, G, D, H, F, A, J, E, I, B. (3-5.23) (IEC p. 554)

22.

A. The echo procedure refers to repeating back a transmission for clarification. It is a major component of the feedback loop and essential in emergency communications. The best example is verifying a medication order with the physician prior to administering it. (3-5.25) (IEC p. 555)

23.

A. The written EMS report is not the place to describe personal opinions of any kind. This includes disagreements related to treatments provided or not provided. Issues related to disagreements of a personal opinion should be expressed through an internal communication device such as an "Incident Report." (3-5.8) (IEC p. 545)

24.

C. The Federal Communications Commission is the government agency responsible for assigning frequencies, regulating all radios, and controlling all radio communications in the United States. (3-5.17) (IEC p. 557)

25.

A. The Federal Communications Commission controls and regulates radio communications through allocating frequencies and establishing technical standards for radio equipment. (3-5.17) (IEC p. 557)

26.

B. The Federal Communications Commission has numerous responsibilities regarding radio frequencies used by EMS personnel. They do not, however, require that a particular set of codes or signals be used. That decision is left up to the local EMS provider. (3-5.17) (IEC p. 557)

27.

C. The primary reason the physician would want that information is so that he can prepare to assume treatment on your arrival. That information may also be useful for ensuring proper care delivery, but that is more the role of the Quality Improvement Committee and not the physician directly.

Billing comes after the trip is completed. (3-5.15) (IEC p. 545)

28.

D. Notifying the family of the seriousness of the illness is not a link in EMS communication. Communication with dispatch, other crews, other public safety services, and the receiving hospital are all appropriate links in an EMS event. (3-5.3) (IEC p. 546)

29.

C. The emergency medical dispatcher is the first person to offer any type of emergency care for the patient prior to the arrival of any first responder or EMS unit. (*) (IEC p. 547)

30.

B. A copy of the EMS report must be filed with the hospital to ensure a proper continuum of care. The report is also used in billing and for other administrative reasons. The data collected from the EMS report is used in medical audits and is a major component in quality assurance and continuous quality improvement programs. (3-5.9) (IEC p. 545)

UNIT

6 Documentation

unit objectives

Questions in this unit relate to DOT Objectives 3-6.1 to 3-6.23. The objectives are listed in the Appendix.

DIRECTIONS
Each of the questions or incomplete statements below is followed by suggested answers or completions. Select the **one answer** that is best in each case.

1. The prehospital care report is likely to be reviewed by which of the following?
   A. surgical team
   B. insurance providers
   C. emergency department staff
   D. all of the above

2. Which of the following is **not** a time commonly recorded on the PCR?
   A. call received
   B. unit alerted
   C. arrival at patient side
   D. departure from scene

3. When is the ideal time to complete your PCR?
   A. en route to the hospital
   B. immediately after the call
   C. at the station
   D. at the end of the shift

4. If you misspell a word or check the wrong box on your PCR, you should
   A. scribble the correction over the mistake.
   B. draw one line through it and initial.
   C. blacken out the entire mistake.
   D. place parentheses around the mistake.

5. If you detect an error after you have submitted your PCR to the hospital, you should
   A. write an addendum.
   B. call the hospital and have the clerk make the correction.

C. do nothing.
D. none of the above

6. Which of the following statements could place you in danger of being sued for libel?
   A. "The patient smelled of alcohol."
   B. "The patient walked with a staggering gait."
   C. "The patient used abusive language."
   D. "The patient was an obnoxious drunk."

7. Which of the following is included in the subjective narrative?
   A. history of present illness
   B. vital signs
   C. HEENT exam
   D. labs and ECG

8. SOAP stands for
   A. **S**cene—**O**bjective—**A**ssessment—**P**ostcall.
   B. **S**ubjective—**O**bjective—**A**ssessment—**P**lan.
   C. **S**ystems—**O**bservation—**A**nterior—**P**osterior.
   D. **S**tatus—**O**ngoing—**A**rrival—**P**ast history.

9. In general, a patient who refuses your care demonstrates mental competence by
   A. understanding the circumstances.
   B. understanding the risks associated with refusing care.
   C. accepting the risks and responsibility.
   D. all of the above

10. If you are canceled as you arrive on an emergency call, you should
   A. return to the station or post.
   B. document "canceled en route" on your PCR.
   C. document the canceling authority.
   D. get the patient's name and vital signs.

Provide the abbreviation for each of the following medical terms (items 11–75):

11. coronary artery bypass graft _____
12. atherosclerotic heart disease _____
13. against medical advice _____
14. blood sugar _____
15. body surface area _____
16. bag-valve-mask _____
17. birth control pills _____
18. cubic centimeter _____
19. chief complaint _____
20. centimeter _____
21. congestive heart failure _____
22. complains of _____
23. carbon monoxide _____
24. carbon dioxide _____
25. chronic obstructive pulmonary disease _____
26. chest pain _____
27. cerebrospinal fluid _____
28. carotid sinus massage _____
29. cerebrovascular accident _____
30. discontinue _____
31. dyspnea on exertion _____
32. deep-vein thrombosis _____
33. estimated date of confinement _____
34. alcohol (ethanol) _____
35. occasional _____
36. fracture _____
37. gastrointestinal _____

38. gunshot wound _____
39. hour _____
40. headache _____
41. history _____
42. intramuscular _____
43. intraosseous _____
44. jugular venous distention _____
45. potassium _____
46. kilogram _____
47. keep vein open _____
48. deciliter _____
49. laceration _____
50. lactated Ringer's _____
51. moves all extremities well _____
52. microgram _____
53. milliequivalent _____
54. milligram _____
55. milliliter _____
56. morphine sulfate _____
57. sodium _____
58. sodium chloride _____
59. no known allergies _____
60. nitroglycerin _____
61. nausea/vomiting _____
62. organic brain syndrome _____
63. penicillin _____
64. hydrogen ion concentration _____
65. pelvic inflammatory disease _____
66. as needed _____
67. patient _____
68. every _____
69. rule out _____
70. range of motion _____
71. positive end-expiratory pressure _____
72. signs/symptoms _____
73. subcutaneous _____
74. sublingual _____
75. within normal limits _____

76. You are treating a patient who has a history of hepatitis. This patient is suffering from
    A. disease of the hepatic duct.
    B. inflammation of the liver.
    C. disease of the kidneys.
    D. inflammation of the kidneys.

77. In reference to the lower extremity, the knee lies _____ to the ankle.
    A. medial
    B. lateral
    C. proximal
    D. distal

78. You are transporting a patient from a nursing home to the hospital. The patient's chart indicates that this patient has a history of RHD. RHD is the medical abbreviation for
    A. rheumatic heart disease.
    B. right-heart disease.
    C. right-hand deficit.
    D. regular history of diabetes.

79. You are online with the medical direction physician. She asks if the patient presents with circumoral cyanosis. She wants to know if the patient has
    A. bluish color to the fingernail beds.
    B. difficulty speaking.
    C. swelling of the face.
    D. blueness around the mouth.

80. You are dispatched to a local nursing home for an elderly patient who is having difficulty speaking. You would document this as
    A. dysphagia.
    B. dyspnea.
    C. dysphasia.
    D. polyphagia.

81. You are treating a patient who has a history of urinary bladder inflammation. Which medical term pertains to this patient's history?
    A. cholecystitis
    B. cystitis
    C. otitis
    D. phlebitis

82. You are transporting a patient to the emergency department for difficulty breathing. While obtaining the patient's medical history, you find he or she is taking a well-known antibiotic t.i.d. The abbreviation t.i.d. means
    A. four times a day.
    B. three times a day.
    C. takes as needed.
    D. two times a day.

83. While transporting a 43-year-old female patient, she informs you she is being treated for nephritis. You associate this term with which organ?
    A. the liver
    B. the kidneys
    C. the stomach
    D. the intestines

84. You are treating a gentleman who started having problems breathing after he went to bed for the evening. He has problems breathing only when lying flat. What term best describes this patient's complaint?
    A. hypopnea
    B. cyanosis
    C. hypoxia
    D. orthopnea

85. The use of appropriate medical terminology would **not** be appropriate when communicating with

    A. the patient.
    B. the patient's sister who is a nurse.
    C. the ED physician.
    D. the medical dispatcher.

86. Which of the following statements is correct regarding the position of the trachea to other thoracic structures?

    A. The trachea is posterior to the esophagus.
    B. The trachea is lateral to the carina.
    C. The trachea is inferior to the diaphragm.
    D. The trachea is medial to the lungs.

87. While reviewing a prehospital care report, you encounter the abbreviation "gtt." This refers to

    A. Glasgow trauma total.
    B. milliliter.
    C. drop.
    D. none of the above

88. While assessing a male patient with diffuse abdominal pain, he tells you he was recently diagnosed with "cholecystitis." You identify this as an inflammation of the

    A. gallbladder.
    B. spleen.
    C. kidney.
    D. nerves.

89. Which of the following suffixes refers to weakness?

    A. -plegia
    B. -paresis
    C. -phagia
    D. -pathy

90. While assessing a patient involved in a diving accident, you note an absence of motor function on the right side and extreme weakness on the left. Which of the following statements represents the most appropriate documentation of this condition?

    A. right hemiplegia and left hemiparesis
    B. left hemiplegia and right-sided weakness
    C. right quadriplegia and left-sided paresis
    D. left quadriplegia and right-sided paresis

91. While assessing a 72-year-old female patient who fell, you note that her left leg seems rotated outward. When communicating with online medical direction, how would you correctly describe the left lower extremity?

    A. flexed
    B. laterally rotated
    C. adducted
    D. medially rotated

92. At a nursing home, a staff RN informs you that your patient's chief complaint is hyperpyrexia and was just given 750 mg of Tylenol p.o. You recognize this as

    A. Tylenol by mouth.
    B. Tylenol per order of physician.
    C. Tylenol by suppository.
    D. Tylenol followed by water.

93. A 76-year-old female suffers from dysphagia. This pertains to

    A. without speech.
    B. without eating.
    C. difficulty swallowing.
    D. difficulty speaking.

94. Your adult patient is breathing 40 times a minute. This is known as
    A. tachycardia.
    B. bradycardia.
    C. tachypnea.
    D. bradypnea.

95. While assessing your patient, she states that she had an oophorectomy last month. You know this to be
    A. visual examination of the airway.
    B. inflammation of the vocal cords.
    C. surgical removal of cataracts.
    D. surgical excision of the ovary.

96. Your patient states he is experiencing pain when he urinates. The medical term is
    A. dysuria.
    B. polyuria.
    C. hematuria.
    D. lipoiduria.

97. Your patient has a GSW below the shoulder blade. You document this on your medical report as
    A. intercostal.
    B. supraclavicular.
    C. infrascapular.
    D. intralobar.

98. Your patient's pupils are equal and reactive to light. Which of these is an acceptable medical abbreviation?
    A. pupils E/R
    B. pupils ERL
    C. PERL
    D. PEARTL

99. The nurse is giving you a report on a patient you will be transporting. He states the patient is medicated q.i.d. How often does the patient receive medication?
    A. once a day
    B. twice a day

C. three times a day
D. four times a day

100. Which of the following root words describes a muscle that closes an opening when it contracts?
    A. sphincter
    B. asthenia
    C. glomerulus
    D. cochlea

101. Which of the following prefixes refers to the blood vessels?
    A. cerebro-
    B. hemato-
    C. pulmo-
    D. angio-

102. Macro- is to micro- as hyper- is to
    A. hyster-.
    B. dys-.
    C. orchi-.
    D. hypo-.

103. Supine is to prone as medial is to
    A. lateral.
    B. ventral.
    C. dorsal.
    D. superior.

104. A fracture at the upper end of the upper arm bone would be described as a
    A. proximal tibial fracture.
    B. distal tibial fracture.
    C. distal humerus fracture.
    D. proximal humerus fracture.

105. An imaginary vertical line that separates the anterior lateral chest from the posterior lateral chest is called the
    A. anterior axillary line.
    B. midaxillary line.
    C. scapular line.
    D. posterior axillary line.

106. Which medical abbreviation is **incorrectly** defined?
   A. GI—gastrointestinal
   B. Dx—dyspnea
   C. cc—cubic centimeter
   D. c/o—complains of

107. Which medical abbreviation is **incorrectly** defined?
   A. L—liter
   B. RBC—red blood cell
   C. WNL—within normal limits
   D. q—drop

108. Which root word is **incorrectly** defined?
   A. stern—chest
   B. pod—back
   C. rhin—nose
   D. xen—foreign

109. Which prefix is **incorrectly** defined?
   A. cephal—large
   B. neo—new
   C. epi—upon
   D. auto—self

110. Which of the following terms are opposites?
   A. anterior—ventral
   B. lateral—medial
   C. posterior—dorsal
   D. superior—cranial

111. A patient who is complaining of shortness of breath is said to have
   A. dyspnea.
   B. dystachea.
   C. apnea.
   D. tachypnea.

112. The portion of the humerus that is closest to the shoulder is the
   A. distal end of the humerus.
   B. medial end of the humerus.
   C. inferior end of the humerus.
   D. proximal end of the humerus.

113. Your partner tells you that the patient has a large open laceration to the occipital portion of her head. The laceration is located on the
   A. top of the head.
   B. side of the head.
   C. back of the head.
   D. front of the head.

114. Dispatch informs you that you have a patient with hematemesis. You know this as
   A. coughing up blood.
   B. urinating blood.
   C. vomiting blood.
   D. blood in the stool.

115. Which of the following prefixes refers to the head?
   A. cerebr-
   B. cephal-
   C. cyan-
   D. cerv-

116. You are reviewing a run sheet in which the EMT-Intermediate used the abbreviation "CHF." You know this means
   A. chronic heart flutter.
   B. chronic hepatic failure.
   C. congestive heart failure.
   D. calcified humoral fracture.

117. In describing the location of a laceration that is located between the elbow and wrist, which of the following statements is most correct?

   A. The laceration is proximal to the elbow.

   B. The laceration is lateral to the pelvis.

   C. The laceration is distal to the elbow.

   D. The laceration is medial to the wrist.

118. Which of the following terms means an abnormally slow heart rate?

   A. bradycardia

   B. bradycephalia

   C. bradypnea

   D. bradykinin

119. Which of the following terms are opposites?

   A. hypopnea—hypoventilation

   B. medial—midline

   C. superior—cephalad

   D. proximal—distal

120. You want to use an abbreviation on your run sheet that represents someone who has difficulty breathing with any physical activity. This abbreviation would be

   A. DOA.

   B. DOE.

   C. MAE.

   D. Dx.

121. You are transferring a patient from the emergency department to another hospital. The physician tells you the patient is NPO. This means the patient

   A. cannot receive oxygen by mask.

   B. is allergic to nitroglycerin.

   C. should not be resuscitated.

   D. cannot have anything by mouth.

122. You are assessing a patient who states he has had hemiparesis for the past few days. He is complaining of which of the following?

   A. paralysis to his lower legs

   B. weakness to one side of his body

   C. tingling to one side of his body

   D. weakness to the lower part of his body

123. Which of the following medical terms would describe a patient who complains of very frequent and excessive urination?

   A. oliguria

   B. hematuria

   C. polyuria

   D. dysuria

124. A patient with a history of PND

   A. has had frequent pelvic infections.

   B. has premature heartbeats.

   C. is awakened at night with difficulty breathing.

   D. is an insulin-dependent diabetic.

125. Translate the following medical report into everyday English:

   Pt is a 45 y.o. male, AO × 4, c/o sudden onset CP and SOB × 2h. Pt also c/o DOE, N/V, and weakness. Pt has Hx of ASHD and AMI × 2 with CHF, and TIA × 1. He takes NTG 0.4 mg SL PRN for CP. NKA. VS as follows: BP 170/80, pulse 80, respirations 28, BS clear bilaterally, skin WNL. ECG shows NSR with PVC's. BS is 120. R/O AMI. Plan—O_2 or 10 lpm, NTG 0.4 mg SL q5 minutes PRN, MS 2 mg IV repeat PRN.

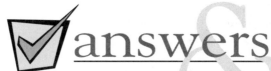

answers & rationales

Following each rationale, you will find a reference to the corresponding objective in the DOT National Standard EMT-Intermediate curriculum. An asterisk denotes material that is supplemental to the DOT curriculum. Page numbers after a rationale indicate where the question topic may be discussed in the Brady text *Intermediate Emergency Care* (Bledsoe, Porter, Cherry).

1.

D. The prehospital care report (PCR) is likely to be reviewed by the emergency department staff, surgical staff, floor or intensive care unit personnel, EMS administrators, billing department, researchers, insurance providers, and lawyers. Your PCR is a direct reflection of your care. (3-6.1) (IEC p. 560)

2.

C. The times commonly recorded on the PCR include call received, crew alerted, en route to scene, arrival at scene, departure from scene, arrival at hospital, in service, and in quarters. One major omission is the actual time of arrival at the patient's side, which gives a false impression of the true response time. (3-6.4) (IEC p. 563)

3.

B. The best time to complete your PCR is at the hospital immediately following the call, when the information is fresh in your mind. En route to the hospital, generally you should be attending to your patient, not filling out your PCR. (*) (IEC p. 570)

4.

B. If you make a mistake—and you will—simply place a line through the mistake, initial it, and make the correction. Never try to cover up a mistake. If you are early in the report, simply start over. (3-6.20) (IEC p. 570)

5.

A. If you detect a mistake or receive additional information after you have submitted your PCR to the hospital, you should write an addendum, noting the reason, the date and time, and the pertinent information. (3-6.21) (IEC p. 570)

6.

D. Always be objective and describe your patient's behavior. Avoid subjective opinions and comments that may damage your patient's character. Even if accurate, a comment such as "The patient was an obnoxious drunk" is still just your opinion and is a potentially libelous statement. (3-6.7) (IEC p. 571)

7.

A. The subjective narrative includes all the information elicited during the history: the chief complaint, history of present illness, past history, current health status, and review of systems. (3-6.8) (IEC p. 571)

8.

B. SOAP stands for **S**ubjective (the history), **O**bjective (the physical exam), **A**ssessment (your field diagnosis), **P**lan (treatment). This mnemonic is commonly used to document your patient assessment. (3-6.14) (IEC p. 574)

9.

D. A patient who refuses care and transportation must demonstrate competence by understanding the circumstances and the risks of refusing care and by accepting the risks of and responsibility for his actions. (3-6.13) (IEC p. 576)

10.

C. Sometimes your services are not needed, and you will be canceled by the on-scene command officer. In this case, document the name of the person and agency canceling your services and document that you never made patient contact. (*) (IEC p. 577)

Fill-ins (3-6.3) (IEC pp. 564–567)

11. coronary artery bypass graft	CABG
12. atherosclerotic heart disease	ASHD
13. against medical advice	AMA
14. blood sugar	BS
15. body surface area	BSA
16. bag-valve-mask	BVM
17. birth control pills	BCP

18. cubic centimeter	cc
19. chief complaint	CC
20. centimeter	cm
21. congestive heart failure	CHF
22. complains of	c/o
23. carbon monoxide	CO
24. carbon dioxide	CO_2
25. chronic obstructive pulmonary disease	COPD
26. chest pain	CP
27. cerebrospinal fluid	CSF
28. carotid sinus massage	CSM
29. cerebrovascular accident	CVA
30. discontinue	D/C
31. dyspnea on exertion	DOE
32. deep-vein thrombosis	DVT
33. estimated date of confinement	EDC
34. alcohol (ethanol)	ETOH
35. occasional	occ
36. fracture	Fx
37. gastrointestinal	GI
38. gunshot wound	GSW
39. hour	h
40. headache	H/A
41. history	Hx
42. intramuscular	IM
43. intraosseous	IO
44. jugular venous distention	JVD
45. potassium	K^+
46. kilogram	kg
47. keep vein open	KVO
48. deciliter	dL
49. laceration	lac

50. lactated Ringer's | LR

51. moves all extremities well | MAEW

52. microgram | mcg

53. milliequivalent | mEq

54. milligram | mg

55. milliliter | ml, mL

56. morphine sulfate | MS

57. sodium | Na$^+$

58. sodium chloride | NaCl

59. no known allergies | NKA

60. nitroglycerin | NTG

61. nausea/vomiting | N/V

62. organic brain syndrome | OBS

63. penicillin | PCN

64. hydrogen ion concentration | pH

65. pelvic inflammatory disease | PID

66. as needed | prn

67. patient | Pt

68. every | q

69. rule out | R/O

70. range of motion | ROM

71. positive end-expiratory pressure | PEEP

72. signs/symptoms | S/S

73. subcutaneous | SC, SQ

74. sublingual | SL

75. within normal limits | wnl

76.

B. This patient has an inflammation of the liver. The prefix *hepat-* means liver, and the suffix *-itis* means inflammation. (3-6.2)

77.

C. The knee is closer to the heart than the ankle. This would make it proximal. (3-6.2)

78.

A. The medical abbreviation RHD stands for rheumatic heart disease. (3-6.3) (IEC p. 564)

79.

D. Circumoral cyanosis means a blue discoloration around the mouth. (3-6.2)

80.

C. The patient is suffering from dysphasia. The prefix *dys-* means difficulty, and the suffix *-phasia* means speech. The suffix *-phagia* means eating, and *-pnea* means breathing. (3-6.2)

81.

B. An inflammation of the urinary bladder is cystitis. The prefix *cyst-* means bladder, and the suffix *-itis* means inflammation. The prefix *cholecyst-* means gallbladder, *ot-* refers to the ear, and *phleb-* is a vein. (3-6.2) (IEC pp. 1049, 1116)

82.

B. The abbreviation t.i.d. means three times a day. A medication taken two times a day is abbreviated b.i.d. and four times a day is q.i.d. PRN means as needed. (3-6.3)

83.

B. *Nephr-* refers to the kidney, *enter-* refers to the intestines, *gastr-* refers to the stomach, and *hepat-* refers to the liver. (3-6.2)

84.

D. Orthopnea is the best term for documentation because it refers to being unable to breathe while lying flat. Cyanosis and hypoxia may result from the scenario but are not adequate terms to describe this patient. Hypopnea is inadequate ventilatory volume. (3-6.2) (IEC pp. 412, 810, 1283)

85.

A. It would be best to talk to the patient in words he or she can understand. Rarely will patients have a good grasp on medical terminology, so they should receive information in a way that they can understand. Medical terminology should be used when conversing with other people involved in caring for a patient both outside and inside the hospital. The use of medical terminology ensures better communication, and it lessens the opportunity for statements to be ambiguous. (*)

86.

D. The location of the trachea can be defined by its medial positioning between each lung. Integral to properly communicating data to the emergency staff is the ability to describe anatomical injuries or landmarks appropriately. This ability will come only from the working knowledge of anatomical terms used in emergency medicine. All other descriptions for the position of the trachea are incorrect. (3-6.2) (IEC pp. 145, 153–154, 203–204)

87.

C. The abbreviation "gtt" refers to "drop." Having a thorough understanding of common medical abbreviations will allow you to prepare a more concise written report quickly. However, using the abbreviations appropriately is a must. (3-6.3) (IEC p. 566)

88.

A. Cholecystitis refers to an inflammation of the gallbladder. *Cholecyst-* means gallbladder, and *-itis* means inflammation. Root words are the portions of the medical term that define the basic meaning of the word. The root words can then be modified by prefixes and suffixes. (3-6.2)

89.

B. The suffix *-paresis* refers to weakness. You may see the same suffix on the end of various root words. For example, paraparesis and hemiparesis refer to weakness of the legs or one half of the body, respectively. The suffix *-phagia* refers to swallowing, and *-pathy* refers to disease. (3-6.2)

90.

A. This patient presents with right hemiplegia (half paralysis) and left hemiparesis (half weakness). The prefix *quad-* refers to all four extremities. (3-6.2)

91.

B. The patient's left leg is laterally rotated or turned away from the midline of the body. (3-6.2)

92.

A. The abbreviation p.o. refers to anything given by mouth. None of the other options represents this definition. (3-6.3) (IEC p. 566)

93.

C. The patient has dysphagia. The prefix *dys-* translates to difficulty, while *-phagia* refers to eating or swallowing. (3-6.2) (IEC p. 1264)

answers & rationales

94.

C. The patient's condition is called tachypnea: *tachy-* is the prefix for fast, and *-pnea* is the common root word for breathing. *Brady-* is the prefix for slow, and *-cardia* is the root word for heart, thus slow heart rate. (3-6.2) (IEC pp. 424, 813)

95.

D. An oophorectomy is the surgical removal of the ovary. *Oophor-* is the prefix for ovary, and *-ectomy* is the suffix meaning to cut out or excise. (3-6.2)

96.

A. Painful urination is dysuria. *Dys-* is with pain or difficulty, and *-uria* has to do with urine. Polyuria is many urinations or frequent urination. Hematuria is blood in the urine. Lipoiduria is lipids or fats in the urine. (3-6.2)

97.

C. Document the GSW (gunshot wound) as being infrascapular. *Infra-* is below, and *-scapular* is scapula or shoulder blade. Intercostal is between the ribs. Supraclavicular is above the clavicle. Intralobar is within a lobe. (3-6.3)

98.

C. The correct medical abbreviation for pupils that are equal and reactive to light is PERL (or PEARL). (3-6.3) (IEC p. 565)

99.

D. The abbreviation q.i.d. is four times a day. Twice a day is b.i.d., and three times a day is t.i.d. (3-6.3)

100.

A. Sphincter describes a muscle that closes an opening when it contracts. This type of muscle can be found in the bladder, stomach, and rectum. (3-6.2)

101.

D. *Angio-* refers to the blood vessels. An example of this is angioplasty, which is repairing a blood vessel. *Cerebro-* refers to the brain, and *hemato-* refers to the blood. *Pulmo-* refers to the lungs. (3-6.2)

102.

D. *Macro-* is a prefix that means large, and *micro-* is a prefix that means small. *Hyper-* means over or excessive, and *hypo-* means under or deficient. *Dys-* translates as with difficulty, *orchi-* is testicle, and *hyster-* pertains to the uterus. (3-6.2)

103.

A. Supine is lying face up, while prone is lying face down. Medial is toward the midline, and lateral is away from the midline. Ventral is toward the front, and dorsal is toward the back. Superior is toward the top. (3-6.2)

104.

D. The humerus is the upper arm bone, and proximal means closer to the top or origin, so this injury would best be described as a proximal humoral fracture. The tibia is the anterior bone of the lower leg, and distal means away from the point of attachment. (3-6.2)

105.

B. The midaxillary line separates the anterior chest from the posterior chest. This is a vertical line located at the midline of the axilla or the armpit. (3-6.2)

106.

B. Dx is the abbreviation for diagnosis. (3-6.3)

107.

D. *q-* means every or four. The abbreviation for drop is gtt. (3-6.3) (IEC p. 566)

108.

B. *Pod-* refers to foot. (3-6.2)

109.

A. *Cephal-* refers to the head. The suffix -*megaly* refers to large. (3-6.2)

110.

B. Lateral and medial are the opposite terms. Lateral means away from the midline of the body, while medial means toward the midline of the body. (3-6.2)

111.

A. The term dyspnea refers to shortness of breath. The prefix *dys-* means difficulty, and -*pnea* is the common root word for breathing. (3-6.2) (IEC p. 412)

112.

D. The part of the humerus that is closest to the shoulder is the proximal end. Proximal is the term that refers to being closest to the heart, while distal is farthest from the heart. The

distal end of the humerus is near the elbow. (3-6.2)

113.

C. The occipital area of the skull is at the back of the head. The frontal refers to the front (forehead), temporal is the side, and parietal is the top. (3-6.2)

114.

C. Hematemesis is defined as vomiting up blood, while hemoptysis is defined as coughing up blood. Blood found in the urine is called hematuria. (3-6.2)

115.

B. The prefix referring to the head is *cephal-*. *Cerebr-* generally refers to the brain. *Cerv-* refers to the cervical region of the spinal column, and *cyan-* means bluish color. (3-6.2)

116.

C. CHF stands for the medical condition known as congestive heart failure. All of the other answers are fictitious names using the abbreviation CHF. (3-6.3) (IEC p. 564)

117.

C. A laceration between the elbow and wrist could be phrased as a laceration occurring distal to the elbow. In describing injury locations, the EMT-Intermediate needs to know appropriate terminology to describe locations. Distal means away from the heart, and proximal means closer to the heart. Lateral means to the sides, and medial means toward the midline. (3-6.2)

118.

A. Bradycardia is an abnormally slow heart rate: *brady-* means slow, and *-cardia* is the root word for heart. Bradypnea refers to an abnormally slow respiratory rate, and *-pnea* is the root word for breathing. (3-6.2) (IEC p. 424)

119.

D. Proximal and distal are opposite terms and are used for referencing locations on the body. Hypopnea and hypoventilation refer to abnormally shallow breathing. Medial means toward the midline. Superior means a position above another, and cephalad means toward the head. (3-6.2)

120.

B. DOE stands for dyspnea on exertion. This is the abbreviation that should be used for a patient who is having difficulty breathing with any physical activity. (3-6.3) (IEC p. 564)

121.

D. The medical abbreviation NPO means nothing by mouth. (3-6.3) (IEC p. 566)

122.

B. The patient has weakness to one side of his body. The prefix *hemi-* refers to half of the body if split into a right and a left side; *-paresis* means weakness. (3-6.2)

123.

C. A patient with polyuria is suffering from frequent and excessive urination. *Poly-* means many or excessive, and *-uria* refers to urine. (3-6.2) (IEC p. 412)

124.

C. A patient who is awakened at night with difficulty breathing is said to have paroxsysmal (sudden onset) nocturnal (nighttime) dyspnea (difficulty breathing). It is a common complaint of patients with congestive heart failure. They often sleep with their upper bodies propped up on pillows. For example, a patient can have three-pillow orthopnea. (3-6.3) (IEC p. 810)

125.

The patient is a 45-year-old male, alert and oriented to person, place, and time, who complains of a sudden onset of chest pain and shortness of breath that began 2 hours ago. The patient also complains of dyspnea on exertion, nausea, vomiting, and weakness. The patient has a history of atherosclerotic heart disease and has had two heart attacks with congestive heart failure and one transient ischemic attack. He takes nitroglycerine 0.4 mg sublingually as needed for chest pain. He has no known allergies. His vital signs are as follows: blood pressure 170/80, pulse 80, respirations 28, breath sounds clear bilaterally, skin within normal limits. His electrocardiogram shows normal sinus rhythm with premature ventricular contractions. Blood sugar is 120. Rule out acute myocardial infarction. Plan—oxygen at 10 lpm, nitroglycerine 0.4 mg sublingually every 5 minutes as needed; morphine sulfate 2 mg intravenously, repeat as needed. (3-6.2, 3-6.3) (IEC p. 564-567)

UNIT
1A
Trauma and Trauma Systems

unit objectives

Questions in this unit relate to DOT Objectives 4-1.1 and 4-1.10. The objectives are listed in the Appendix.

DIRECTIONS Each of the questions or incomplete statements below is followed by suggested answers or completions. Select the **one answer** that is best in each case.

1. Serious and life-threatening injuries occur in _____% of trauma patients.
   A. <10
   B. 15–25
   C. 30–40
   D. >50

2. In 1990, the American College of Surgeons worked to pass the _____, which helped develop trauma systems.
   A. Highway Safety Act
   B. EMS Systems Act
   C. COBRA
   D. Trauma Care Systems Act

3. Guidelines to aid the prehospital provider in determining which patients require immediate transport to a trauma center are known as
   A. mechanism of injury standards.
   B. injury severity indexes.
   C. standing orders.
   D. trauma triage criteria.

4. Which of the following adult patients require rapid transport to a trauma center?
   A. adult who falls 10 feet
   B. passenger in a car in which driver died
   C. patient ejected from vehicle
   D. motorcycle driver thrown from bike
   E. passenger in a compartment intruded by 24 inches
   F. victim with flail chest
   G. victim with femur fracture
   H. victim with respirations of 24, systolic BP of 98, pulse of 110
   I. victim shot in the wrist
   J. patient with systolic BP of 88 and pulse of 130
   K. ambulatory patient from rollover with no signs of serious impact
   L. patient with extrication time of 35 minutes
   M. patient with unstable pelvis
   N. patient with facial burns
   O. patient with lower-extremity paralysis

5. Which of the following children requires rapid transport to a trauma center?
   A. child who fell from 12-foot roof
   B. child in bicycle/vehicle collision
   C. unrestrained child in vehicle collision at medium speed
   D. all of the above

6. The Golden Hour begins at the time of _____ and ends at the time of _____.
   A. dispatch, arrival at the hospital
   B. injury, surgery
   C. arrival at the scene, departure to the hospital
   D. none of the above

7. Disdvantages to using an air medical service (helicopter) include
   A. limited space for in-flight care.
   B. distracting engine noise.
   C. expense.
   D. all of the above

8. "Let's Not Meet by Accident" is a(n)

    A. ad campaign by NHTSA.

    B. public television documentary.

    C. public education program for high schools.

    D. pamphlet denouncing drunk driving.

9. Which of the following technical developments has played a major role in reducing highway deaths?

    A. better highway design

    B. air bag restraint systems

    C. vehicles designed to absorb impact

    D. all of the above

10. Your patient presents with slight tachycardia and cool skin following blunt abdominal trauma in a motor vehicle crash. There are no obvious signs of serious injury, but your "gut" tells you that, because of the mechanism of injury and her vital signs, she may have an abdominal bleed, so you decide to transport her to a Level I trauma center. This is an example of

    A. overtriage.

    B. diversion.

    C. false imprisonment.

    D. misuse of resources.

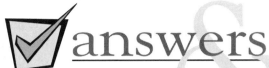
answers & rationales

Following each rationale, you will find a reference to the corresponding objective in the DOT National Standard EMT-Intermediate curriculum. An asterisk denotes material that is supplemental to the DOT curriculum. Page numbers after a rationale indicate where the question topic may be discussed in the Brady text *Intermediate Emergency Care* (Bledsoe, Porter, Cherry).

1.

A. Serious and life-threatening injuries occur in fewer than 10% of trauma patients. That's the good news. The bad news is that prehospital care providers can do little to stabilize these patients because they involve major head injury or body cavity hemorrhage. In these cases, the best care includes rapid transport to a trauma center. (*) (IEC p. 583)

2.

D. In 1990, the American College of Surgeons worked to achieve passage of the Trauma Care Systems Act, which helped establish guidelines, funding, and state-level leadership and support for the development of trauma systems. (4-1.1) (IEC p. 584)

3.

D. Trauma triage criteria are guidelines that help prehospital personnel determine which patients require immediate transportation to a trauma center. They identify the mechanism of injury that can cause serious internal trauma, and they establish the physical or clinical findings that reflect serious internal injury. (4-1.3) (IEC p. 588)

4.

The following mechanisms of injury and physical findings indicate rapid transportation to a trauma center: B, C, D, E, F, J, L, M, N, O (4-1.3) (IEC pp. 589, 822)

Falls greater than 20 feet

Death of a car occupant

Pedestrian/bicyclist struck by a vehicle traveling over 5 mph

Ejection from the vehicle

Severe vehicle impact

Rollover with signs of serious impact

Motorcycle impact greater than 40 mph

Extrication time greater than 20 minutes

Revised trauma score less than 11

Glasgow Coma Score less than 14

Pulse greater than 120 or less than 50

Systolic blood pressure less than 90

Respiratory rate less than 10 or greater than 29

Penetrating trauma except for distal extremities

Two or more proximal long-bone fractures

Flail chest

Pelvic fractures

Limb paralysis

Burns to more than 15% of body surface area

Burns to the face or airway

5.

D. Significant mechanism of injury considerations with infants and children include the following: (4-1.3) (IEC pp. 488, 588, 822)

Falls of greater than 10 feet

Bicycle/vehicle collisions

Vehicle collisions at medium speed

Unrestrained child in vehicle collisions

6.

B. The Golden Hour begins at the time of injury and ends with the time of surgery. Trauma research done at the University of Maryland concluded that critical trauma victims survived if surgical repair of their injuries occurred within 1 hour. (*) (IEC p. 588)

7.

D. Air medical services are a valuable patient transportation option, but there are disdvantages. These include limited space for in-flight care, engine noise, expense, adverse weather conditions, and the unpredictable nature of combative patients. (4-1.4) (IEC p. 588)

8.

C. "Let's Not Meet by Accident" is a public education program aimed at high school children that reinforces safe driving. The program is taught in hospital emergency departments by prehospital personnel, nurses, and physicians who stress the results of unsafe driving practices. (*) (IEC p. 590)

9.

D. Technical developments such as air bag restraint systems, better highway design, and vehicles constructed to better absorb impact have all helped reduce the number of yearly highway deaths. (*) (IEC p. 590)

10.

A. Trauma triage criteria are designed for the "overtriage" of trauma patients. They ensure that patients with very subtle signs and symptoms yet with serious injuries are not missed during assessment. Yes, you will transport some patients to trauma centers needlessly. But this is far better than not transporting a patient who needs that level of care. (4-1.3) (IEC p. 589)

1B Mechanism of Injury

unit objectives

Questions in this unit relate to DOT Objectives 4-1.7 to 4-1.9 and 4-1.11 to 4-1.14. The objectives are listed in the Appendix.

DIRECTIONS Each of the questions or incomplete statements below is followed by suggested answers or completions. Select the **one answer** that is best in each case.

1. A car traveling at 55 mph will tend to remain traveling at 55 mph until something stops it or slows it down. This is known as the law of
   A. kinetics.
   B. inertia.
   C. energy.
   D. motion.

2. Which of the following will generate the greatest amount of kinetic energy?
   A. 20-lb. object traveling at 50 mph
   B. 30-lb. object traveling at 40 mph
   C. 40-lb. object traveling at 30 mph
   D. 50-lb. object traveling at 20 mph

3. In an automobile collision, there are five events that occur. Place them in chronological order:
   A. body collision
   B. additional impacts
   C. secondary collision
   D. organ collision
   E. vehicle collision

4. During your scene assessment, you learn that the driver wore a lap belt only. Based on this information, what types of injuries would you expect?
   A. head and neck
   B. chest
   C. intraabdominal or lower spine
   D. pelvic and femur fractures

5. Your patient was a restrained driver in a two-car frontal impact collision. You notice also that his air bag was deployed. He complains only of a burning in his eyes. What is the most likely cause of his complaint?
   A. a preexisting eye problem
   B. residue from the air bag
   C. corneal abrasion from the air bag
   D. increasing intracranial pressure

6. The recommended child safety seat position for infants and small children is the
   A. front seat facing the front.
   B. front seat facing the rear.
   C. backseat facing the front.
   D. backseat facing the rear

7. In the urban setting, which of the following types of impact is most common?
   A. frontal
   B. lateral
   C. rotational
   D. rear end

8. Axial loading occurs when
   A. the shoulder strikes the side window.
   B. the head strikes the front windshield.
   C. the knee strikes the lower dashboard.
   D. the chest strikes the steering wheel.

9. Injuries from the paper bag syndrome include
   A. subdural hematoma.
   B. pericardial tamponade.
   C. lacerated trachea.
   D. pneumothorax.

10. Which of the following statements is true regarding lateral impact collisions?
    A. The greater amount of passenger protection in these collisions lessens the injury pattern.
    B. These collisions account for the smallest percentage of vehicular deaths.
    C. The amount of vehicular damage exaggerates the injury pattern.
    D. none of the above

11. The most commonly seen injury associated with rear-impact collisions is
    A. kidney laceration.
    B. lumbar spine fracture.
    C. cervical spine injuries.
    D. cardiac contusion.

12. Which body area is associated with the highest mortality from motor vehicle trauma?
    A. head
    B. chest/abdomen
    C. lower extremities
    D. pelvis

13. Which of the following injury patterns is most associated with frontal motorcycle collisions in which the driver is ejected?
    A. lateral pelvis dislocations
    B. bilateral femur fractures

C. spleen and liver lacerations
D. crushing injuries

14. Which of the following statements is true regarding auto-pedestrian collisions?
    A. Adults tend to turn away from the oncoming car prior to impact.
    B. Children tend to face the oncoming car prior to impact.
    C. Adults are often thrown up and over the bumper.
    D. all of the above

15. Primary injuries from a blast include
    A. extremity fractures.
    B. liver lacerations.
    C. lung injuries.
    D. impaled objects.

16. Secondary injuries from a blast include
    A. extremity fractures.
    B. liver lacerations.
    C. lung injuries.
    D. impaled objects.

17. Tertiary injuries from a blast include
    A. extremity fractures.
    B. liver lacerations.
    C. lung injuries.
    D. impaled objects.

18. When assessing falls, you should focus your attention on
    A. the height of the fall.
    B. the surface the victim fell onto.
    C. the body part that hit first.
    D. all of the above

19. The recommended method for immobilizing a football player's head and neck on a long board is to

    A. keep both helmet and shoulder pads on.

    B. remove helmet, keep shoulder pads on.

    C. remove shoulder pads, keep helmet on.

    D. remove both helmet and shoulder pads.

    E. A or D

20. If you double the speed of an object, its kinetic energy increases by

    A. half.

    B. double.

    C. fourfold.

    D. eightfold.

21. The study of projectiles in motion and their interactions with the gun, the air, and the objects they contact is known as

    A. trajectory.

    B. ballistics.

    C. profile.

    D. caliber.

22. As a rifle bullet hits the body, what generally happens to its profile?

    A. It stays on the same straight path.

    B. It tumbles and rotates 180°.

    C. It breaks apart like shrapnel.

    D. It remains in a gyroscopic motion.

23. A hunting rifle produces much greater kinetic energy because of its

    A. heavy projectile.

    B. high speed.

    C. bullets that expand on impact.

    D. all of the above

24. Which of the following statements is true regarding knife injuries?

    A. Men attackers usually stab downward.

    B. Women attackers usually stab upward and outward.

    C. Impaled knives should always be removed in the field.

    D. none of the above

25. According to the projectile injury process, which tissue suffers the most damage?

    A. tissue that is stretched from the cavitational wave

    B. tissue in the direct pathway

    C. adjacent tissue

    D. all of the above

26. Which of the following impaled objects should be removed?

    A. lodged in the cheek, causing airway obstruction

    B. lodged in the trachea, causing airway obstruction

    C. lodged in such a way as to prevent CPR

    D. all of the above

27. Which of the following statements is true regarding penetrating injuries?

    A. Solid organs have the resiliency of muscle and other connective tissues.

    B. Muscles, the skin, and other connective tissues are thin and delicate.

    C. When muscle is penetrated, the wound track closes, and serious injury is limited.

    D. Penetrating injury to the lung is generally less extensive than in other body tissue.

28. Which of the following statements is true regarding penetrating trauma to a hollow organ?

    A. If the organ is filled with fluid, it can tear apart explosively.

    B. If it is filled with fluid, the energy is dissipated in the fluid with minimal damage.

    C. Injury to an air-filled organ results in explosive tissue damage and hemorrhage.

    D. Pericardial tamponade results from rupture of the heart's contents into the thorax.

29. Which of the following statements is true regarding penetrating trauma to the abdomen?

    A. The area is well protected by skeletal structures.

    B. Projectiles rarely produce a cavitational wave.

    C. The intestines tolerate stretching and compression well.

    D. Serious peritoneal irritation may result from bowel perforation with immediate signs and symptoms.

30. Which of the following statements is true regarding a bullet's entrance wound?

    A. It matches the size of the bullet's profile.

    B. It will often have a "blown out" appearance.

    C. If the bullet is fired at close range, subcutaneous emphysema will be present.

    D. It accurately portrays the potential for damage.

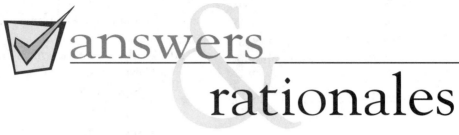

answers & rationales

Following each rationale, you will find a reference to the corresponding objective in the DOT National Standard EMT-Intermediate curriculum. An asterisk denotes material that is supplemental to the DOT curriculum. Page numbers after a rationale indicate where the question topic may be discussed in the Brady text *Intermediate Emergency Care* (Bledsoe, Porter, Cherry).

1.

B. Sir Isaac Newton described the law of inertia. It states that an object at rest tends to remain at rest, while an object in motion tends to remain in motion unless acted on by an external force. Therefore, a car traveling at 55 mph will tend to remain traveling at 55 mph until something stops it (i.e., another car, tree, telephone pole, wall) or slows it down (i.e., brakes, road friction, gravity). (4-1.6) (IEC p. 594)

2.

A. Kinetic energy is the energy of motion. It can be measured by the following formula:

$$\frac{\text{Mass (weight)} \times \text{Velocity}^2}{2}$$

Using this formula, speed becomes the most important factor. Even the lightest object (20 lbs.) traveling at the fastest speed (50 mph) will generate the greatest amount of kinetic energy. (4-1.6) (IEC p. 594)

3.

First, you have the vehicle collision (car hits tree), then the body collision (body hits dash and windshield), then the organ collision (internal organs hit sternum and rib cage), then the secondary collisions (backseat grocery bags hit front-seat passengers), and, finally, any additional impacts (another car fails to break and hits you). E, A, D, C, B (4-1.9) (IEC p. 597)

4.

C. When the lap belt is worn without the shoulder straps, the victim suffers a sudden folding of the body at the waist, resulting in intraabdominal and lower-spine injuries. (4-1.10) (IEC p. 599)

5.

B. The residue from the air bag deployment may cause eye irritation. This can be relieved by gentle irrigation with sterile water. (4-1.10) (IEC p. 600)

6.

D. With infants and very small children, the child safety seat should be positioned in the backseat facing the rear. As the child grows, the seat can be turned to face the front. (4-1.10) (IEC p. 601)

7.

C. In a rotational impact, the auto is struck from an oblique angle and rotates as the collision forces are expended. Rotational impacts account for 38% of all motor vehicle collisions in the urban setting. In the rural setting, anticipate a greater percentage of frontal impacts. (4-1.7) (IEC p. 605)

8.

B. Axial loading is the application of forces of trauma along the axis of the spine. When the head hits the windshield, that force is transmitted down the cervical spine, often causing compressions of those vertebrae. (4-1.7) (IEC p. 604)

9.

D. The paper bag syndrome is a common injury process associated with steering wheel impact. The driver takes a deep breath in anticipation of the collision. When the chest impacts the steering wheel, lung tissue ruptures, much like an inflated paper bag caught between clapping hands. Pneumothorax and pulmonary contusion may result. (4-1.7) (IEC p. 602)

10.

D. Lateral impacts account for 15% of all auto accidents, yet they are responsible for 22% of vehicular fatalities. The amount of structural steel between the impact side and the vehicle interior is greatly reduced. When a lateral impact occurs, the index of suspicion for serious internal injuries should be higher than vehicle damage alone suggests. (4-1.7) (IEC p. 604)

11.

C. In rear-end impact, the collision force pushes the auto forward, while the vehicle seat propels the occupant forward. If the headrest is not up, the head is unsupported and remains stationary. The neck extends severely, while the head rotates backward. Cervical spine injuries are common with rear-end collisions. (4-1.7) (IEC p. 605)

12.

A. Trauma to the head (47.7%) and body cavity (37.3%) accounts for 85% of vehicular mortality. This is why you focus on the head, neck, chest, abdomen, and pelvis during your rapid trauma assessment. (4-1.7) (IEC p. 609)

13.

B. In frontal or head-on motorcycle collisions, the impact often propels the rider upward and forward. Occasionally, the rider traps both femurs at the handlebars, causing bilateral fractures. (4-1.7) (IEC p. 610)

14.

B. In contrast to adults, children turn toward an oncoming vehicle. Because they are smaller, the injury is located anatomically higher, as the bumper fractures the femur or pelvis. (*) (IEC p. 611)

15.

C. Primary blast injuries are caused by the initial air blast and pressure wave. Injuries resulting from the compression of hollow organs, such as the lungs, include pneumothorax and alveolar rupture. (4-1.13) (IEC p. 616)

16.

D. Secondary blast injuries are caused by flying debris propelled by the force of the blast. Impacting debris may produce blunt or penetrating trauma. (4-1.13) (IEC p. 616)

17.

A. Tertiary blast injuries propel the victim away from the blast and into objects or the ground. Injuries are similar to those found in auto ejection. (4-1.13) (IEC p. 616)

18.

D. When assessing the mechanism of injury of falls, you should evaluate the following aspects: the height of the fall, the landing surface, and the part of the body that impacted first. (4-1.13) (IEC p. 866)

19.

E. When immobilizing the head and neck of a football player, you should either remove both helmet and shoulder pads or leave them both on in order to maintain the head and neck in a neutral position. (*) (IEC p. 621)

20.

C. The speed of an object has a squared relationship to its kinetic energy. If you double the speed of an object, its kinetic energy increases by fourfold ($2^2 = 4$). As in blunt trauma, speed kills. (4-1.6) (IEC p. 625)

21.

B. The study of projectiles in motion and their interactions with the gun, the air, and the object they contact is known as ballistics. (4-1.6) (IEC p. 626)

22.

B. Since a rifle bullet has its center of gravity farther back from the leading edge, it is likely to tumble once it hits the body. It generally rotates 180° and continues its travel base-first, causing massive damage. (4-1.5) (IEC p. 627)

23.

D. High-powered rifles produce tremendous kinetic energy because of their high muzzle velocity (speed) and their heavy projectiles (bullets) that expand dramatically on impact. Domestic hunting ammunition is especially lethal. (4-1.5, 4-1.6) (IEC p. 629)

24.

D. Knife-wielding males usually strike with a forward, outward, or crosswise stroke. Females usually strike with an overhand and downward blow. (4-1.13) (IEC p. 869)

25.

B. Tissue in the direct pathway of the bullet suffers most. It is severely contused and likely to have been torn from its attachments. (4-1.5) (IEC p. 632)

26.

D. In general, you want to immobilize an impaled object to prevent further injury except in the following cases: an object lodged in the cheek or trachea, causing an airway obstruction, or one preventing you from performing CPR. (*) (IEC p. 640)

27.

D. Because the lung tissue consists of millions of small, air-filled sacs that slow down and limit the transmission of the cavitational wave, penetrating trauma to the lungs generally causes less damage than trauma to other body tissues. (4-1.12) (IEC p. 634)

28.

A. Since fluid is noncompressible and rapidly transmits the impact energy outward, the energy released can tear the organ apart explosively. This is true of the bladder, stomach, intestines, and heart. (4-1.12) (IEC p. 634)

29.

C. The major occupant of the abdomen, the bowel, is very tolerant of compression and stretching. The liver, kidneys, spleen, and pancreas, however, are highly susceptible to injury and life-threatening hemorrhage. (4-1.12) (IEC p. 636)

30.

A. Entrance wounds are generally the size of the bullet's profile and quickly close because of the skin's natural elasticity. (4-1.12) (IEC p. 637)

Hemorrhage and Shock

unit objectives

Questions in this unit relate to DOT Objectives 4-2.1 to 4-2.39. The objectives are listed in the Appendix.

DIRECTIONS
Each of the questions or incomplete statements below is followed by suggested answers or completions. Select the **one answer** that is best in each case.

1. Which of the following factors does **not** affect the heart's stroke volume?
   A. heart rate
   B. preload
   C. afterload
   D. contractile force

2. Stroke volume could be increased by all of the following **except**
   A. increasing venous return.
   B. increasing contractile force.
   C. decreasing afterload.
   D. venous dilation.

3. The amount of blood pumped from the heart in one contraction is called
   A. preload.
   B. afterload.
   C. stroke volume.
   D. tidal volume.

4. Which of the following statements best illustrates Starling's law of the heart?
   A. The greater the afterload, the greater the stroke volume.
   B. The less the stroke volume, the less the afterload.
   C. The greater the preload, the greater the stroke volume.
   D. The less the preload, the greater the afterload.

5. The amount of blood pumped by the heart in 1 minute is called
   A. minute volume.
   B. stroke volume.
   C. cardiac output.
   D. contractile volume.

6. The amount of resistance against which the heart must pump in order to eject blood is called
   A. stroke volume.
   B. end-diastolic volume.
   C. afterload.
   D. pulse pressure.

7. The muscular layer of an artery is called the tunica
   A. intima.
   B. media.
   C. adventitia.
   D. arteriole.

8. Which of the following blood vessels has the greatest ability to vary the size of its internal lumens?
   A. artery
   B. arteriole
   C. capillary
   D. venule

9. Which of the following statements is true regarding capillaries?
   A. They lack tunica media.
   B. Their tunica adventitia is very thin.
   C. The walls are only two cells thick.
   D. They contain over 20% of the vascular volume.

10. The majority of blood volume consists of
    A. red blood cells.
    B. plasma.
    C. platelets.
    D. white blood cells.

11. The percentage of red blood cells in the blood is called
    A. homeostasis.
    B. hematocrit.
    C. hemoglobin.
    D. hematoma.

12. Red blood cells make up what percentage of total blood volume in the healthy adult?
    A. 20
    B. 45
    C. 55
    D. 60

13. Which of the following is **not** a phase of clotting?
    A. vascular phase
    B. platelet phase
    C. coagulation phase
    D. autonomic phase

14. Clotting normally takes _____ minutes.
    A. 7–10
    B. 10–20
    C. 20–30
    D. >30

15. Your patient has attempted suicide by slitting his wrists. You notice that he has run the knife across his wrist, perpendicular to the arm, and that the wound is rather deep. Which of the following statements is true regarding the likelihood for serious blood loss?
    A. You should expect severe blood loss.
    B. There is most likely tremendous internal blood loss.
    C. Blood loss is probably not life threatening.
    D. A tourniquet will probably be necessary.

16. Which of the following would **not** adversely affect the clotting process?
    A. aggressive fluid therapy
    B. immobilization of the wound site
    C. hypothermia
    D. administration of an NSAID

17. Which of the following techniques is **not** recommended for external hemorrhage control?
    A. venous constricting band
    B. direct pressure
    C. pressure points
    D. tourniquet

18. Epistaxis can be caused by
    A. hypertension.
    B. a strong sneeze.
    C. direct trauma.
    D. all of the above

19. Hemoptysis is best described as
    A. coughing up bright red blood.
    B. vomiting up dark brown blood.
    C. blood in the urine.
    D. blood in the stool.

20. Your patient presents with melena. This is best described as
    A. bright red blood from rectal hemorrhoids.
    B. massive vaginal hemorrhage.
    C. anemic blood.
    D. black, tarry stools.

21. Your patient presents with profound hypotension from external and internal hemorrhage. How much blood do you estimate he has already lost?

    A. <15%

    B. 15–25%

    C. 25–35%

    D. >35%

22. Which of the following factors renders the elderly more susceptible to the adverse effects of hemorrhage?

    A. lower fluid volume reserve

    B. beta blockers and anticoagulant medications

    C. less responsive compensatory mechanisms

    D. all of the above

23. Pelvic fractures can account for blood loss of _____ ml.

    A. up to 500

    B. 500–750

    C. up to 1500

    D. more than 2000

24. Your patient complains of rectal bleeding. On examination of the toilet immediately following his bowel movement, you note the presence of bright red blood in the water. This type of bleeding is known as

    A. hematochezia.

    B. melena.

    C. hematemesis.

    D. hemostasis.

25. A positive tilt test occurs when the pulse rate _____ by 10–20 beats per minute or the BP _____ by 10–20 mm Hg when a patient moves from a supine position to a sitting position.

    A. increases, increases

    B. decreases, increases

    C. increases, decreases

    D. decreases, decreases

26. The process known as glycolysis requires _____ oxygen and generates _____ energy.

    A. no, a small amount of

    B. a small amount of, no

    C. adequate, normal

    D. adequate, a great amount of

27. In the second stage of cellular metabolism, what is added to complete the Krebs cycle?

    A. fats

    B. glucose

    C. oxygen

    D. carbohydrates

28. Which of the following increases the flow of blood through a capillary bed?

    A. histamine release

    B. a rise in pH

    C. an increase in oxygen supply

    D. a decrease in carbon dioxide

29. The body can quickly increase its circulating blood volume by _____ the precapillary sphincters and _____ the postcapillary venule.

    A. opening, closing

    B. opening, opening

    C. closing, closing

    D. closing, opening

30. Blood is returned to the heart via the venous system. This flow is aided by

    A. skeletal muscle contractions.

    B. respirations.

    C. valves in the veins.

    D. all of the above

31. Baroreceptors constantly monitor for changes in
    A. oxygen levels.
    B. carbon dioxide levels.
    C. heart rate.
    D. blood pressure.

32. Stimulation of the baroreceptors causes all of the following **except**
    A. peripheral vasodilation.
    B. increased cardiac output.
    C. increased heart rate.
    D. bronchodilation.

Match the following agents and hormones with their respective roles in influencing operations of the cardiovascular system:

33. _____ epinephrine
34. _____ ADH
35. _____ angiotensin II
36. _____ aldosterone
37. _____ glucagon
38. _____ ACTH
39. _____ growth hormone
40. _____ erythropoietin

    A. increases red blood cell production
    B. reduces inflammation, increases clotting time
    C. increases cardiac output, vasoconstricts
    D. reduces urine output
    E. promotes glucose uptake and protein synthesis
    F. potent vasoconstrictor
    G. converts glycogen to glucose
    H. maintains ion balance in the kidneys

41. Anaerobic metabolism results in which of the following?
    A. inefficient energy
    B. increased pyruvic acid formation

C. continued glycolysis
D. all of the above

42. Tachycardia; cool, clammy, and pale skin; and a stable blood pressure describe a patient in
    A. compensated shock.
    B. decompensated shock.
    C. irreversible shock.
    D. none of the above

43. Which of the following happens in decompensated shock?
    A. Precapillary sphincters open.
    B. Rouleaux are formed.
    C. Blood pressure falls.
    D. all of the above

Match the following types of shock with their respective examples:

44. _____ hypovolemic
45. _____ anaphylactic
46. _____ septic
47. _____ obstructive
48. _____ cardiogenic
49. _____ respiratory
50. _____ neurogenic

    A. pulmonary embolus
    B. spinal cord injury
    C. third-space fluid loss
    D. flail chest
    E. myocardial infarction
    F. massive infection
    G. massive histamine release

51. A drop in cardiac output from volume loss would initially be detected by
    A. chemoreceptors.
    B. baroreceptors.
    C. pressoreceptors.
    D. adenoreceptors.

52. Which of the following contributes most to diminished coronary artery perfusion in hypovolemic shock states?

    A. diminished preload

    B. shortened diastole

    C. increased systemic vascular resistance

    D. increased glomerular filtration

53. You are treating a 37-year-old male who was struck by an automobile while jogging. Your partner estimates that the patient lost a significant amount of blood, but you note that there is still a radial pulse present. This finding means

    A. the cardiovascular system is still able to perfuse distal extremities.

    B. the patient has not really lost very much blood.

    C. the heart is not compromised.

    D. the arterial oxygen saturation is still adequate.

54. What negative feedback mechanism will become activated to maintain blood pressure when circulating volume is lost?

    A. precapillary sphincters close

    B. arterio-venule shunts close

    C. precapillary sphincters relax

    D. postcapillary sphincters relax

55. A patient was attacked and stabbed several times in the chest. A drop in pulmonary perfusion occurs as a result of the injuries. Which of the following is most likely the cause?

    A. an increase in arterial tone

    B. venous vasospasms

C. a lengthened diastole

D. a drop in stroke volume

56. A 45-year-old man was stabbed with an ice pick that penetrated the heart. The patient is presenting with severe dyspnea and pulmonary edema. Which heart valve is most likely affected by this injury?

    A. pulmonic valve

    B. mitral valve

    C. tricuspid valve

    D. aortic valve

57. An increase in the force of contraction of the myocardium will cause

    A. an increase in the heart rate.

    B. a decrease in afterload.

    C. an increase in blood pressure.

    D. none of the above

58. You are treating a patient with hypotension and severe dyspnea. Which of the following assessment findings would be most consistent with dyspnea caused by a left-ventricular failure?

    A. acute excessive peripheral edema

    B. decreased breath sounds

    C. jugular venous distention

    D. crackles on auscultation

59. The best estimate of systemic vascular resistance is provided by the

    A. pulse pressure.

    B. diastolic pressure.

    C. presence of a radial pulse.

    D. systolic pressure.

60. A woman informs you that her grandfather has been vomiting heavily for the past 3 days. In addition, the patient has had a decreased level of consciousness and intermittent convulsions. You suspect this individual is suffering from
    A. respiratory alkalosis.
    B. metabolic acidosis.
    C. hypervolemia.
    D. metabolic alkalosis.

61. Baroreceptor reflexes cause a change primarily in which of these components of the cardiovascular system?
    A. vena cava
    B. venules
    C. arterioles
    D. capillaries

62. The first step in glucose metabolism results in the formation of pyruvic acid. This is a(n)
    A. lactate process.
    B. anaerobic process.
    C. aerobic process.
    D. gluconeogenic process.

63. Hypovolemia impacts cardiac output by
    A. reducing preload, thus decreasing cardiac output.
    B. increasing afterload, thus increasing cardiac output.
    C. reducing afterload, thus decreasing cardiac output.
    D. increasing preload, thus increasing cardiac output.

64. The body compensates for shock in all of the following ways **except**
    A. vasoconstriction of the arterioles and venules of the skin.
    B. initiation of the renin-angiotension pathway to increase blood pressure.
    C. intravascular clotting maintains blood volume by limiting blood loss.
    D. increased reabsorption of sodium and water to restore blood volume.

65. Which of the following will reverse anaerobic metabolism?
    A. a decrease in perfusion and an increase in oxygenation
    B. an increase in perfusion and a decrease in hypoxia
    C. an increase in perfusion and a decrease in oxygenation
    D. a decrease in perfusion and an increase in hypoxia

66. Which of the following will improve cardiac output?
    A. an increase in stroke volume and an increase in heart rate
    B. a decrease in stroke volume and a decrease in heart rate
    C. an increase in systemic vascular resistance
    D. a reduction in preload

67. Constriction of the venous side of the vascular system will result in
    A. decreased cardiac preload.
    B. increased cardiac preload.
    C. decreased afterload.
    D. decreased blood pressure.

68. Which of the following best describes the physiology of decompensated shock?

    A. Precapillary sphincters relax, postcapillary sphincters remain closed, and capillary pressure diminishes.

    B. Cardiac preload is reduced, and heart rate and peripheral vascular resistance increase to maintain blood pressure and perfusion.

    C. Prolonged inadequate tissue perfusion results in cellular death; the result is the same even if perfusion and vital signs return.

    D. The venous system constricts, reducing the vascular container size, and blood is directed away from noncritical areas such as the skin.

69. The body responds to shock by improving cardiac output. This can occur by

    A. decreasing heart rate and decreasing stroke volume.

    B. decreasing heart rate and increasing stroke volume.

    C. increasing heart rate and decreasing stroke volume.

    D. increasing heart rate and increasing stroke volume.

70. When the baroreceptors in the carotid bodies and the aortic arch detect a decrease in blood pressure, which of the following occurs?

    A. stimulation of the parasympathetic nervous system resulting in a decreased heart rate

    B. stimulation of the parasympathetic nervous system resulting in an increased heart rate

    C. stimulation of the sympathetic nervous system resulting in a decreased heart rate

    D. stimulation of the sympathetic nervous system resulting in an increased heart rate

71. Which stage of shock is characterized by a drop in blood pressure?

    A. compensated shock

    B. fatal shock

    C. irreversible shock

    D. decompensated shock

72. Which statement best describes shock and its relationship to the body's metabolic process?

    A. Low perfusion results in anaerobic metabolism, which leads to excessive lactic acid production.

    B. Low perfusion results in aerobic metabolism, which leads to excessive lactic acid production.

    C. Low perfusion pressure results in anaerobic metabolism, which leads to reduced lactic acid production.

    D. High perfusion pressure results in anaerobic metabolism, which leads to reduced lactic acid production.

73. Appropriate tissue oxygenation depends on adequate perfusion. Three primary factors influence perfusion. These factors are

    A. adequate heart rate, adequate fluid, and an intact vascular system.

    B. adequate pump, adequate fluid, and an intact vascular system.

    C. adequate pump, adequate fluid, and a dilated vascular system.

    D. adequate heart rate, adequate fluid, and a dilated vascular system.

74. Which statement best describes why it is important for the EMT-Intermediate to adequately ventilate a patient with hypoperfusion or shock?

    A. Increasing the oxygen concentration improves cerebral blood flow.

    B. Increasing the oxygen concentration causes arterial vasoconstriction.

    C. Removal of carbon dioxide is important in reducing the accumulation of body acids.

    D. Removal of carbon dioxide will increase the acid and reduce the pH.

75. An increase in peripheral vascular resistance with compensated shock will be measured by a(n)

    A. increase in systolic blood pressure.

    B. increase in diastolic blood pressure.

    C. decrease in systolic blood pressure.

    D. decrease in diastolic blood pressure.

76. What effect does peripheral vasodilation have on blood return to the heart?

    A. Blood return to the heart is decreased.

    B. Blood return to the heart is increased.

    C. Blood return to the heart is unchanged.

    D. Blood return to the heart is minimally increased.

77. Hypoperfusion or shock may result in cerebral hypoxia. Which of the following is an early sign of cerebral hypoxia?

    A. a slowing pulse rate

    B. restlessness or anxiety

    C. presence of decerebrate posturing

    D. presence of decorticate posturing

78. Which of the following signs would be consistent with decompensated shock?

    A. pink color skin

    B. strong regular pulse of 90

    C. narrow pulse pressure

    D. warm, dry skin

79. One principal problem for a patient in shock is the excessive production of acid. This production of acid is primarily a result of

    A. decreased production of pyruvate.

    B. increased activity of the sodium/potassium pump.

    C. the liberation of lysosomes.

    D. a shift to anaerobic metabolism.

80. A patient has sustained a laceration to the forearm from a bar fight. When you arrive, the patient is still bleeding profusely. You quickly control the bleed, and during your assessment you find the following vitals: HR 110, RR 30, BP 110/88. Skin is cool, diaphoretic, and pale to the extremities. Your patient is in what stage of shock?

    A. irreversible shock

    B. progressive shock

    C. compensated shock

    D. decompensated shock

81. When a person is suffering from distributive shock, the blood pressure characteristically drops because of

    A. an increase in the heart rate.

    B. a drop in the cardiac preload.

    C. severe vasoconstriction.

    D. an increase in stroke volume.

82. Anaerobic metabolism may be reduced by

    A. decreasing cardiac preload.

    B. decreasing afterload.

    C. widening the pulse pressure.

    D. improving the FiO_2.

83. The most reliable indicator of cerebral perfusion status in shock is
    A. the level of consciousness.
    B. a Glasgow Coma Score over 8.
    C. a normal pupillary response.
    D. moist mucosal membranes.

84. The baroreceptors monitor
    A. carbon dioxide levels.
    B. oxygen levels.
    C. blood pressure.
    D. the heart rate.

85. A significant increase in hydrostatic pressure in the pulmonary capillary network will have which of the following effects on oxygenation?
    A. It will improve oxygenation of tissue because of an increase in perfusion pressures.
    B. Hypoxia will occur from leakage of fluid into the alveolar-capillary interface, interfering with gas diffusion.
    C. It will reduce the amount of gas flowing into the alveoli from the terminal bronchiole.
    D. Oxygen diffusion is improved because of the increased number of red blood cells in the alveolar capillary interface.

86. You arrive on-scene and find a patient with a suspected intraabdominal bleed from blunt trauma. The blood pressure is 102/84 mmHg. The skin is pale, cool, and clammy. The diastolic blood pressure reflects
    A. decompensatory shock.
    B. an increase in cardiac output.

    C. an increase in systemic vascular resistance.
    D. a widening in the pulse pressure.

87. Which of the following is an early sign of an increase in systemic vascular resistance?
    A. an increase in heart rate
    B. a decreased mental status
    C. pale, cool, clammy skin
    D. a decrease in systolic blood pressure

88. A decrease in venous volume will
    A. increase stroke volume.
    B. trigger peripheral vasodilation.
    C. increase cerebral perfusion pressure.
    D. reduce preload in the left ventricle.

89. Eventually, the normal saline or lactated Ringer's that was infused in a trauma patient will move out of the vascular space. This is primarily because of
    A. diffusion of the charged particles.
    B. osmosis of the plasma proteins.
    C. active transport of dextrose molecules.
    D. nonpermeable capillary membranes.

90. The immediate response of the body to a decrease in blood pressure is innervated through which of the following?
    A. hormonal response from the sympathetic nervous system
    B. vagal nerve impulses
    C. direct neural stimulation from the sympathetic nervous system
    D. parasympathetic nervous stimulation and release of acetylcholine

91. The cascade effect of nervous system innervation and the hormonal response seen in the compensatory phase of shock is initiated primarily by
    A. an increase in systemic vascular resistance.
    B. a decrease in the PaO_2 recognized by the medullary chemoreceptor.
    C. a change in the perfusion pressure in the kidney.
    D. a decrease in the volume of blood and pressure found in the aortic arch and carotid bodies.

92. An increase in the stretch of the baroreceptor would cause which of the following effects?
    A. an increase in the heart rate and stroke volume
    B. a decrease in peripheral vascular resistance
    C. vasoconstriction of the systemic vessels
    D. an increase in stroke volume and peripheral resistance

93. The best clinical indicator of early peripheral vasoconstriction is measured by assessing the
    A. heart rate.
    B. skin color, temperature, and condition.
    C. systolic blood pressure.
    D. pupillary response to light.

94. Diaphoretic skin found in shock patients is typically a result of
    A. alpha properties stimulation of the sweat glands.
    B. antidiuretic hormone effect on sodium reabsorption.
    C. beta receptor stimulation.
    D. an increase in cardiac output.

95. During the ischemic phase of shock, what occurs in the microcirculation?
    A. The precapillary sphincters open, and the postcapillary venules close.
    B. The arteriovenular shunts close, and the precapillary sphincters close.
    C. The precapillary sphincters close, and the postcapillary venules close.
    D. The precapillary spincters open, and the postcapillary venules open.

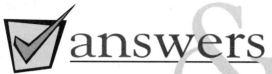

answers & rationales

Following each rationale, you will find a reference to the corresponding objective in the DOT National Standard EMT-Intermediate curriculum. An asterisk denotes material that is supplemental to the DOT curriculum. Page numbers after a rationale indicate where the question topic may be discussed in the Brady text *Intermediate Emergency Care* (Bledsoe, Porter, Cherry).

1.

A. The amount of blood ejected by the heart at one contraction is referred to as the stroke volume. Stroke volume is determined by preload, afterload, and contractile force. (*) (IEC p. 840)

2.

D. Preload could be increased by increasing venous return, by increasing the contractile force of the heart, and by decreasing the afterload. (*) (IEC p. 840)

3.

C. The amount of blood pumped from the heart in one contraction is called stroke volume. (*) (IEC p. 196)

4.

C. The greater the volume of the preload is, the more the ventricles are stretched. The greater the stretch, up to a certain point, the greater the subsequent cardiac contraction. This is referred to as Starling's law of the heart (also called the Frank Starling mechanism). (*) (IEC pp. 197, 840)

5.

C. The amount of blood pumped from the heart in 1 minute is called cardiac output. Cardiac output is calculated by stroke volume times heart rate. (*) (IEC p. 198)

6.

C. The amount of resistance against which the heart must pump is called afterload. The heart must overcome this resistance in order to eject blood. Afterload is determined by the degree of peripheral vascular resistance. Peripheral resistance is determined by the degree of vasoconstriction present on the arterial side. (*) (IEC pp. 197, 840)

7.

B. Arteries consist of three distinct layers: the tunica intima (innermost), tunica media (muscular), and tunica adventitia (outer covering). The tunica media allows the vessel to regulate blood flow by increasing or decreasing its lumen through muscle constriction and dilation. In fact, arterioles can change their size by a factor of 6. (*)

8.

B. Arterioles have the greatest ability to vary the size of their inner lumen via constriction or dilation. (*)

9.

A. The capillaries are microscopic vessels that lack the muscular and connective layers of arteries and veins. They are one cell thick and contain 7% of the vascular volume. (*)

10.

B. Plasma makes up approximately 55% of the total blood volume. It consists of 92% water, 6–7% proteins, and a small portion consisting of electrolytes, lipids, enzymes, clotting factors, glucose, and other dissolved substances. (*) (IEC p. 106)

11.

B. The percentage of blood occupied by red blood cells is referred to as the hematocrit. Normal hematocrit in the healthy person is approximately 45%. (*) (IEC p. 106)

12.

B. Red blood cells account for approximately 45% of the total blood volume. This percentage is known as the patient's hematocrit. (*) (IEC p. 106)

13.

D. There are three phases of clotting: the vascular phase (where the vessel constricts), the platelet phase (where platelets adhere to blood vessel walls), and the coagulation phase (where fibrin forms a network around the wound for protection). (*) (IEC p. 644)

14.

A. The clotting mechanism normally takes between 7 and 10 minutes to stop the flow of blood. The nature of the wound and other factors affect how rapidly and well the clotting mechanisms respond to hemorrhage. (*) (IEC p. 644)

15.

C. A clean, lateral cut of a blood vessel allows the vessel to retract and thicken its wall. This reduces the lumen, reduces blood flow, and assists in the clotting mechanism. In this type of case, blood loss usually will not be life threatening. A longitudinal cut to a vessel would cause the wound to open wider as the vessel constricts in an attempt to control the bleeding. This would lead to more severe bleeding. (4-2.4) (IEC p. 644)

16.

B. The clotting process normally works very well unless inhibited by the following factors: movement of the wound site (tears the clot loose), aggressive fluid therapy (increases pressure and dilutes clotting factors), hypothermia (slows the process), and medications (such as aspirin, NSAIDs, warfarin). (4-2.7) (IEC pp. 645–646)

17.

A. External hemorrhage should be controlled in the following manner: direct pressure over the wound site and elevation, pressure point compression, and, as a last resort, application of an artery-constricting tourniquet. (4-2.7) (IEC pp. 646–647)

18.

D. A moderate to severe nosebleed, known as epistaxis, can be caused by direct trauma, hypertension, a strong sneeze, or dry air. (*) (IEC p. 649)

19.

A. Hemoptysis, coughing up bright red blood, is due to a disruption in the alveolar-capillary membrane. This is caused by certain degenerative diseases, such as tuberculosis or cancer, or by chest trauma. (4-2.4) (IEC p. 649)

20.

D. Melena is black, tarry feces due to gastrointestinal bleeding, usually indicating digested blood. (4-2.4) (IEC p. 649)

21.

D. At greater than 35% blood loss, a person will present with profound hypotension because he has lost the massive vasoconstriction that helped maintain the blood pressure. As the precapillary sphincters reopened, the blood pressure dropped. This marks the beginning of decompensated shock. (4-2.11, 4-2.30) (IEC p. 651)

22.

D. The elderly are more adversely affected by blood loss because of their lower fluid volume reserve, slower and less responsive compensatory mechanisms, reduced perception of pain, and lower levels of mental acuity and because of the presence of medications such as beta blockers and anticoagulants. (4-2.1, 4-2.3) (IEC p. 652)

23.

D. Pelvic fractures can account for more than 2 liters of blood loss. If you suspect a fracture, always maintain the stability and integrity of the pelvic ring to minimize the possibility of lacerating a major blood vessel. (4-2.3) (IEC p. 654)

24.

A. Hematochezia is the passage of stools containing red blood. This usually represents active bleeding in the colon or rectum or internal hemorrhoids. (4-2.4) (IEC p. 655)

25.

C. A positive tilt test occurs when the pulse rate increases by 10–20 beats per minute or the BP decreases by 10–20 mm Hg when a patient moves from a supine to a sitting position. This is known as orthostatic hypotension and is the result of relative hypovolemia. When assessing for orthostatic hypotension, you must understand that a large percentage of the population, especially the elderly, will experience a drop in systolic blood pressure of 10–20 mm Hg when normovolemic. Thus, a drop in the systolic blood pressure is not a sensitve test when assessing for orthostatic hypotension. The most sensitive variable is an increase in the heart rate. An increase in the heart rate of 30 beats per minute or greater is a good indication that the patient has lost a significant amount of volume. (4-2.4) (IEC p. 655)

26.

A. Glycolysis is the first stage of the process in which the cell breaks apart an energy source and releases a small amount of energy. It requires no oxygen at this stage. (*)

27.

C. The Krebs cycle, also known as the citric acid cycle, is the second stage of metabolism, requiring the presence of oxygen, in which the breakdown of glucose yields a great amount of energy. This is also known as aerobic metabolism. (*)

28.

A. The precapillary sphincters regulate the flow of blood into a capillary bed. They will open when the oxygen supply decreases, the carbon dioxide level increases, the pH falls, or histamine is released. This process is just one component of the homeostatic control process. (4-2.20)

29.

D. The interstitial and intracellular spaces represent 88% of the body's total fluid volume. In a crisis, the body can draw on this reservoir by closing the precapillary sphincters, drawing fluid from the interstitial spaces and cells into the capillary bed, and returning this fluid to the general circulation through the opened postcapillary venule. (4-2.20)

30.

D. Venous return is aided by skeletal muscle contractions (help push the blood against gravity), valves in the veins (prevent backflow), and respirations (create negative pressure in the chest). (4-2.20)

31.

D. Baroreceptors are located in the carotid bodies and the arch of the aorta. These baroreceptors closely monitor pressure. (4-2.20)

32.

A. Baroreceptors are stretch receptors that stretch with increased pressure. When they detect reduced flow and pressure, they send messages to the brain to stimulate the sympathetic nervous system. This results in increased heart rate and cardiac output to increase circulation and bronchodilation. (4-2.20)

Matching (4-2.20)

33.   C epinephrine
34.   D ADH
35.   F angiotensin II
36.   H aldosterone
37.   G glucagon
38.   B ACTH
39.   E growth hormone
40.   A erythropoietin

41.

D. During periods of inadequate tissue perfusion, cell metabolism switches from an aerobic to an anaerobic mode. Results of this process are inefficient energy, an increase in pyruvic acid formation, and continued glycolysis as long as glucose remains available. (4-2.20)

42.

A. Following the onset of inadequate tissue perfusion, various compensatory mechanisms of the body are stimulated. The heart rate and strength of cardiac contractions increase. There will be an increase in systemic vascular resistance to assist in maintaining the blood pressure. These compensatory changes will continue until the body is unable to maintain blood pressure and tissue perfusion. Your patient in compensatory shock will exhibit tachycardia, cool, clammy, and pale skin with a stable blood pressure. (4-2.21) (IEC p. 661)

43.

D. In the later stages of shock, the blood pressure begins to fall, and blood supply to essential organs diminishes. As a result, the precapillary sphincters open, while the postcapillary sphincters remain closed. This results in sludging of red blood cells and the formation of rouleaux. (4-2.24) (IEC p. 660)

Matching (4-2.2)

44.	C	hypovolemic
45.	G	anaphylactic
46.	F	septic
47.	A	obstructive
48.	E	cardiogenic
49.	D	respiratory
50.	B	neurogenic

51.

B. Baroreceptors are special pressure receptors found only in the aortic arch and carotid bodies. These sensors monitor the degree of arterial pressure and provide feedback to the vasomotor center in the medulla regarding the degree of arterial tone. Chemoreceptors monitor O_2, CO_2, and hydrogen levels for respiratory efficiency. (4-2.20)

52.

A. A decrease in preload decreases coronary artery perfusion, which occurs only during diastole. (4-2.3)

53.

A. As long as there is a radial pulse, perfusion pressures are considered to generally be at a resuscitation level that is acceptable. If, however, the patient continues to lose blood to the point where compensatory mechanisms fail, the radial pulse will disappear. If this happens, it generally correlates with the patient progressing from compensatory shock to decompensatory shock. (4-2.21)

54.

A. A negative feedback system for shock patients is closure of precapillary sphincters. This will direct blood away from the nonessential vascular beds of the periphery back to core perfusion. This effectively decreases the size of the vascular "container," which brings the amount of volume and the "container" size closer to normal proportions. The body tries, as long as possible, to maintain perfusion to the heart, lungs, brain, and kidneys. (4-2.20)

55.

D. Because of a diminishment in preload (presumably caused by pulmonary vessel damage from the assault), there will be less blood for the heart to pump out. This will result in a drop in stroke volume that will subsequently cause a drop in cardiac output and blood pressure. (4-2.3)

56.

B. Damage to the mitral valve will allow regurgitation of blood backward through the left atrium, pulmonary veins, and into the perialveolar capillary beds. Here, hydrostatic pressure will increase to a point where fluid is forced into the alveoli, causing pulmonary edema. (4-2.4)

57.

C. An increase in the force of ventricular contraction will cause improvement in the stroke volume. This leads to better cardiac output and an increased systolic blood pressure. (4-2.20)

58.

D. Dyspnea associated with inspiratory crackles is very characteristic of pump failure. One role of the EMT-Intermediate is to delineate the different presentations of shock—either a volume, a pump, or a container problem. There may be associated hypotension, which is not treated with fluid bolus. (4-2.4)

59.

B. Systemic vascular resistance relates to the degree of pressure that exists in the peripheral vasculature when not influenced by cardiac output. Therefore, an appropriate measure of this pressure can be estimated by using the diastolic number obtained in the blood pressure. Consequently, the systolic pressure is incorrect in that this is a measurement of pressure created by actual cardiac output. Also, the palpation of a radial pulse is a function of cardiac output and is incorrect. The pulse pressure is an indicator of the degree to which a body is compensating during illness or injury. (4-2.4)

60.

D. Extensive vomiting results in a loss of hydrogen cations from the body. Such a loss causes an increase in pH and results in metabolic alkalosis. Respiratory alkalosis is a result of a disproportionate loss of CO_2

through the respiratory system. Metabolic acidosis would indicate the loss of a base or an unbuffered increase in the hydrogen cation. Hypervolemia is incorrect in that this suggests an overloading of fluid. (4-2.4)

61.

C. Neural stimuli initiated by the baroreceptors causes pronounced smooth-muscle contraction or relaxation of the arterioles, resulting in changes in the blood pressure. The vena cava, venules, and capillaries contain little to no smooth muscle, so minimal or no contraction/relaxation occurs. (4-2.20)

62.

B. The initial step in glucose metabolism by the cell (glycolysis) is an anaerobic process that results in the formation of pyruvic acid. If oxygen is not available to continue the process, pyruvic acid will convert to lactic acid. (*)

63.

A. Cardiac output is decreased when hypovolemia reduces preload, the blood available to the pump. Adequate tissue perfusion is dependent on a functional and well-oxygenated pump (heart), adequate volume (blood), and an intact container (blood vessels). The fluid-container-volume ratio must match. (4-2.3)

64.

C. Compensatory mechanisms for shock are mediated by the sympathetic nervous system, and the release of various substances after the decrease in blood volume is recognized by baroreceptors. These mechanisms include vasoconstriction of the arterioles and venules of the skin, initiation of the renin-angiotension pathway to increase blood pressure, and increased reabsorption of sodium and water to restore blood volume. (4-2.20)

65.

B. In poor perfusion states and hypoxia, an inadequate amount of oxygen is available to the cells, resulting in anaerobic metabolism. You can increase perfusion by positioning the patient, replacing the lost volume, and hemorrhage control. Hypoxia can be decreased by administering oxygen and ensuring adequate alveolar ventilation. (4-2.3)

66.

A. An increase in either stroke volume or heart rate will improve the patient's cardiac output. Decreasing the stroke volume or the heart rate will cause a decrease in cardiac output. Decreased preload and an increase in systemic vascular resistance will decrease cardiac output. (4-2.20) (IEC pp. 198, 840)

67.

B. Cardiac preload is increased when the venous side of the vascular system contracts, decreasing capacitance (the size of the container). (4-2.20) (IEC p. 197)

68.

A. All of these are associated with decompensated shock. Also, blood supply to essential organs diminishes, and blood pressure falls. (4-2.20)

69.

D. An increase in stroke volume or heart rate or both can increase cardiac output. In the early

(compensated) stage of shock, increased cardiac output can be detected by an increasing pulse rate. (4-2.20) (IEC pp. 198, 840)

70.

D. If the blood pressure falls, the baroreceptors stimulate the sympathetic nervous system. Both the heart rate and cardiac contractility are increased along with an increase in systemic vascular resistance. (4-2.20)

71.

D. In decompensated shock, the blood supply— and consequently the oxygen supply—to the organs decreases, and the blood pressure begins to fall. The pulse and respirations continue to increase. The patient's level of consciousness deteriorates to confusion and eventually coma. (4-2.24) (IEC pp. 661-662)

72.

A. Low perfusion states (hypoperfusion) or shock leads to a reduction in oxygen transported to body cells. Normal metabolic processes utilize oxygen to degrade pyruvic acid into carbon dioxide, water, and energy. In low perfusion states where oxygen is not present, the pyruvic acid is not degraded. The pyruvic acid collects and degrades into lactic acid. The accumulation of lactic acid and other metabolic acids results in cellular death. Cellular death leads to tissue death, tissue death leads to organ death, organ death leads to system death, and system death leads to the death of the patient. (4-2.3)

73.

B. The movement and utilization of oxygen is dependent on factors that make up what is called the "Fick Principle." The factors are adequate oxygen in the inspired air, oxygen "loaded" on red blood cells, adequate tissue perfusion, and oxygen "off-load" at the body tissues. The three factors required for adequate tissue perfusion are functioning pump, adequate fluid levels, and an intact container. All three must be working appropriately to produce adequate perfusion pressures. Failure of any one will result in hypoperfusion. Hypoperfusion will yield inadequate oxygenation of body cells or tissues. (*) (IEC pp. 195-199)

74.

C. It is important to adequately ventilate shock patients in order to reduce the acidotic state. Lactic acid production results in the accumulation of hydrogen ions. The more hydrogen ions present in a solution, the more acidic the solution. Ensuring adequate ventilation reduces the number of hydrogen ions present and reduces the total accumulated acids in the patient's body. Make sure the shock patient's ventilations are adequately supported. (4-2.6)

75.

B. Peripheral vascular resistance or afterload is reflected by the diastolic blood pressure. As the peripheral vascular resistance increases, the diastolic blood pressure increases. The reverse occurs as well: when the peripheral vascular resistance decreases, the diastolic blood pressure decreases. You would expect to see a slight increase in the diastolic blood pressure as the body's compensatory mechanisms adjust to the diminished perfusion. An early reaction during compensated shock is to increase the peripheral vascular resistance. (4-2.21)

76.

A. Blood return, or what is called preload, is decreased with vasodilation. The "container"

size is increased with peripheral vasodilation. If the amount of fluid in the body remains constant, the amount of fluid available to return to the heart is reduced. The container becomes larger than the available fluid. Some conditions that cause peripheral vasodilation include decompensated shock, anaphylaxis, septic shock, and vasogenic shock. (4-2.24) (IEC pp. 198-199)

77.

B. Restlessness or anxiety is an early sign of cerebral hypoxia. This is a result of diminished perfusion and oxygenation of cerebral tissue. An alteration in the patient's level of consciousness, disorientation, and confusion are signs of cerebral hypoperfusion and hypercapnea. (4-2.4) (IEC p. 663)

78.

C. Signs of decompensated shock would include an increase in the pulse rate and a decrease in the pulse amplitude. A falling systolic blood pressure is a late sign that is observed in decompensated shock. The skin color would be pale or cyanotic, cool, and moist. The pulse pressure will become more narrow as the condition progresses. (4-2.25)

79.

D. Anaerobic metabolism occurs when there is a lack of sufficient oxygen for cellular metabolism. This leads to production of lactic acid. Failure of the sodium/potassium pump from hypoxemia causes cells to rupture and the liberation of lysosome. (4-2.3)

80.

C. There are three clinical stages of shock: compensatory, decompensatory, and irreversible. This patient is exhibiting signs of the first stage. (4-2.21) (IEC p. 661)

81.

B. During distributive shock, there is profound peripheral vasodilation, causing blood pooling in the extremities and promoting hypotension. This will decrease the amount of blood returning to the heart, causing a diminished preload. The decreased preload will decrease cardiac output and blood pressure. (4-2.2, 4-2.3)

82.

D. Anaerobic metabolism occurs when there is an insufficient supply of oxygen available to meet the demands of the tissues. Constantly ensure that the patient is receiving an appropriate amount of oxygen (increase FiO_2, or the fraction of inspired oxygen). (4-2.6)

83.

A. During shock, the brain is also affected by hypoperfusion. The best indicator of poor cerebral perfusion is decreased mental status. Pupillary response will usually be altered also by hypoperfusion, but it is not as reliable as the level of consciousness. (4-2.4)

84.

C. Baroreceptors are specialized sensors located in the aortic arch and carotid bodies. These unique sensors monitor blood pressure in these arterial blood vessels and feed this information to the vasomotor center in the medulla. Peripheral chemoreceptors are sensors that monitor oxygen levels, and central chemoreceptors are sensors that monitor hydrogen levels and are located on the medulla. There are no specific receptors for monitoring the heart rate. (4-2.3)

85.

B. An increase in pulmonary capillary hydrostatic pressure will cause fluid to leak out of the capillary and fill the space between the alveoli and the capillary, interfering with oxygen and carbon dioxide diffusion. This will eventually lead to hypoxia. (4-2.3)

86.

C. The diastolic blood pressure is a measurement of the systemic vascular resistance. The narrow pulse pressure (systolic minus the diastolic) and pale, cool, clammy skin are indicative of peripheral vasoconstriction, which causes an increased systemic vascular resistance. (4-2.4)

87.

C. The earliest sign of an increase in systemic vascular resistance is pale, cool, clammy skin. This sign results from a decreased perfusion of peripheral skin and subcutaneous tissue. (4-2.4)

88.

D. A decrease in venous volume will directly result in a reduction in the preload or the amount of blood in the left ventricle at the end of diastole. (4-2.3) (IEC pp. 197, 840)

89.

A. Diffusion of the charged particles out of the vascular space will cause a change in the osmotic pressure inside the vessel and will allow the fluid to leave with the electrolytes. (*)

90.

C. An immediate response to a drop in blood pressure causes a direct neural response from the sympathetic nervous system. A nerve fiber stimulates the adrenal medulla to release catecholamines, epinephrine, and norepinephrine. It takes a few minutes for the hormonal response to be activated. (4-2.3)

91.

D. A decrease in the blood volume and pressure in the aortic arch and carotid bodies cause a decrease in the stretch of the baroreceptor. The baroreceptor initiates the cascade effect of compensatory mechanisms seen in shock. (4-2.20)

92.

B. An increase in the stretch of the baroreceptor indicates an increase in pressure. To reduce the pressure, the body's response will be to reduce heart rate, stroke volume, and peripheral vascular resistance by vasodilation. (4-2.3)

93.

B. Pale, cool, clammy skin provides the earliest sign of peripheral vasoconstriction. Since the skin is the most nonessential organ, its perfusion is reduced first through peripheral vasoconstriction. The blood is shunted away from the periphery and toward the core circulation. (4-2.21)

94.

A. Patients in shock commonly present with diaphoretic skin. This results from stimulation of the sweat glands by alpha properties found in epinephrine and norepinephrine. Diaphoresis also results as a neural response from direct nerve fiber stimulation of the sweat glands. (4-2.3)

95.

C. During the ischemic phase of shock, the precapillary sphincters close, the arteriovenular shunt opens, and the postcapillary venules close. This allows the blood to be directed away from the capillary bed and back into the core circulation. (4-2.3) (IEC p. 660)

UNIT

3 Burns

unit objectives

Questions in this unit relate to DOT Objectives 4-3.1 to 4-3.58. The objectives are listed in the Appendix.

DIRECTIONS Each of the questions or incomplete statements below is followed by suggested answers or completions. Select the **one answer** that is best in each case.

1. The extent of burn injury depends on which of the following factors?
   A. temperature
   B. concentration of heat energy
   C. length of contact time
   D. all of the above

2. According to Jackson's theory of thermal wounds, which of the following zones suffers the greatest amount of tissue damage?
   A. zone of stasis
   B. zone of coagulation
   C. zone of hyperemia
   D. zone of emergence

3. Which of the following lists the phases of a thermal burn in their proper chronological order?
   A. resolution, emergent, hypermetabolic, fluid shift
   B. hypermetabolic, fluid shift, resolution, emergent
   C. emergent, fluid shift, hypermetabolic, resolution
   D. fluid shift, resolution, emergent, hypermetabolic

4. Liquefaction necrosis is caused by
   A. acid burns.
   B. alkali burns.
   C. either A or B.
   D. neither A nor B.

5. Which of the following types of radiation emits the most powerful rays?
   A. alpha
   B. beta
   C. delta
   D. gamma

6. The extent of radiation depends on which of the following factors?
   A. duration of exposure
   B. distance from the source
   C. shielding from the source
   D. all of the above

7. Cumulative radiation exposure is measured with a(n)
   A. dosimeter.
   B. radmeter.
   C. Gray device.
   D. Geiger counter.

8. Any patient who has been in an enclosed area during combustion should be suspected of having
   A. pulmonary embolism.
   B. pulmonary edema.
   C. carbon monoxide poisoning.
   D. hyponatremia.

9. Which of the following is most likely to cause subglottic burns?
   A. hot air
   B. flame
   C. steam
   D. hot gases

10. Your patient, who presents with dyspnea and hoarseness following the inhalation of superheated steam, is in danger of developing
    A. pulmonary embolism.
    B. complete upper-airway obstruction.
    C. anaphylaxis.
    D. bronchospasm.

11. A burn involving the epidermis and dermis, producing blisters and pain, is classified as
    A. first degree.
    B. second degree.
    C. superficial.
    D. full thickness.

12. An adult with burns to both arms, chest, abdomen, and entire back has a _____% BSA burn.
    A. 36
    B. 45
    C. 54
    D. 63

13. An infant with burns to both legs has a _____% BSA burn.
    A. 9
    B. 14
    C. 18
    D. 27

14. Which of the following is a complication of a burn injury?
    A. hypothermia
    B. hypovolemia
    C. eschar
    D. all of the above

15. The major complication of circumferential burns is the
    A. fluid loss in the burn area.
    B. loss of a barrier against infection.
    C. tourniquet effect, cutting off distal circulation.
    D. anaerobic metabolism proximal to the burn site.

16. According to the American Burn Association, which of the following patients should be evaluated in a burn center?
    A. partial thickness burn to >15% of BSA
    B. full-thickness burn to >5% of BSA
    C. high-voltage electrical injuries
    D. all of the above

17. What percentage of partial thickness burns can be safely cooled with water?
    A. <15%
    B. 15–20%
    C. 20–25%
    D. 25–50%

18. Partial thickness burns over 15% or full-thickness burns over 5% of BSA should be managed by
    A. rapid cooling with water.
    B. water and fanning.
    C. applying ice to the burned area.
    D. dry, sterile dressings.

19. Standard management of chemical burns includes
    A. rinsing the area with ice water.
    B. using a neutralizing agent.
    C. leaving any corrosive materials on the skin.
    D. irrigating vigorously with cool water.

20. Which of the following substances can you safely irrigate?
    A. sodium
    B. phenol
    C. lye
    D. dry lime

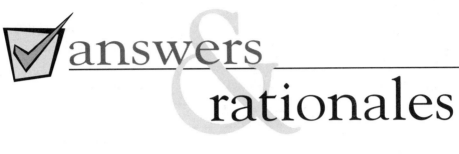

answers & rationales

Following each rationale, you will find a reference to the corresponding objective in the DOT National Standard EMT-Intermediate curriculum. An asterisk denotes material that is supplemental to the DOT curriculum. Page numbers after a rationale indicate where the question topic may be discussed in the Brady text *Intermediate Emergency Care* (Bledsoe, Porter, Cherry).

1.

D. The extent of burn injury depends on the amount of heat energy transferred to the patient's body. When assessing the severity of a burn injury, focus on three important factors: the temperature, the concentration of heat energy, and the length of contact time. (4-3.7) (IEC p. 673)

2.

B. According to Jackson's theory on thermal wounds, the zone of coagulation suffers the most damage because it is the nearest to the source. Cell membranes rupture and are destroyed, blood coagulates, and structural proteins denature. (4-3.16) (IEC p. 674)

3.

C. The body's response to burns includes the following stages in order: emergent (catecholamine release), fluid shift (massive external plasma losses), hypermetabolic (major need for nutrients for tissue repair), and resolution (scarring and rehabilitation). (4-3.16) (IEC p. 674)

4.

B. Liquefaction necrosis is the process by which an alkali dissolves and liquefies tissue. The alkali quickly penetrates the skin and causes progressively deeper burns. Acid burns are generally less severe because they result in coagulation necrosis, which forms a protective layer that limits further damage. (4-3.32) (IEC p. 677)

5.

D. Gamma radiation, also known as X-rays, is the most powerful ionizing radiation. It has the ability to travel through the entire body or ionize any atom within. It is the most dangerous and most feared type of radiation because it is difficult to protect against. (4-3.48) (IEC p. 678)

6.

D. The extent of a radiation injury depends on three important factors: the duration of the exposure, the distance from the source, and the shielding from the source. (4-3.50) (IEC p. 679)

7.

A. A Geiger counter measures immediate radiation exposure, while a dosimeter measures cumulative exposure. (4-3.51) (IEC p. 679)

8.

C. Any patient who has been in an enclosed area during combustion should be suspected of having carbon monoxide poisoning. Carbon monoxide is a by-product of incomplete combustion. Poisoning occurs because the hemoglobin of the blood has a much greater affinity for carbon monoxide than it does for oxygen. If your patient inhales carbon monoxide, it will displace oxygen, resulting in hypoxemia. (4-3.28) (IEC p. 681)

9.

C. Superheated steam has a greater heat content than air, flame, or gas and can cause subglottic (below the glottis) burns. (4-3.25) (IEC p. 681)

10.

B. A patient who inhales superheated steam and presents with shortness of breath, difficulty breathing, and hoarseness is in danger of developing a complete airway obstruction. Superheated steam contains enough energy to severely burn the upper airway. If damaged, this tissue will swell rapidly and seriously reduce the size of the airway lumen. The patient who presents with minor hoarseness may develop a complete airway obstruction later on. (4-3.27) (IEC p. 681)

11.

B. A second-degree, or partial thickness, burn involves the epidermis and the dermis. It produces blisters and is extremely painful. (4-3.5) (IEC p. 681)

12.

C. The rule of nines states that in the adult patient, the arms are worth 9% each, the chest and abdomen 18%, and the entire back 18%. This patient, therefore, has a 54% body surface area (BSA) burn. (4-3.6) (IEC p. 683)

13.

D. In the child, the rule of nines differs slightly. The head, being larger in proportion to the rest of the body, is worth 18%. The legs, therefore, are 13.5% each. So a child with burns to both legs has a 27% BSA burn. (4-3.6) (IEC p. 683)

14.

D. Some complications of burns include hypothermia (loss of body heat through the burn area), hypovolemia (plasma loss through the burn area), and eschar (destruction of skin cells). (4-3.10) (IEC p. 684)

15.

C. A circumferential burn encircles the complete exterior of an extremity. In these types of burns, the constriction may be severe enough to occlude all blood flow into the distal extremity. In the case of a thoracic burn, it may drastically reduce chest expansion, reducing respiratory tidal volume. (4-3.10) (IEC p. 684)

16.

D. According to the American Burn Association, the following burn injuries should be evaluated in a burn center: (4-3.13) (IEC p. 690)

- Partial thickness burn >15% BSA
- Full-thickness burn >5% BSA
- Significant face, feet, hands, perineal burns
- High-voltage electrical injuries
- Inhalation injuries
- Chemical burns causing progressive tissue destruction
- Associated significant injuries

17.

A. Use local cooling to treat minor soft-tissue burns that involve only a small portion of the body surface area at partial thickness. Care for only those burns that involve less than 15% of the body surface area in this way. (4-3.13) (IEC p. 692)

18.

D. Use dry sterile dressings to treat partial thickness burns over 30% of the body or full-thickness burns over 5% of the body surface area. This will reduce air movement past the sensitive first- and second-degree burns and provide padding against minor bumping. In the third-degree burn, they provide a barrier to possible contamination. (4-3.13) (IEC p. 693)

19.

D. Prehospital management of most chemical burns includes rinsing the area with large volumes of cool water. The water not only rinses away the offending material but also dilutes any water-soluble agents. The cooling effect of the water also reduces the heat and the rate of chemical reaction. (4-3.37) (IEC p. 696)

20.

C. Some substances either do not dissolve in water or may react violently with it. Phenol, dry lime, and sodium are three of those substances. In these cases, you should try to remove as much of the substance as possible before applying water. All others should be irrigated with copious amounts of water. (4-3.37) (IEC p. 697)

Thoracic Trauma

unit objectives

Questions in this unit relate to DOT Objectives 4-4.1 and 4-4.38. The objectives are listed in the Appendix.

DIRECTIONS Each of the questions or incomplete statements below is followed by suggested answers or completions. Select the **one answer** that is best in each case.

1. The uppermost part of the sternum is the
   A. mediastinum.
   B. manubrium.
   C. sternal body.
   D. xiphoid process.

2. The heart is suspended in the chest by the aortic arch and the ligamentum
   A. arteriosum.
   B. cardiosum.
   C. teres.
   D. pericardium.

3. Which of the following statements is true regarding multiple high-rib fractures (1–3)?
   A. They are the most commonly fractured.
   B. They are the least protected.
   C. They have an associated mortality of <15%.
   D. You should suspect severe intrathoracic injuries.

C. traumatic asphyxia.
D. hemothorax.

5. The paradoxical movement is due to
   A. the instability of the chest wall.
   B. air in the pleural space.
   C. blood in the pleural space.
   D. paralysis of the respiratory muscles.

6. The major complication from this injury is
   A. bleeding into the pericardial space.
   B. air leaking into the subcutaneous tissues.
   C. decreased tidal volumes.
   D. rib displacement.

7. Prehospital management of this patient includes
   A. positive pressure ventilation.
   B. emergency chest decompression.
   C. pericardiocentesis.
   D. having the patient breathe into a paper bag.

Scenario

Questions 4–7 refer to the following scenario:

Your patient is a 15-year-old male who fell off his bicycle and hit the ground very hard. He presents with paradoxical chest movement on the right side, dyspnea, and guarded respirations. His vital signs are BP 140/80, pulse 100, respirations 30 and shallow, and diminished breath sounds on both sides.

4. Your field diagnosis is
   A. pneumothorax.
   B. flail chest.

Scenario

Questions 8–10 refer to the following scenario:

Your patient is a 35-year-old female who was stabbed in the right chest after a quarrel with her girlfriend. You quickly discover a sucking wound in the right chest. She presents with diminished breath sounds on the right side, hyperresonance to percussion on the right side, ecchymosis from T-5 to T-8 on the right side, and dyspnea. BP is 120/70, pulse is 90, and respirations are 26 and shallow.

8. In addition to the sucking wound, your field diagnosis is
   A. massive hemothorax.
   B. pneumothorax.
   C. pericardial tamponade.
   D. tension pneumothorax.

9. Her condition is due to
   A. blood in the pleural space.
   B. air in the pleural space.
   C. blood in the pericardial sac.
   D. air in the pericardial sac.

10. Your initial management of this patient is to
    A. intubate the trachea.
    B. ventilate with 100% oxygen.
    C. seal the open wound with an occlusive dressing.
    D. decompress the chest immediately.

Scenario

Questions 11–13 refer to the following scenario:

Your patient is a 26-year-old who was shot with a small-caliber handgun in the right chest. She presents with dyspnea, distended neck veins, absent breath sounds on the right side, diminished breath sounds on the left side, hyperresonance on both sides, and tracheal deviation toward the left side. Her vital signs are BP 70/30, pulse 120 and weak, and respirations 30 and shallow.

11. Your field diagnosis is
    A. simple pneumothorax.
    B. tension pneumothorax.
    C. pericardial tamponade.
    D. massive hemothorax.

12. Her hypotension could be caused by
    A. decreased venous return.
    B. tamponade effect on the heart.
    C. blood loss.
    D. all of the above

13. Emergency field management of this patient includes
    A. pneumatic antishock garment.
    B. needle chest decompression.
    C. pericardiocentesis.
    D. none of the above

Scenario

Questions 14–15 refer to the following scenario:

Your patient is a 67-year-old female who was struck by a car and lies on the ground. She presents with dyspnea, pain to the right chest, dull percussion on the right side, and diminished breath sounds on the right side. Her vital signs are BP 80/60, pulse 110, respirations 30, skin cool and clammy, and flat neck veins.

14. Your field diagnosis is
    A. tension pneumothorax.
    B. hemothorax.
    C. pericardial tamponade.
    D. traumatic asphyxia.

15. Emergency field management of this patient includes
    A. rapid IV fluid replacement.
    B. pericardiocentesis.
    C. needle decompression.
    D. pneumatic antishock garment.

Scenario

Questions 16–18 refer to the following scenario:

Your patient is a 35-year-old unbelted male driver who hit the steering wheel and windshield in a one-car accident. He presents unconscious with the following vital signs: BP 110/90, pulse 120 and weak, respirations 28 and shallow, lungs equal and clear, distant heart sounds, skin cool and clammy, and distended neck veins. His only external sign of trauma is a midsternal bruise.

16. Your field diagnosis is
    A. tension pneumothorax.
    B. massive hemothorax.
    C. traumatic asphyxia.
    D. pericardial tamponade.

17. This patient's primary problem is
    A. air filling the pleural space.
    B. fluid in the pericardial sac.
    C. severe crushing injury to the chest.
    D. blood in the pleural space.

18. Emergency management of this patient includes
    A. needle decompression.
    B. chest tube.
    C. pneumatic antishock garment.
    D. pericardiocentesis.

Scenario

Questions 19–20 refer to the following scenario:

Your patient is a 45-year-old who presents with a bluish discoloration above the nipple line, absent vital signs, bloodshot eyes, and distended neck veins. He was pinned for a short time underneath his car following a rollover accident.

19. He is most likely suffering from
    A. tension pneumothorax.
    B. traumatic asphyxia.
    C. massive hemothorax.
    D. pericardial tamponade.

20. The bluish discoloration is caused by
    A. lack of oxygen in the tissues.
    B. low PaO_2.
    C. the bursting of capillaries.
    D. high $PaCO_2$.

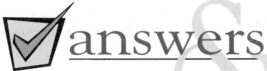

answers & rationales

Following each rationale, you will find a reference to the corresponding objective in the DOT National Standard EMT-Intermediate curriculum. An asterisk denotes material that is supplemental to the DOT curriculum. Page numbers after a rationale indicate where the question topic may be discussed in the Brady text *Intermediate Emergency Care* (Bledsoe, Porter, Cherry).

1.

B. The sternum is divided into three parts. The uppermost part is a triangular-shaped bone called the manubrium. The manubrium is the attaching point for the clavicles and first ribs. (4-4.2) (IEC p. 708)

2.

A. The heart is suspended in the chest by the aortic arch and the ligamentum arteriosum. The ligamentum arteriosum is the remnant of the fetal vessel that connected the pulmonary artery to the aorta. At birth, this vessel closes to redirect blood flow to the lungs. (4-4.2) (IEC p. 719)

3.

D. It takes a tremendous force to fracture ribs 1–3 because they are well protected by the shoulder girdle and heavy musculature of the upper chest. Their fracture is frequently associated with severe intrathoracic injuries, such as aortic rupture, tracheobronchial tears, and other vascular injuries. (4-4.9) (IEC p. 708)

4.

B. Paradoxical chest movement is a classic sign of a flail chest. Flail chest occurs when three or more ribs are fractured in multiple places, causing a floating segment and reducing the stability of the chest wall. (4-4.10) (IEC p. 709)

5.

A. The paradoxical movement is due to the instability of the chest wall. During inspiration, the negative pressures within the chest wall cause the flail segment to suck in. On exhalation, the positive intrathoracic pressures cause the flail segment to bow out. These movements are the opposite of how the rest of the chest wall moves. (4-4.9) (IEC p. 709)

6.

C. Flail chest can result in severe respiratory compromise. The hypoventilation results in decreased air available for gas exchange, leading to hypoxia and hypercarbia. Broken rib pieces can also cause penetrating injuries to the lungs. (4-4.9) (IEC p. 709)

7.

A. Prehospital management of a patient suspected of having a flail chest includes positive pressure ventilation to ensure good ventilation and stabilizing the loose flail segment. (4-4.12) (IEC p. 710)

8.

B. This patient's presentation of diminished breath sounds on the right side with hyperresonance and ecchymosis indicates pneumothorax. (4-4.14) (IEC p. 711)

9.

B. A pneumothorax is caused by a tear in the pleura. Air enters the pleural space, collapsing the lung in that particular area. (4-4.13) (IEC p. 711)

10.

C. Initial management of this patient is aimed at sealing the wound with an occlusive dressing during exhalation. At the end of exhalation, cover the wound and tape it on three sides to prevent air from entering on inhalation but allowing air to escape during exhalation. (4-4.15) (IEC p. 729)

11.

B. This patient who presents with absent lung sounds on one side and decreased sounds on the other, with hyperresonance, jugular venous distention, and a deviated trachea, has a tension pneumothorax. (4-4.14) (IEC p. 713)

12.

D. Her hypotension could be the result of a combination of factors. The high intrathoracic pressures caused by the injury may decrease venous return. The tension could produce a tamponade effect on the heart, severely decreasing cardiac output. She may have blood loss from bleeding within the chest or other injuries. (4-4.13) (IEC p. 713)

13.

B. Emergency management of this patient includes immediate and rapid evacuation of the air trapped in the pleural space. Needle decompression is done by placing a large-bore IV catheter into the chest at the second intercostal space, midclavicular line. Then remove the needle and attach a one-way valve device, allowing air to escape but not to enter. (4-4.15) (IEC p. 713)

14.

B. This patient's presentation of dyspnea, pain to the right chest, diminished breath sounds on the right side, dull to percussion on the right side, and shock indicate hemothorax. A hemothorax is caused by bleeding into the pleural space. (4-4.14) (IEC p. 713)

15.

A. Emergency field management of this patient includes treating for shock by replacing blood fluid volume rapidly. (4-4.15) (IEC p. 731)

16.

D. This patient's presentation of distant heart sounds, distended neck veins, and a narrow pulse pressure indicates pericardial tamponade. This is the classic Beck's triad. (4-4.18) (IEC p. 717)

17.

B. Pericardial tamponade is the filling of the pericardial sac with fluid, which in turn limits the filling of the heart. (4-4.17) (IEC p. 717)

18.

D. Definitive emergency management of this patient includes pericardiocentesis. This procedure involves the insertion of a large-bore spinal needle into the pericardial sac and aspirating the excess blood. This procedure has many complications and is seldom performed by EMT-Intermediates in the field. This patient requires rapid transport. (4-4.19) (IEC p. 732)

19.

B. Sudden compression of the chest from a crushing injury can lead to traumatic asphyxia. The compression severely limits chest excursion and results in hypoventilation. It may also cause a backup of venous blood within the head and neck, causing the classic bloodshot eyes, bulging blue tongue, distended neck veins, and cyanotic upper body, the classic "hood sign." (4-4.34) (IEC p. 721)

20.

C. Backflow of venous blood through the jugular veins into the head causes tremendous pressures in the capillaries, resulting in bursting. The result is petechiae, which gives the patient a purplish look above the nipples. (4-4.33) (IEC p. 721)

5A Head, Face, Neck, Spine, Extremity, and Abdominal Trauma

unit objectives

Questions in this unit are supplemental to the DOT curriculum.

DIRECTIONS Each of the questions or incomplete statements below is followed by suggested answers or completions. Select the **one answer** that is best in each case.

SECTION 1: HEAD, FACE, AND NECK TRAUMA

1. Which of the following is **not** a component of the scalp?
   A. skin
   B. aponeurotica
   C. cranium
   D. periosteum

2. The irregular bone at the base of the skull is the
   A. falx cerebri.
   B. central sulcus.
   C. cribriform plate.
   D. tentorium.

3. The three meningeal layers of the brain from the inside out are the
   A. dura mater, pia mater, arachnoid membrane.
   B. pia mater, dura mater, arachnoid membrane.
   C. arachnoid membrane, pia mater, dura mater.
   D. pia mater, arachnoid membrane, dura mater.

4. Cerebrospinal fluid circulates through which meningeal layer?
   A. epidural space
   B. cerebellar space
   C. subarachnoid space
   D. intracerebral space

5. The area of the brain that is the center of conscious thought is the
   A. cerebrum.
   B. cerebellum.

C. central sulcus.
D. falx cerebri.

6. The cerebrum is separated from the cerebellum by the
   A. falx cerebri.
   B. central sulcus.
   C. cribriform plate.
   D. tentorium.

Match the following components of the brain with the functions they control:

7. _____ frontal lobe
8. _____ parietal lobe
9. _____ temporal lobe
10. _____ occipital lobe
11. _____ cerebellum
12. _____ hypothalamus
13. _____ reticular activating system
14. _____ medulla oblongata

   A. fine motor coordination
   B. sight
   C. personality
   D. endocrine function
   E. cardiorespiratory centers
   F. motor and sensory function
   G. speech
   H. consciousness

15. Cerebral perfusion pressure is the difference between the mean arterial pressure and the _____ pressure.
   A. mean venous
   B. capillary wedge
   C. pulse
   D. intracranial

16. The ascending reticular activating system is responsible for
    A. the sleep–wake cycle.
    B. endocrine function.
    C. voluntary muscle control.
    D. maintenance of cerebral perfusion pressure.

17. The prominent bone of the cheek is known as the
    A. mandible.
    B. maxilla.
    C. sphenoid.
    D. zygoma.

18. Which of the following statements is true regarding scalp lacerations?
    A. They tend to bleed profusely.
    B. They result in severe bleeding that can lead to shock.
    C. The blood vessels lack effective muscular control.
    D. all of the above

19. Battle's sign and periorbital ecchymosis are classic signs of a(n)
    A. intracerebral hemorrhage.
    B. basilar skull fracture.
    C. depressed skull fracture.
    D. subdural hematoma.

20. A brain injury occurring on the opposite side of the side of impact is known as a
    A. concussion.
    B. contusion.
    C. contrecoup.
    D. cochlea.

21. A patient who has sustained a closed head injury with a brief loss of consciousness but no tissue damage and who experiences a complete recovery of function has suffered a
    A. concussion.
    B. contusion.
    C. contrecoup.
    D. cochlea.

22. A patient who has sustained a closed head injury with resulting tissue damage has suffered a
    A. concussion.
    B. contusion.
    C. contrecoup.
    D. cochlea.

23. A person who cannot remember the events that occurred before the trauma that caused the condition is said to have _____ amnesia.
    A. anterograde
    B. retrograde
    C. posttraumatic
    D. concussive

24. A patient who complains of sudden painless loss of vision in one eye has most likely suffered a
    A. retinal detachment.
    B. retinal artery occlusion.
    C. hyphema.
    D. blowout fracture.

25. Which of the following is a complication of jugular vein laceration?
    A. pulmonary embolism
    B. air embolism
    C. hemorrhagic shock
    D. all of the above

26. Which of the following is **not** part of Cushing's response?
    A. hypertension
    B. bradycardia
    C. altered respirations
    D. hypothermia

27. A patient who responds only to deep pain by abnormally flexing the arms has a Glasgow Coma Score of
    A. 3.
    B. 5.
    C. 7.
    D. 9.

Scenario

Questions 28–36 refer to the following scenario:

Your patient is a 25-year-old boxer who was knocked out with a left hook to the side of the head and now lies in the dressing room fully awake. His initial vital signs are BP 130/80, pulse 80, respirations 18, and pupils equal and reactive to light. En route to the hospital, he begins to lose consciousness and complains of being sleepy. His breathing becomes erratic, his pulse slows to 60, and his blood pressure rises to 180/90. His left pupil is larger than the right and is slow to react to light.

28. This patient is probably suffering from a(n)
    A. epidural hematoma.
    B. subdural hematoma.
    C. basilar skull fracture.
    D. concussion.

29. The rapid onset of signs and symptoms is most likely due to the
    A. fracture of the cribriform plate.
    B. rupture of the middle meningeal artery.

C. leakage of CSF into soft tissues.
D. jarring of the reticular activating system.

30. This patient also shows the classic signs and symptoms of
    A. increasing intracranial pressure.
    B. decreasing cerebral blood volume.
    C. basilar skull fracture.
    D. contrecoup injury.

31. These signs and symptoms are caused by
    A. brain shrinkage.
    B. cerebral blood flow interruption.
    C. brain-stem herniation.
    D. abnormally low carbon dioxide levels.

32. His abnormal breathing pattern is caused by
    A. high levels of carbon dioxide.
    B. pressure on the medulla oblongata.
    C. the leakage of cerebrospinal fluid into the nasal cavity.
    D. foramen magnum collapse.

33. This patient may hyperventilate in an attempt to
    A. vasodilate the brain vasculature.
    B. vasoconstrict the brain vasculature.
    C. increase carbon dioxide levels.
    D. cause a metabolic alkalosis.

34. The larger left pupil is caused by compression of the
    A. third cranial nerve.
    B. reticular activating system.
    C. extraoccular muscles.
    D. iris muscle.

35. This patient may vomit without accompanying nausea because of
    A. high levels of carbon dioxide.
    B. brain hypoxia.
    C. Cushing's reflex.
    D. pressure on the medulla oblongata.

36. Prehospital management of this patient includes all of the following **except**
    A. prophylactic hyperventilation with 100% oxygen.
    B. maximizing oxygen concentration.
    C. spinal immobilization.
    D. all of the above

Scenario

Questions 37–39 refer to the following scenario:

Your patient is a 75-year-old nursing home resident who presents with a decreased level of response. The staff claims he began acting strangely hours before calling you. He has no history of diabetes or CNS disease. His only history is that of a minor fall he took 1 week ago. He presents with a slow bounding pulse; a systolic blood pressure of 170, which is high for him; an erratic breathing pattern; and a slightly larger right pupil. His blood sugar is 120, and there is no history or evidence of substance abuse.

37. This patient has probably suffered a(n)
    A. epidural hematoma.
    B. subdural hematoma.
    C. basilar skull fracture.
    D. concussion.

38. The signs and symptoms of this type of injury often present themselves hours or days following the injury because
    A. significant brain swelling takes that long to develop.
    B. the bleeding is from a small vein.
    C. the bleeding is from a large artery.
    D. there is no real tissue damage.

39. High-risk factors for this type of injury include
    A. alcoholism.
    B. the elderly.
    C. recent head injuries.
    D. all of the above

SECTION 2: SPINAL TRAUMA

1. Which mechanism of injury causes the majority of spinal cord injuries?
    A. penetrating trauma
    B. sports-related trauma
    C. falls
    D. motor vehicle crashes

2. Approximately how many spinal cord injuries result from improper handling after the incident?
    A. 5%
    B. 25%
    C. 50%
    D. 75%

3. The fingerlike process of the second vertebra around which the first cervical vertebra rotates is the
    A. atlas.
    B. axis.
    C. odontoid.
    D. mastoid.

4. The opening on the vertebrae through which the spinal cord passes is the
    A. foramen magnum.
    B. odontoid process.
    C. spinal canal.
    D. dura mater.

5. Cerebrospinal fluid circulates through which meningeal space?

A. epidural space

B. subdural space

C. subarachnoid space

D. intracerebral space

6. The first spinous process that you can palpate just above the shoulders is

A. C-2.

B. C-4.

C. C-7.

D. T-1.

7. Which section of the spinal canal has the largest foramen?

A. cervical

B. thoracic

C. sacral

D. lumbar

8. Bundles of nerves that transmit impulses from the body to the brain are known as

A. descending tracts.

B. ascending tracts.

C. anterior medial fissures.

D. posterior medial sulci.

9. The phrenic nerve is comprised of peripheral nerve roots

A. C-1–C-8.

B. C-3–C-5.

C. T-1–T-3.

D. L-1 and below.

10. Topographical regions of the body innervated by specific nerve roots are known as

A. dermatomes.

B. cauda equina.

C. neurilemma.

D. axons.

Match the following mechanisms of injury with their respective example (a term can be used more than once):

11. _____ flexion

12. _____ compression

13. _____ hyperextension

14. _____ distraction

15. _____ rotation

A. hanging

B. axial loading

C. whiplash

D. left hook

E. in-line impacts

16. If your patient presents with loss of motor function and sensation to pain, light touch, and temperature below T-1 while retaining positional and vibration sense, he has most likely sustained a(n)

A. complete cord transection.

B. central cord syndrome.

C. Brown-Séquard's syndrome.

D. anterior cord syndrome.

Scenario

Questions 17–21 refer to the following scenario:

Your patient is a 45-year-old male who was ejected from a vehicle in a one-car rollover accident. He presents on the ground complaining of the inability to move his arms and legs. His airway is clear, and his vital signs are respirations 18 with no chest rise, BP 70/30, pulse 50, and skin warm and dry. He also presents with priapism and the hands in the "hold-up" position.

17. Your field diagnosis of this patient should include
    A. neurogenic shock.
    B. cervical spinal cord interruption.
    C. bilateral paralysis.
    D. all of the above

18. His unusual vital sign presentation is due to
    A. peripheral nerve interruption.
    B. loss of sympathetic nervous system control.
    C. loss of parasympathetic nervous system control.
    D. blood loss below the injury.

19. The priapism is caused by
    A. parasympathetic stimulation.
    B. sympathetic stimulation.
    C. total autonomic nervous system dysfunction.
    D. none of the above

20. The absence of chest rise is due to
    A. intercostal muscle paralysis.
    B. rupture of the diaphragm.
    C. damage to the third cranial nerve.
    D. Cushing's reflex.

21. Prehospital management includes which of the following procedures?
    A. IV fluid replacement
    B. atropine IV
    C. spinal immobilization
    D. all of the above

SECTION 3: EXTREMITY TRAUMA

1. Which of the following is **not** part of the axial skeleton?
   A. skull
   B. pelvis
   C. vertebral column
   D. thorax

Match the following components of long bones with their definitions:

2. _____ diaphysis
3. _____ epiphysis
4. _____ metaphysis
5. _____ periosteum
6. _____ haversian canal

   A. intermediate transition region
   B. passage for blood vessels and nerves
   C. the wide end of a long bone
   D. long cylindrical shaft
   E. tough outer bone layer

7. Connective tissue that provides the articular surfaces of the skeletal system is called
   A. cartilage.
   B. synovium.
   C. ligament.
   D. fossa.

8. The connective tissue band that holds joints together is called a
   A. fossa.
   B. ligament.
   C. cartilage.
   D. synovium.

9. The oily, viscous fluid that lubricates articular surfaces is known as
   A. fossa.
   B. ligaments.
   C. cartilage.
   D. synovium.

10. The most commonly fractured bone in the human body is the
    A. scapula.
    B. humerus.
    C. femur.
    D. clavicle.

11. The proximal humerus articulates with the
    A. radius.
    B. ulna.
    C. glenoid fossa.
    D. clavicle.

12. The act of turning the palm or foot upward
    is called
    A. pronation.
    B. abduction.
    C. adduction.
    D. supination.

13. The metacarpal bones articulate with the
    A. radius.
    B. ulna.
    C. phalanges.
    D. all of the above

14. The hollow surface of the pelvis into which
    the head of the femur fits is the
    A. glenoid fossa.
    B. calcaneus.
    C. acetabulum.
    D. tibial plateau.

15. The distal femur articulates with the
    A. pelvis.
    B. tibia.
    C. fibula.
    D. radius.

16. The medial malleolus is formed by the
    A. tibia.
    B. fibula.
    C. calcaneus.
    D. tarsal bones.

17. _____ is the only muscle over which we
    have control.
    A. Cardiac muscle
    B. Smooth muscle

C. Skeletal muscle
D. none of the above

18. The Achilles is an example of a
    A. ligament.
    B. tendon.
    C. cartilage.
    D. long bone.

19. Blunt trauma causing bleeding and
    discoloration underneath the skin is a(n)
    A. laceration.
    B. contusion.
    C. abrasion.
    D. subluxation.

20. The overstretching of a muscle is called a
    A. strain.
    B. sprain.
    C. subluxation.
    D. dislocation.

21. The overstretching of a ligament is known
    as a(n)
    A. strain.
    B. sprain.
    C. abduction.
    D. adduction.

22. A partial separation of a joint is called
    a(n)
    A. dislocation.
    B. subluxation.
    C. pronation.
    D. insufflation.

23. The biceps/triceps relationship is an
    example of
    A. opposition.
    B. synergism.
    C. direct articulation.
    D. indirect articulation.

24. The origin point for the biceps muscle is the
    A. humerus.
    B. radius.
    C. clavicle.
    D. scapula.

25. You learn that 3 days after hip fracture surgery, your 34-year-old patient went into cardiac arrest and died. The most likely cause for his sudden death was
    A. acute myocardial infarction.
    B. fat embolism.
    C. cardiac tamponade.
    D. massive hemorrhage and internal blood loss.

26. In pediatrics, an epiphyseal fracture is especially worrisome because of the
    A. threat of fat embolism.
    B. increased incidence of osteomyelitis.
    C. damage to the growth plate.
    D. increased angulation that inhibits proper healing.

27. Which of the following is **not** one of the six Ps in evaluating a limb injury?
    A. paralysis
    B. paresthesia
    C. pressure
    D. pruritis

28. Which of the following statements is true regarding the management of musculoskeletal injuries?
    A. Always splint the joints above and below the fracture site.
    B. Always splint the bones above and below a dislocated joint.
    C. Always perform distal neurovascular tests before and after any splinting.
    D. all of the above

29. The best position for an injured limb is
    A. halfway between flexion and extension.
    B. fully extended.
    C. fully flexed.
    D. in the deformed position.

30. Which of the following statements best describes the proper use of heat and ice for musculoskeletal injuries?
    A. ice for the first 24 hours, followed by heat
    B. heat for the first 24 hours, followed by ice
    C. ice for the first 48 hours, followed by heat
    D. ice only

31. In which of the following situations should you attempt to reduce a dislocation in the field?
    A. There is a significant neurovascular deficit.
    B. Transport time is very short.
    C. You are unsure of your diagnosis.
    D. There are other significant injuries.

32. The management of a pelvic fracture includes which of the following procedures?
    A. pneumatic antishock garment
    B. IV fluid replacement
    C. rapid transport
    D. all of the above

33. Traction splinting is indicated in which of the following conditions?
    A. isolated midshaft femur fracture
    B. disease-induced proximal femur fracture
    C. bilateral femur fractures with profound shock
    D. all of the above

34. A Colles' fracture involves which bone?
    A. proximal ulna
    B. proximal radius
    C. distal radius
    D. distal ulna

35. Often you may not be able to differentiate a proximal femur fracture from a(n)
    A. posterior hip dislocation.
    B. anterior hip dislocation.
    C. pelvic fracture.
    D. acetabulum fracture.

36. Your patient presents with her foot turned outward and the head of her femur palpable in the inguinal area. Your field diagnosis and management include
    A. anterior hip dislocation—immediate reduction.
    B. anterior hip dislocation—immobilization.
    C. proximal femur fracture—traction splint.
    D. posterior hip dislocation—reduction.

SECTION 4: ABDOMINAL TRAUMA

1. The kidneys, spleen, and part of the pancreas are located within the _____ cavity.
    A. peritoneal
    B. retroperitoneal
    C. pleural
    D. pericardial

2. The sigmoid colon is located in the
    A. right upper quadrant.
    B. left upper quadrant.
    C. right lower quadrant.
    D. left lower quadrant.

3. The appendix is located in the
    A. right upper quadrant.
    B. left upper quadrant.
    C. right lower quadrant.
    D. left lower quadrant.

4. The gallbladder is located in the
    A. right upper quadrant.
    B. left upper quadrant.
    C. right lower quadrant.
    D. left lower quadrant.

5. The stomach is located in the
    A. right upper quadrant.
    B. left upper quadrant.
    C. right lower quadrant.
    D. left lower quadrant.

6. The continuous tube that extends from the esophagus to the rectum is the
    A. duodenal canal.
    B. digestive tract.
    C. parenteral canal.
    D. peritoneal tract.

7. The wavelike muscular motion of the intestines is known as
    A. alimentation.
    B. peristalsis.
    C. omentum.
    D. mesentery action.

8. Which of the following is a function of the liver?
    A. detoxifying blood from the intestines
    B. storing body energy reserves
    C. producing plasma proteins
    D. all of the above

9. Bile is stored in the
    A. liver.
    B. gallbladder.
    C. pancreas.
    D. spleen.

10. The small bowel consists of which following three sections in order?
    A. ileum, duodenum, jejunum
    B. jejunum, omentum, duodenum
    C. duodenum, jejunum, ileum
    D. omentum, ileum, jejunum

11. The liver is suspended in the abdomen by the
    A. ligamentum teres.
    B. bundle of Kent.
    C. isle of Langerhans.
    D. mesentery.

12. Bile is produced in the
    A. stomach.
    B. liver.
    C. gallbladder.
    D. pancreas.

13. The pancreas
    A. produces glucagon and insulin.
    B. secretes digestive enzymes.
    C. is a solid, encapsulated organ.
    D. all of the above

14. The most delicate and fragile abdominal organ is the
    A. pancreas.
    B. spleen.
    C. duodenum.
    D. gallbladder.

15. Pregnancy affects maternal circulation by
    A. decreasing blood volume.
    B. decreasing heart rate.
    C. increasing cardiac output.
    D. increasing hematocrit.

16. The abdominal aorta bifurcates into two _____ arteries.
    A. femoral
    B. iliac
    C. mesentery
    D. pelvic

17. The secondary circulatory system that transports intestinal blood to the liver for detoxification is known as the _____ system.
    A. mesentery
    B. omentum
    C. peritoneal
    D. portal

18. Which of the following organs is located in the retroperitoneal space?
    A. small intestine
    B. mesentery
    C. pancreas
    D. stomach

19. Your patient is a 24-year-old male who was stabbed in the left upper quadrant. He presents alert and oriented in moderate respiratory distress and with minor external blood loss. His airway is clear, but his breathing is shallow at a rate of 36 per minute. He has good peripheral pulses, and his skin is warm and pink. He complains of pain on inspiration in the left chest. On auscultation, you hear what sounds like bowel sounds in the left lower lobes. The right lungs are clear. Your likely field diagnosis is
    A. tension pneumothorax.
    B. massive hemothorax.
    C. cardiac tamponade.
    D. diaphragmatic herniation.

20. Which of the following is **not** a sign of a hollow abdominal organ rupture?

A. hematochezia

B. hemoptysis

C. hematuria

D. hematemesis

21. Rebound tenderness is a classic sign that suggests

A. diaphragmatic tear.

B. hypovolemic shock.

C. peritoneal irritation.

D. aortic aneurysm.

22. Abdominal guarding usually indicates

A. diaphragmatic tear.

B. hypovolemic shock.

C. peritoneal irritation.

D. aortic aneurysm.

23. Your patient is a 57-year-old female who was a passenger in a two-car accident. She was ejected from the vehicle and lies on the ground next to the car. She presents unconscious with no obvious signs of trauma. Her vital signs are BP 50/30, pulse 120 and weak, respirations 38 and shallow, lungs equal and clear, and flat neck veins. On examination, you find discoloration around the umbilicus and abdominal guarding. Your field diagnosis is

A. tension pneumothorax.

B. pericardial tamponade.

C. intraabdominal hemorrhage.

D. ruptured diaphragm.

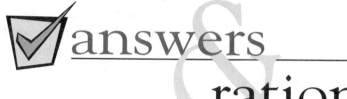

answers & rationales

Following each rationale, you will find an asterisk indicating that the material (for all questions in this unit) is supplemental to the DOT curriculum. Page numbers after a rationale indicate where the question topic may be discussed in the Brady text *Intermediate Emergency Care* (Bledsoe, Porter, Cherry).

ANSWERS AND RATIONALES FOR SECTION 1: HEAD, FACE, AND NECK TRAUMA

1.

C. The scalp, which helps protect and insulate the skull and brain, is comprised of **S**kin, **C**onnective tissue, **A**poneurotica, **L**ayer of areolar tissue, and **P**eriosteum—SCALP. (*) (IEC pp. 134–135)

2.

C. The cribriform plate is an irregular and bony plate at the base of the skull. It has surfaces against which the brain may abrade, lacerate, or contuse in severe deceleration injuries. This is the location of the common basilar skull fracture. (*) (IEC p. 136)

3.

D. The meninges are a group of three tissues between the skull and the brain and between the inside of the spinal foramen and the cord. The outermost layer is the dura mater. The layer closest to the brain and spinal cord is the pia mater, and separating the two layers is connective tissue called the arachnoid membrane. From the inside out, they form a "PAD" for the brain and spinal cord. (*) (IEC p. 136)

4.

C. Beneath the arachnoid membrane is the subarachnoid space, which is filled with cerebrospinal fluid. Cerebrospinal fluid is the medium that surrounds the central nervous system and acts to absorb the shock of minor deceleration. (*) (IEC p. 137)

5.

A. The cerebrum is the largest of the brain regions and occupies most of the cranial cavity. It is the center of conscious thought, personality, speech, motor control, and visual, auditory, and tactile perception. (*) (IEC p. 137)

6.

D. The tentorium is an extension of the dura mater separating the cerebrum from the cerebellum. It is a fibrous sheet and runs at right angles to the falx cerebri. (*) (IEC p. 137)

Matching (*) (IEC pp. 137–138)

7. C frontal lobe
8. F parietal lobe
9. G temporal lobe
10. B occipital lobe
11. A cerebellum
12. D hypothalamus
13. H reticular activating
14. E medulla

15.

D. Cerebral perfusion pressure is the pressure moving blood through the brain. It is the difference between the mean arterial pressure and intracranial pressure. When brain swelling or bleeding increases intracranial pressure, the brain signals the cardiovascular system to raise the mean arterial pressure in order to perfuse the brain. (*) (IEC p. 139)

16.

A. The ascending reticular activating system is responsible for the sleep–wake cycle. It is our on–off switch for consciousness. (*) (IEC p. 139)

17.

D. The zygoma is the prominent bone of the cheek. It protects the eyes and the muscles controlling eye and jaw movement. (*) (IEC p. 139)

18.

D. The scalp is an area frequently subjected to soft-tissue injury. Because this area is extremely vascular and because the scalp vessels are larger and not quite as muscular as other vessels, blood loss can be rapid and difficult to control. Severe and persistent bleeding from scalp lacerations can contribute to shock. (*) (IEC p. 790)

19.

B. Battle's sign is a black-and-blue discoloration over the mastoid process just behind the ear. Bilateral periorbital ecchymosis is a black-and-blue discoloration of the area surrounding the eyes. Both of these signs are normally associated with a basilar skull fracture. (*) (IEC p. 519)

20.

C. A contrecoup injury occurs on the opposite side of the side of impact. The brain impacts the interior of the skull on the opposite side, causing soft-tissue injury such as contusions, lacerations, and hemorrhages. (*)

21.

A. A person who has sustained a closed head injury with a brief loss of consciousness but no tissue damage and who experiences a complete recovery of function has suffered a concussion. (*)

22.

B. A contusion is a more significant jarring than a concussion and results in cell damage. It is a closed wound in which the skin is unbroken, although damage has occurred to the tissue beneath. If the loss of consciousness is longer than 5 minutes, the patient is usually admitted to the hospital. (*)

23.

B. A patient who cannot recall the events that occurred before the trauma that caused his condition is said to have retrograde amnesia.

If he cannot recall the events that occurred after the trauma, he is said to have anterograde amnesia. Both are signs of brain injury. (*)

24.

B. Retinal artery occlusion is a vascular emergency in which an embolus, or traveling clot, blocks the blood supply to the eye. The patient complains of sudden and painless loss of vision in one eye. (*)

25.

D. Jugular veins at times maintain a pressure less than atmospheric pressure. An open wound may draw air into a vessel, affecting the heart or pulmonary circulation. Jugular veins, although rather low-pressure vessels, still carry large volumes of blood and will bleed profusely. (*) (IEC pp. 752–753)

26.

D. In cases of increasing intracranial pressure, the brain displaces away from the side of the hematoma toward the foramen magnum. This movement pushes the medulla oblongata into the foramen magnum, producing changes in vital signs. The pulse rate slows, respirations become erratic, and the blood pressure rises. This collective change in vital signs is called Cushing's response. (*) (IEC pp. 1015–1016)

27.

B. The Glasgow Coma Scale objectively rates your patient in three categories: eye opening, best verbal response, and best motor response. Since this patient does not open his eyes, he gets a score of 1 in the first category. Since he does not respond to verbal commands, he gets a 1 in the second category.

He flexes abnormally to pain, earning a score of 3 in the last category, making his total score 5. (*) (IEC pp. 1015–1016)

28.

A. An epidural hematoma is an accumulation of blood between the dura mater and the cranium. (*)

29.

B. The rapid onset of signs and symptoms following an epidural hematoma occurs because the bleeding involves arterial vessels, often the middle meningeal artery. The condition progresses rapidly while the patient moves quickly toward unconsciousness. Since the bleeding is arterial, intracranial pressure builds rapidly, compressing the cerebrum and increasing the pressure within the skull. (*)

30.

A. This patient shows the classic signs and symptoms of increasing intracranial pressure: an altered respiratory pattern, bradycardia, hypertension, unequal pupils, and a decreasing level of consciousness. (*)

31.

C. These signs and symptoms are caused by brain-stem herniation. As the pressure in the cranium increases, the brain is pushed downward through the tentorium toward the brain stem. Because the brain stem houses our cardiac and respiratory centers, these vital signs are affected. (*)

32.

B. Pressure on the medulla oblongata causes alterations in respiratory control. Your patient may hyperventilate, exhibit Cheyne-Stokes respirations, and eventually stop breathing altogether. (*)

33.

B. High levels of carbon dioxide cause the brain vasculature to dilate. This results in increased blood volume, which in turn increases the pressure within the skull. In an attempt to vasoconstrict these vessels and reverse the process, the body may begin to hyperventilate. (*)

34.

A. Pressure on the third cranial nerve, the occulomotor nerve, causes the pupil on that side to dilate. An early indicator of increasing intracranial pressure is a slightly larger pupil that reacts slowly to light. As the pressure increases, the pupil will become fixed and totally dilated. (*)

35.

D. The vomit center is located in the medulla oblongata. Pressure on this center will cause immediate vomiting without accompanying nausea. The vomiting is usually forceful and known as "projectile vomiting." (*)

36.

A. Prehospital management of a patient with increasing intracranial pressure includes the following: spinal immobilization, elevation of the head of the stretcher to maximize venous drainage, aggressive airway management and intubation as soon as possible to protect the airway from the eventual vomiting, and high-flow O_2 to maximize brain oxygenation and prevent tissue swelling. Only in the event of severe

deterioration from brain swelling should you perform hyperventilation. (*) (IEC p. 753)

37.

B. A subdural hematoma is a collection of blood directly beneath the dura mater. (*)

38.

B. The signs and symptoms following a subdural hematoma occur very slowly and are subtle in presentation because blood loss is usually due to rupture of a small venous vessel. (*)

39.

D. You will frequently encounter subdural hematomas in elderly patients or chronic alcoholics. Because the aging process and chronic alcoholism shrink the brain, both groups are prone to this condition following even seemingly minor head injuries. Your patient's altered behavior pattern may be caused by a subdural hematoma. (*)

ANSWERS AND RATIONALES FOR SECTION 2: SPINAL TRAUMA

1.

D. The majority of spinal cord injuries (48%) are the result of motor vehicle crashes, most commonly in young men ages 16–30. (*)

2.

B. As many as 25% of all spinal cord injuries result from improper handling of the spinal column (and the patient) after an injury. This is often caused by bystanders. (*)

3.

C. The second cervical vertebra, the axis, has a small fingerlike upper projection, called the odontoid process, which forms the pivot point around which the head rotates. The first cervical vertebra, the atlas, sits atop this protrusion. (*) (IEC pp. 148, 149)

4.

C. The spinal canal (or foramen) is the opening in the vertebrae through which the spinal cord passes. The cord travels from the skull to the second lumbar vertebra. This tube must remain aligned to prevent injury to the spinal cord. (*) (IEC p. 147)

5.

C. Beneath the arachnoid membrane is the subarachnoid space, which is filled with cerebrospinal fluid. Cerebrospinal fluid is the medium that surrounds the central nervous system and acts to absorb the shock of minor deceleration. (*)

6.

C. The last cervical vertebra (C-7) is the first bony prominence you can feel just above the shoulders. It is an important landmark when counting vertebrae. (*) (IEC pp. 149–150)

7.

D. The lumbar spine has the largest vertebral bodies, the thickest intervertebral disks, and the largest foramen (spinal canal). (*) (IEC p. 150)

8.

B. Bundles of axons that transmit sensory impulses from the body to the brain are known as the ascending tracts. These tracts are paired with the descending tracts (which carry motor impulses from the brain to the body) on each side of the spinal cord. Injury may affect one, some, or all of these tracts. (*) (IEC p. 162)

9.

B. The phrenic nerve is comprised of peripheral nerve roots C-3 through C-5. It innervates the diaphragm, the main muscle for breathing. (*) (IEC p. 164)

10.

A. Dermatomes are body regions corresponding to various nerve routes. As these peripheral routes branch off the spine, they perceive sensation lower and lower on the body. (*) (IEC p. 164)

Matching (*)

11.	E	flexion
12.	B, E	compression
13.	C	hyperextension
14.	A	distraction
15.	D	rotation

16.

D. Anterior cord syndrome is caused by bony fragments or pressure compressing the arteries that perfuse the anterior cord. This causes a loss of motor function and sensation to pain, light touch, and temperature below the injured site. Potential for recovery is poor. (*)

17.

D. Your prehospital diagnosis of this patient should include cervical spinal cord interruption, bilateral paralysis, and neurogenic shock. (*)

18.

B. Patients in shock usually present with hypotension, tachycardia, and cool, clammy skin. These signs indicate that the sympathetic nervous system compensatory mechanism has been activated. Your patient's unusual vital sign presentation (i.e., hypotension, bradycardia, warm and dry skin) indicates the loss of sympathetic nervous system control. (*)

19.

A. Priapism is a painful penile erection. In this case, it is caused by the loss of sympathetic nervous system tone, allowing parasympathetic stimulation to dominate. (*)

20.

A. Interruption of the spinal cord in the cervical region will cause the intercostal muscles of the chest to become dysfunctional. Patients with this problem exhibit "belly breathing," characterized by movement of the diaphragm. (*)

21.

D. Prehospital management of this patient includes spinal immobilization, IV fluid replacement with normal saline or lactated Ringer's, and atropine to raise the heart rate. Other interventions include a steroid, such as methylprednisolone or dexamethasone, to decrease cord swelling and dopamine to raise the blood pressure if atropine fails to improve cardiac output. (*) (IEC pp. 756–767)

ANSWERS AND RATIONALES FOR SECTION 3: EXTREMITY TRAUMA

1.

B. The axial skeleton consists of the skull, the vertebral column, and the thorax. The upper and lower extremities, the shoulder girdle, and the pelvis make up the appendicular skeleton. (*) (IEC p. 116)

Matching (*) (IEC pp. 113–115)

2.	D	diaphysis
3.	C	epiphysis
4.	A	metaphysis
5.	E	periosteum
6.	B	haversian canal

7.

A. A layer of connective tissue called cartilage covers the epiphyseal surface. It is a smooth, strong, flexible material that functions as the actual surface of articulation between bones. It allows for easy movement between the ends of adjacent bones, such as the femur and tibia. It also absorbs some of the impact associated with walking, running, or other jarring activities. (*) (IEC p. 115)

8.

B. Ligaments are connective tissues connecting bone to bone and holding the joints together. Ligaments will stretch to allow joint movement while holding the bone ends firmly in place. (*) (IEC p. 115)

9.

D. The ligaments surrounding a joint form the synovial capsule. This chamber holds a small amount of fluid to lubricate the articular surfaces. The oily, viscous fluid assists joint motion by reducing friction. (*) (IEC p. 116)

10.

D. The clavicle, which is anterior to the scapula and not very well protected, is the most commonly fractured bone in the human body. (*) (IEC p. 778)

11.

C. The humerus is the single bone of the proximal upper extremity. It is secured against the glenoid fossa of the shoulder joint proximally. The humerus articulates with the radius and ulna at the elbow. (*) (IEC p. 123)

12.

D. The act of turning the palm or foot upward is called supination. The opposite movement, turning the hand or foot downward, is called pronation. (*)

13.

C. The metacarpal bones articulate with the phalanges of the fingers and the carpal bones. (*) (IEC p. 118)

14.

C. The actual articular surface for the femur is the acetabulum. It is a hollow depression in the lateral pelvis into which the head of the femur fits. (*) (IEC pp. 126, 128)

15.

B. The distal femur articulates with the tibia. (*) (IEC pp. 126, 127)

16.

A. The distal tibia forms the medial malleolus or the protuberance of the ankle, while the fibula forms the lateral malleolus. (*) (IEC p. 124)

17.

C. Skeletal muscles are muscles over which we have conscious control. They are necessary to move the extremities and the body in general. The largest component of the muscular system, they are the muscles most commonly traumatized. (*) (IEC p. 130)

18.

B. The Achilles is an example of a tendon. A tendon is a specialized connective tissue band that accomplishes the insertion and in some cases the origin of muscles. They are extremely strong and will not stretch. They often will break an area of bone loose rather than tear. (*) (IEC p. 133)

19.

B. Trauma frequently causes contusions. As with all contusions, small blood vessels rupture, causing dull pain, leakage of fluid into the interstitial spaces, and the classical discoloration. (*)

20.

A. A strain is an overstretching of the muscle and presents as pain. (*)

21.

B. A sprain is a tearing of the connective tissue of the joint capsule—specifically, a ligament or ligaments. This injury causes exquisite pain at the site, followed shortly by inflammation and swelling. (*)

22.

B. A subluxation is an incomplete dislocation of the joint. The surfaces remain in contact, while the joint is partially deformed. (*)

23.

A. The biceps muscle group allows us to flex our elbow. The triceps muscle group allows us to extend our elbow. This is known as opposition because while one contracts, the other relaxes. (*) (IEC p. 130)

24.

D. The origin of a muscle is the point of attachment that remains stationary as the muscle contracts. The origin of the biceps muscle is at two points on the scapula—the acromion and coracoid processes. The other attachment point is known as the insertion. (*)

25.

B. An infrequent but serious complication from a fracture is a fat embolism that enters the venous system and travels to the heart and then the lungs, where it lodges. If it is large enough, it can cause cardiac arrest. (*) (IEC p. 618)

26.

C. The epiphyseal plate is another term for the growth plate. Damage to this area may inhibit proper bone growth, usually of the proximal tibia. (*) (IEC pp. 114, 1193, 1249)

27.

D. The six Ps constitute a helpful mnemonic to remember key elements when evaluating a limb injury. They include **P**ain (on palpation or movement), **P**allor (pale skin), **P**aralysis (immobility), **P**aresthesia (numbness or tingling), **P**ressure (inner tension), and **P**ulses (absence or weakness). (*)

28.

D. Always splint the joints above and below the fracture site and the bones above and below a dislocated joint. Before and after any splinting, always perform distal neurovascular checks for circulation, sensory, and motor function. (4-5.14) (IEC p. 771)

29.

A. To best maintain proper neurovascular function, you should immobilize an injured limb halfway between flexion and extension, also called the position of function. In this position, you place the least amount of stress on the joint ligaments and the muscles and tendons surrounding the injury. (4-5.14) (IEC p. 771)

30.

C. The standard mnemonic for musculoskeletal injuries is RICE. This stands for **R**est, **I**ce, **C**ompression, and **E**levation. Heat may be applied 48 hours after the injury to promote healing and circulation. (*)

31.

A. Because reducing a dislocation is risky, you should attempt to reduce a dislocated joint in the field only if there is a significant neurovascular deficit, there is a prolonged extrication or transport time, there are no other associated serious injuries, and you are sure the injury is a dislocation. (*) (IEC p. 771)

32.

D. Fractures to the pelvic ring are especially worrisome because of the danger of severe bleeding and associated injuries to the reproductive, digestive, and urinary organs. Management of a pelvic fracture includes immobilization of the pelvic ring with the pneumatic antishock garment, IV fluid replacement, and rapid transport to a trauma center. (4-5.14) (IEC p. 777)

33.

A. The traction splint is the best device to splint the hemodynamically stable patient with an isolated femur fracture. (4-5.14) (IEC p. 777)

34.

C. Commonly, fractures will occur at the distal end of the radius, breaking it just above the articular surface. This is known as a Colles' fracture and presents with the wrist turned up at an unusual angle. (*) (IEC p. 783)

35.

B. Fracture of the femur near the hip may be difficult to differentiate from an anterior hip dislocation. While you may expect a broken leg to be slightly shorter than the unbroken one, the difference may be slight and unnoticeable if the legs are not straight and parallel. (*) (IEC p. 777)

36.

B. The foot turned outward and the head of the femur palpable in the inguinal region suggest an anterior hip dislocation. Management is aimed at immobilization on a spine board with lots of padding for comfort. Do not attempt to reduce an anterior hip dislocation. (4-5.14) (IEC p. 780)

ANSWERS AND RATIONALES FOR SECTION 4: ABDOMINAL TRAUMA

1.

B. The retroperitoneal space lies behind the layers of the peritoneum. The organs within this space include the kidneys, spleen, and part of the pancreas. (*)

2.

D. The left lower quadrant houses the sigmoid colon as well as portions of the small and large intestines. (*) (IEC p. 217)

3.

C. The right lower quadrant contains the appendix. (*) (IEC p. 217)

4.

A. The right upper quadrant contains the liver, right kidney, gallbladder, duodenum, and part of the pancreas. (*) (IEC p. 217)

5.

B. The left upper quadrant includes the stomach, left kidney, spleen, and most of the pancreas. (*) (IEC p. 217)

6.

B. The digestive tract (alimentary canal) is a continuous tube that begins with the esophagus and ends with the rectum. In this canal, food goes through the digestive process. (*) (IEC p. 216)

7.

B. Peristalsis is the wavelike muscular motion of the esophagus and bowel, moving food through the digestive system. (*) (IEC p. 216)

8.

D. The liver occupies the area below and under the rib cage in the right upper quadrant. A large and vascular organ, it detoxifies the blood coming from the digestive field, stores body energy reserves, produces plasma proteins, and performs many other important functions. (*) (IEC p. 218)

9.

B. Beneath and behind the liver is the gallbladder, a storehouse for bile. Bile is a product of the liver that helps in the digestion of fat. (*) (IEC p. 218)

10.

C. The small intestine consists of three sections. The first section is called the duodenum. The second section is called the jejunum, and the third section is the ileum. (*) (IEC p. 217)

11.

A. The ligamentum teres suspends the liver. In deceleration, the ligament may slice the liver as cheese is sliced by a wire cutter. This laceration is severe, often resulting in rapid hemorrhage. (*) (IEC p. 218)

12.

B. Bile, produced in the liver and stored in the gallbladder, helps the body by emulsifying ingested fats that would otherwise remain in clumps during the digestive process. (*) (IEC p. 218)

13.

D. The pancreas, a solid, encapsulated organ, secretes hormones that regulate blood sugar (insulin and glucagon) and powerful digestive enzymes. (*) (IEC p. 218)

14.

B. The spleen, part of the immune system, is the most delicate abdominal organ. Since it is engorged with blood, it has the potential for life-threatening hemorrhage when injured. Luckily, it is well protected by the ribs, spine, and flank and back muscles. (*) (IEC p. 218)

15.

C. During pregnancy, maternal physiology undergoes significant changes in circulation. By the third trimester, circulating volume increases by 45% with no increase in red blood cell production. The heart rate increases by 15 beats per minute, and cardiac output increases by up to 40%. (*) (IEC p. 1124)

16.

B. The abdominal aorta bifurcates into two iliac arteries. When these arteries pass through the pelvis at the inguinal ligament, they eventually become the femoral arteries. (*) (IEC p. 214)

17.

D. The portal system transports venous blood from the intestines to the liver. Here the liver detoxifies the fluid, stores excess nutrients, adds nutrients when they are deficient, and then sends the blood into the inferior vena cava for a return to the general circulation. When a drug is given orally, it makes this "first pass" through the liver and may lose some of its potency through this detoxifying process. (*)

18.

C. The retroperitoneal space lies behind the peritoneum. Organs within this space include the kidneys, pancreas, posterior portions of the ascending and descending colon, rectum, duodenum, and urinary bladder. (*)

19.

D. Bowel sounds in the chest following penetrating trauma to either the lower chest or the upper abdomen usually indicate a ruptured diaphragm. On inspiration, the negative pressure in the chest draws the intestines through the hole in the diaphragm into the chest, resulting in bowel sounds in the lower lobes. This commonly occurs on the left side, as the right side of the diaphragm is well protected by the massive liver. (*) (IEC p. 720)

20.

B. Hematochezia (frank blood in the stool), hematuria (blood in the urine), and hematemesis (blood in emesis) are all classic signs of a ruptured abdominal organ.

Hemoptysis is the presence of blood in sputum (lungs). (*) (IEC pp. 412, 618, 652)

21.

C. Rebound tenderness is pain on the release of your hand during deep palpation, allowing the patient's abdominal wall to return to its normal position. It is a classic sign of peritoneal irritation and suggests a bacterial or chemical irritation caused by intraabdominal bleeding or hollow organ rupture. (*)

22.

C. The peritoneum can become irritated by the presence of blood. The patient with peritoneal irritation often presents with guarding because it hurts to move. (*)

23.

C. Any patient who presents with signs and symptoms of shock and discoloration around the umbilicus, also known as Cullen's sign, should be suspected of having an intraabdominal hemorrhage. (*) (IEC p. 515)

UNIT
5B

Shock and Trauma Management

unit objectives

Questions in this unit relate to DOT Objectives 4-5.1 to 4-5.24. The objectives are listed in the Appendix.

DIRECTIONS
Each of the questions or incomplete statements below is followed by suggested answers or completions. Select the **one answer** that is best in each case.

Scenario

Questions 1–12 refer to the following scenario:

You are awakened in the middle of the night for a call on a quiet country road. Your patient was the unrestrained driver in a one-car high-speed auto accident involving frontal impact with a telephone pole. He is a 19-year-old male who presents unconscious and partially trapped in the severely deformed vehicle. According to witnesses, he was driving at a high rate of speed. On initial examination, you immediately hear gurgling respirations. Vital signs are weak carotid pulse of 120; BP 70/40; respirations 36 and shallow; skin cool, pale, and clammy; and capillary refill time 4 seconds. Pulse oximetry reads 70%. On physical exam, you discover a bruise to the front chest wall with a loose flail segment and some abdominal guarding. Lung sounds are diminished on the right side with some hyperresonance in that area.

1. Which of the following programs is aimed at preventing such an incident?
   A. fire department explorer program
   B. "Just say no"
   C. OSHA night driving course
   D. "Let's not meet by accident"

2. Your initial management of this patient should be to
   A. perform immediate nasotracheal intubation.
   B. start two large-bore IVs.
   C. manually stabilize his head and neck.
   D. place an oxygen mask on him.

3. The gurgling noise that accompanies his breathing calls for immediate
   A. suctioning.
   B. intubation.
   C. head tilt/chin lift procedure.
   D. chest decompression.

4. You are concerned about the right-sided flail segment because
   A. it indicates lung tissue damage beneath the injury.
   B. it may severely inhibit ventilation and oxygenation.
   C. it is usually accompanied by pericardial tamponade.
   D. underlying damage to the heart is expected.

5. His respiratory status indicates the need for immediate
   A. chest decompression.
   B. Trendelenburg positioning.
   C. intubation.
   D. positive pressure ventilation.

6. Your patient's pulse and blood pressure indicate which stage of shock?
   A. compensated
   B. irreversible
   C. decompensated
   D. none of the above

7. The most likely cause of your patient's shock is
   A. loss of alveolar function.
   B. internal blood loss.
   C. massive vasodilation.
   D. acute myocardial infarction.

8. Peripheral vascular resistance is primarily regulated in which blood vessels?

   A. veins

   B. venules

   C. arteries

   D. arterioles

9. Which of the following statements is **true** regarding this patient?

   A. Anaerobic metabolism is occurring.

   B. Resuscitation is still possible.

   C. Irreversible shock will ensue if left untreated.

   D. all of the above

10. This patient responds to pain stimuli by moaning. He receives a(n) _____ on the AVPU scale.

    A. A

    B. V

    C. P

    D. U

11. Prehospital fluid resuscitation of this patient should include

    A. lactated Ringer's.

    B. 0.45% sodium chloride.

    C. 5% dextrose and water.

    D. any of the above

12. Which of the following IV equipment would best help this patient?

    A. 20-gauge, 2-inch catheter and 60-drop/ml tubing

    B. 14-gauge, 1-inch catheter and 10-drop/ml tubing

    C. 16-gauge, 3-inch catheter and 60-drop/ml tubing

    D. 22-gauge, $\frac{1}{2}$-inch catheter and 10-drop/ml tubing

13. In general, fluid resuscitation in the field should be limited to

    A. 1 liter.

    B. 2 liters.

    C. 3 liters.

    D. none of the above

14. During a hot load, you should always

    A. approach the helicopter from the rear.

    B. stay clear of the tail rotor.

    C. direct lights directly at the pilot.

    D. use flares instead of flashlights.

15. The appropriate helicopter landing zone for a large aircraft is at least

    A. 60×60 feet.

    B. 75×75 feet.

    C. 120×120 feet.

    D. 200×200 feet.

16. For which of the following patients would a hypertonic intravenous solution be most appropriate?

    A. a dehydrated patient

    B. a congestive heart failure patient

    C. a burn patient

    D. a hypovolemic patient

17. Administering an isotonic crystalloid solution intravenously to a hypovolemic patient will increase the cardiac output primarily by increasing

    A. preload.

    B. heart rate.

    C. contractility.

    D. afterload.

18. You have been administering an isotonic crystalloid solution to an elderly trauma patient. After a period of time, you hear bilateral crackles on auscultation of the lungs. You should
    A. change over to a hypotonic solution and continue fluid administration.
    B. disconnect the IV since there is volume overload.
    C. slow the IV infusion rate and consult medical direction.
    D. leave the infusion running at the current rate and consult medical direction.

19. Which of the following IV solution/equipment setups is most appropriate for a volume-depleted patient?
    A. 0.9% NaCl, 16-gauge angiocath, macrodrip administration set
    B. 5% dextrose in water, 20-gauge angiocath, minidrip administration set
    C. 0.45% NaCl, 14-gauge angiocath, macrodrip administration set
    D. lactated Ringer's, 14-gauge angiocath, microdrip administration set

20. You are treating a multisystem trauma patient who is in cardiac arrest. All of the following treatment considerations for this patient are correct **except**
    A. you should avoid intubation since hypoxemia is probably severe.
    B. you should provide full spinal immobilization prior to transport.
    C. you should utilize the AED if medical direction allows.
    D. you should initiate an IV of normal saline or Ringer's lactate.

21. You are assessing a hypotensive, anxious, tachycardic patient who was struck with a baseball bat in the upper-left quadrant of the abdomen. Which of the following is a first priority in treatment for this patient?
    A. oxygen administration
    B. fluid replacement
    C. full spinal immobilization
    D. drug administration

22. A 17-year-old female has fallen down 14 stairs. In your assessment, you note a large laceration to the posterior head and some deformity to the left tibia. Vitals include BP 88/68, HR 112/regular, RR 32/shallow. The best treatment for this patient prior to transport would include which of the following?
    A. Begin BVM ventilation and immobilize to a backboard.
    B. Place patient in a semi-Fowler's position and begin BVM ventilation.
    C. Apply a traction splint to the left tibia and begin BVM ventilation.
    D. Apply the PASG and a nonrebreather at 15 lpm.

23. You are managing a patient in hemorrhagic shock from a gunshot wound to the chest. After administering 2 liters of lactated Ringer's while en route to the trauma center, the patient regains a radial pulse with a blood pressure of 118/86. You should
    A. continue rapid transport and keep IVs wide open.
    B. back down to a nonemergent transport and set the administration of lactated Ringer's at TKO.
    C. continue rapid transport and set administration of lactated Ringer's at TKO.
    D. begin nonemergent transport and consider the administration of plasma.

24. The best indicator of effective fluid therapy in a hypovolemic patient is
    A. presence of diaphoresis.
    B. regaining radial pulse.
    C. warm skin.
    D. increased blood pressure.

25. The administration of oxygen and ventilatory support are critical to the management of shock by reducing
    A. acidosis and blood loss.
    B. blood loss and respiratory effort.
    C. respiratory effort and hypoxia.
    D. hypoxia and acidosis.

26. Which of the following is the primary reason for not using 5% dextrose in water for fluid resuscitation?
    A. The glucose is quickly metabolized and leaves free water in the intravascular space.
    B. Edema results from the retention of glucose in the intravascular space.
    C. Glucose supplies more calories than are necessary for metabolism.
    D. Alkalosis follows the administration of large volumes of glucose.

27. The flow rate for fluid replacement should be based on the
    A. protocols or online medical direction.
    B. patient's vital signs, mental status, and peripheral pulses.

C. development of peripheral edema and diastolic blood pressure.
    D. transport time and distance.

28. You are treating an unresponsive patient who has been involved in a motor vehicle crash. He has pale, cool, clammy skin; a RR of 42 and shallow; and only a carotid pulse present. What is the most appropriate treatment for this patient?
    A. supine position, oxygen via nonrebreather mask, IV via 22-gauge catheter, transport
    B. elevation of the legs, high-flow oxygen, IV fluids via 14-gauge catheter, rapid transport
    C. Fowler position, ventilation, IV fluids via 20-gauge catheter, rapid transport
    D. positive pressure ventilation, rapid transport, IV fluid initiation en route

29. Which of the following IV solutions will draw water from the intracellular compartment and interstitial space into the intravascular space?
    A. 5% dextrose in water
    B. normal saline
    C. lactated Ringer's
    D. dextran 40

30. Which IV fluid is not compatible with whole blood?
    A. plasmanate
    B. normal saline
    C. lactated Ringer's
    D. 5% dextrose in water

31. While infusing IV fluids, you reassess your patient and find that the patient has developed signs of tachypnea, crackles on ascultation, and jugular venous distention. You recognize these as signs of
    A. thrombophlebitis.
    B. air embolism.
    C. pyrogenic reaction.
    D. circulation overload.

32. Which of the following techniques can be used to check the patentcy of the IV?
    A. Lower the IV bag below the IV site; if blood enters the tubing, the IV is patent.
    B. Compress the bag firmly to force the fluid out; if the fluid drips, the IV is patent.
    C. Replace the constricting band on the arm; if the flow continues, the IV is patent.
    D. Lift the bag above the IV site; if the drip chamber stops flowing, the IV is patent.

33. Which of the following IV catheters provides the greatest volume flow rate?
    A. 20-gauge, 5-cm catheter
    B. 20-gauge, 15-cm catheter
    C. 14-gauge, 5-cm catheter
    D. 14-gauge, 15-cm catheter

34. The ideal replacement fluid for a patient in hemorrhagic shock is
    A. 5% dextrose in water.
    B. lactated Ringer's or normal saline.
    C. plasmanate.
    D. whole blood.

35. You are ordered to administer an IV of a crystalloid solution over 90 minutes at 45 drops per minute using a microdrip administration set. How many milliliters would you deliver to the patient?
    A. 0.5 ml
    B. 2 ml
    C. 67.5 ml
    D. 120 ml

36. You are treating a patient who has experienced considerable blood loss. Which of the following sites would be most appropriate for initiating intravenous therapy?
    A. antecubital fossa
    B. dorsum of the hand
    C. internal jugular vein
    D. ventral forearm

37. All of the following intravenous fluids are correctly paired with their class or form **except**
    A. plasma protein fraction (plasmanate)— colloid.
    B. hetastarch (hespan)—colloid.
    C. normal saline—crystalloid.
    D. lactated Ringer's—colloid.

38. What two parameters are monitored during fluid replacement therapy in an adult patient?
    A. pulse and pupil reaction
    B. blood pressure and pupil reaction
    C. blood pressure and body temperature
    D. pulse and blood pressure

39. You are transporting a patient from a local hospital to a regional trauma center. The patient was struck by a car an hour earlier. An intravenous solution of whole blood is being administered during your transport. The patient suddenly develops hives and palpitations and is nauseated. You should suspect what condition?

    A. fluid overload

    B. pulmonary embolism

    C. transfusion reaction

    D. pulmonary contusion

40. What two factors are most important in determining the speed of flow of intravenous fluids?

    A. the height of the intravenous fluid container and the size of the vein utilized

    B. the size of the vein utilized and the length of the intravenous catheter

    C. the length of the intravenous catheter and the height of the intravenous container

    D. the length of the intravenous catheter and the diameter of the intravenous catheter

41. Which of the following fluids is hypertonic and will cause water to enter the intravascular compartment?

    A. 0.45% NaCl

    B. 0.9% NaCl

    C. 3% NaCl

    D. none of the above

42. Your patient has lost an estimated 1000 ml of blood from a penetrating thoracic injury. What should guide the volume of fluid administered to the patient?

    A. diastolic blood pressure

    B. pulse pressure and heart rate

C. radial pulse and systolic blood pressure

D. carotid pulse and diastolic blood pressure

43. You are providing aggressive fluid resuscitation to a patient who has lost a large amount of blood from multiple gunshot wounds. The volume to be infused is

    A. 20 ml/kg and then reassess.

    B. 2000 ml and then reassess.

    C. 40 ml/kg and then reassess.

    D. 4000 ml and then reassess.

44. Which of the following would allow the fastest administration of solution in a hypovolemic trauma patient?

    A. 14-gauge angio with a microdrip administration set

    B. 22-gauge angio with a microdrip administration set

    C. 16-gauge angio with a macrodrip administration set

    D. 18-gauge angio with a macrodrip administration set

45. When infusing fluids in a trauma patient, there is stretch of the myocardial fibers from the increased preload. As this stretch occurs, the force of contraction _____.

    A. increases

    B. rapidly decreases

    C. progressively decreases

    D. does not change

46. Which of the following fluids would exert a hypertonic effect?

    A. lactated Ringer's

    B. normal saline

    C. packed cells

    D. human serum albumin

47. In the hypovolemic patient who has a suspected intraabdominal hemorrhage, you should run the fluid wide open until
    A. at least 20 ml/kg of fluid are delivered.
    B. you get a systolic blood pressure of at least 90 mm Hg.
    C. the heart rate decreases by 10 beats per minute.
    D. there is no orthostatic drop in blood pressure.

48. You arrive on-scene and find a patient who has sliced his forearm on a piece of glass while replacing a window. He is bleeding profusely on your arrival. You control the bleeding with direct pressure. His vital signs are BP 88/68 mm Hg, HR 118, and RR 22 per minute with good tidal volume. His skin is pale, cool, and clammy. Your treatment should consist of
    A. administering O_2 by nonrebreather, beginning rapid transport, and initiating an IV of normal saline running at 20 ml/kg until the systolic blood pressure returns to greater than 100 mm Hg.
    B. applying a nasal cannula at 6 lpm, initiating an IV of lactated Ringer's, and infusing wide open until the systolic BP reaches 90 mm Hg, then cutting it back to TKO and beginning transport.
    C. inserting an oropharyngeal airway, beginning bag-valve-mask ventilation, initiating an IV of normal saline en route run at a TKO rate and beginning rapid transport.
    D. applying a nonrebreather, initiating an IV of lactated Ringer's running wide open until the radial pulse returns, then cutting it back to TKO and beginning rapid transport.

49. You are instructed by medical direction to infuse 1000 ml of normal saline in a trauma patient as quickly as possible. You would select which of the following equipment?
    A. 18-gauge catheter with a 10-drop macrodrip set
    B. 16-gauge catheter with a 20-drop macrodrip set
    C. 20-gauge catheter with a blood solution set
    D. 14-gauge catheter with a 10-drop macrodrip set

50. You have started an IV line of normal saline in a trauma patient and have it running at a wide-open rate. The patient experiences a sudden onset of fever, chills, headache, and nausea and begins to vomit. You should
    A. suspect the shock is worsening and infuse the fluid faster.
    B. immediately stop the infusion and restart a new IV in the opposite extremity using new tubing, solution, and catheter, suspecting a pyrogenic reaction.
    C. apply pressure to the IV site and remove the catheter because of extravasation of the fluid into the interstitial spaces.
    D. apply warm compresses to the IV site and request antibiotic therapy on your arrival at the hospital for thrombophlebitis.

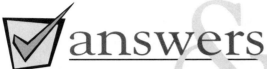

answers & rationales

Following each rationale, you will find a reference to the corresponding objective in the DOT National Standard EMT-Intermediate curriculum. An asterisk denotes material that is supplemental to the DOT curriculum. Page numbers after a rationale indicate where the question topic may be discussed in the Brady text *Intermediate Emergency Care* (Bledsoe, Porter, Cherry).

1.

D. "Let's not meet by accident" is a program developed by a trauma system and prehospital care providers. It is designed to acquaint high school students with EMS and to alert them to the trauma hazards in our society. (*)

2.

C. Always manually stabilize a spine if the mechanism of injury strongly suggests an injury in this area. Assign one of your crew to stabilize the head manually while you continue your primary assessment. Release manual stabilization only after you secure the head to a long spine board. (4-5.16) (IEC p. 739)

3.

A. Always ensure a patent airway immediately. Examine it for fluids, obstruction, or signs of trauma and apply suction as necessary. A noisy airway is an obstructive airway. (*) (IEC pp. 740, 749)

4.

B. Always be concerned about a flail segment because it may severely inhibit ventilation and oxygenation. Your patient may become hypoxic and hypercarbic. (4-5.11) (IEC p. 740)

5.

D. This patient's respiratory status indicates the need for positive pressure ventilation with a bag-valve-mask and supplemental oxygen. (4-5.12) (IEC pp. 740–741)

6.

C. Your patient's blood pressure and pulse indicate that he is in decompensated shock. It is during this stage that the body's normal defense mechanisms are failing. (4-5.5) (IEC pp. 661–662)

7.

B. The most probable cause of this patient's shock is internal blood loss, probably in the abdomen. (4-5.7) (IEC pp. 647–650)

8.

D. Peripheral vascular resistance is primarily regulated in the arterioles. Arterioles have the ability to affect blood pressure and direct blood flow from the heart to various organs. They can open and close with a valvelike function and can vary their inner diameter by as much as a factor of 5. (*)

9.

D. In decompensated shock, anaerobic metabolism occurs. Anaerobic metabolism occurs when there is insufficient oxygen for the cell to function. As a result of this inefficient process, acids accumulate. Resuscitation at this point is still possible, but irreversible shock will ensue if this patient is left untreated. (4-5.5)

10.

C. Since this patient responds only to pain stimuli, he receives a P on the AVPU scale. (4-5.5) (IEC pp. 493–494)

11.

A. Prehospital fluid resuscitation is accomplished using normal saline or lactated Ringer's. These isotonic solutions are ideal for fluid resuscitation because they tend to remain in the intravascular space for a period of time. (4-5.10) (IEC p. 665)

12.

B. In order to maximize fluid flow, use an IV catheter with the largest gauge and shortest length and 10-drop/m/IV tubing. (4-5.10) (IEC pp. 306–308, 666)

13.

C. Fluid resuscitation in the field is very controversial. In general, it should be limited to 3 liters of crystalloid solution. Reasons for the controversy include the loss of two-thirds of the fluid from the vascular space within 1 hour, its inability to transport oxygen to the tissues, and its possible interference with normal clotting. (4-5.2) (IEC p. 667)

14.

B. Hot loading refers to loading a patient into a helicopter while the rotors continue to turn. If you are asked to help load the patient, stay close to the flight crew and avoid the area of the tail rotor. The tail rotor spins at speeds in excess of 2000 rpm and is almost invisible. (*)

15.

C. A landing zone should be a minimum of 60×60 feet for small helicopters, 75×75 feet for medium ones, and 120×120 feet for large ones. (*)

16.

C. A burn patient would benefit from a hypertonic solution because the hypertonicity of the IV fluids would draw water from the interstitial spaces back into the vasculature. Remember also that a burn patient loses a large amount of fluids to the tissues as a result of the burn. A hypertonic solution can also help reduce the swelling seen in severe burn patients. (*) (IEC p. 307)

17.

A. Administering a fluid bolus to a hypovolemic patient will provide more volume in the venous system, which will result in an increased preload. Heart rate and contractility may be moderately enhanced with the increased preload, but that is not the major benefit of IV therapy. Afterload refers to the degree of arterial tone the heart needs to contract against. (*) (IEC p. 307)

18.

C. The treatment is to slow the IV rate down to KVO and consult medical direction. Volume expansion is necessary for a hypovolemic patient in shock. Be careful, however, not to overhydrate the patient. If that occurs, you may note inspiratory crackles. (4-5.2)

19.

A. When providing fluid resuscitation, use the most appropriate equipment that will allow a rapid infusion of volume. This should include a large-bore angiocatheter, an isotonic solution, and macrodrip administration or even a blood solution set. (4-5.2) (IEC pp. 665–667)

20.

A. Any patient who cannot control his or her own airway should have it done artificially by endotracheal intubation in the absence of a gag reflex. Immobilization should always occur on the basis of the mechanism of injury, and medical control may still authorize the use of the AED. Volume expansion should occur with an isotonic volume expander, such as normal saline or lactated Ringer's. (*)

21.

A. High-flow oxygen would be the most beneficial option for this patient. This individual appears to have a lacerated spleen and is becoming hypovolemic. Human cellular function is dependent on adequate oxygenation via the red blood cells (hemoglobin). Because the hemorrhage is internal, hemorrhage control is difficult. Subsequently, the EMT-Intermediate must saturate the remaining red blood cells with oxygen in an attempt to maximize delivery of oxygen to the body tissues. Fluid replacement is important but will not deliver increased amounts of oxygen to the individual cells. (*) (IEC p. 768)

22.

A. Prior to transport, first you must begin bag-valve-mask ventilation with supplemental oxygen connected to the reservoir. Second, the patient must be fully immobilized to a backboard. The fractures will be somewhat splinted by the backboard and are not a major concern. (*) (IEC pp. 752, 756)

23.

C. The continued needs of this patient include rapid transport and the continued administration of lactated Ringer's. The administration of lactated Ringer's with its associated positive effects are only temporary in that only volume expansion has been achieved. Volume expansion does not replace the loss of the red blood cells, which serve to transport oxygen to the individual cells. Once a radial pulse is regained, reduce the fluid administration so as not to promote further bleeding. (4-5.12)

24.

B. Regaining the radial pulse would indicate that the peripheral perfusion is improving. The presence of diaphoresis would suggest continued cellular hypoxia through the innervation of the sympathetic nervous system. Warm skin is not the best indication because this may suggest body-heated volume expansion. This is not a guarantee of alleviated anaerobic metabolism. In addition, the sympathetic nervous system can maintain the blood pressure via vasoconstriction in a compensatory effort. (4-5.12)

25.

D. Administering oxygen and ventilatory support are critical to the management of shock. Hypoxia triggers the release of vasodilators as a compensatory mechanism in shock. This increases localized blood flow but decreases systemic vascular resistance, resulting in low blood pressure. Acidosis causes depression of the central nervous system, including the vasomotor center. (4-5.2) (IEC p. 665)

26.

A. While the administration of any solution will cause an initial increase in circulatory volume, 5% dextrose in water is a poor choice for fluid replacement because the glucose is quickly metabolized, resulting in an increase in free water. This free water is hypotonic, and it will dilute the remaining blood volume and leave the intravascular space quickly. (4-5.2) (IEC p. 307)

27.

B. Although protocols may set parameters for fluid replacement, the flow rate for fluid replacement should be based on the patient's response to treatment as evidenced by improving vital signs, mental status, and return of peripheral pulses. Once stabilized, you should continue to closely monitor your patient's status being alert to the presence of signs and symptoms of developing pulmonary edema. (4-5.2) (IEC pp. 666–667)

28.

D. This patient is in decompensated shock and needs to be rapidly and aggressively managed. This patient needs to be ventilated immediately. Also, this patient will need an intravenous line placed once en route to the trauma center. (4-5.6) (IEC pp. 665–667)

29.

D. Dextran 40 is a colloid solution with large sugar molecules and osmotic properties. Dextran will remain in the intravascular space for an extended period of time. Colloids attract water into the intravascular space by increasing the colloid osmotic pressure, which helps expand the volume. D5W is a hypotonic glucose solution that does not expand the fluid in the intravascular space. (4-5.2) (IEC pp. 306–307)

30.

C. Lactated Ringer's is not compatible with whole blood. Since it is likely that whole blood will be administered at the hospital, it is recommended that two IV lines be started. At least one IV should be normal saline where whole blood can be given if necessary. (4-5.2)

31.

D. All these are signs of circulation overload and can cause great harm or even death to your patient. As soon as you notice these symptoms, immediately adjust the flow rate to a KVO. Thrombophlebitis is inflammation of the vein and is more common when the IV therapy is long term. Air embolism is when air is allowed to enter the vein. (4-5.2) (IEC pp. 319–320)

32.

A. By lowering the bag, gravity will allow the blood to flow from the vein into the tubing, thus confirming that the IV is patent. Compressing the bag will not ensure that the IV is in the lumen of the vein and may cause further damage if the IV has infiltrated. Replacing the constricting band on the arm will not permit you to check for patentcy; furthermore, this will reduce venous flow and cause the flow to cease. If the bag is above the IV site and the flow ceases, the IV is not patent. (4-5.2) (IEC p. 319)

33.

C. The greatest amount of volume can be delivered through the 14-gauge, 5-cm catheter. A lower gauge number represents a larger-diameter catheter that will deliver larger amounts of fluid. A shorter catheter will deliver more fluid than a longer catheter. (4-5.2) (IEC pp. 312, 666)

34.

D. Whole blood is the most desirable fluid replacement. It contains hemaglobin and other essential proteins. However, it is not a practical choice in the prehospital setting. While plasmanate would be the next choice, colloids are not typically used in the prehospital setting because of either their expense or their short shelf life. The solution of choice in the prehospital setting is an isotonic crystalloid. (4-5.2) (IEC p. 307)

35.

C. (4-5.2) (IEC pp. 345–346)

$$\frac{1 \text{ ml}}{60 \text{ gtt}} \times \frac{45 \text{ gtt}}{\text{minutes}} \times 90 \text{ min} = 67.5 \text{ ml}$$

36.

A. The antecubital fossa and external jugular veins are the ideal site for fluid volume replacement. The larger diameter of both of these veins compared to the veins of the hand and distal portion of the arm makes these veins more suitable for resuscitation. (4-5.2) (IEC pp. 312–317)

37.

D. Lactated Ringer's, normal saline, and 5% dextrose in water are all considered crystalloids. Lactated Ringer's solution and normal saline stay in the intravascular compartment longer than does 5% dextrose in water. Normal saline and lactated Ringer's solution will stay in the vascular space for up to 1 hour before moving into the interstitial space. Colloids such as plasmanate, albumin, dextran, and hetastarch contain proteins or large glucose molecules. Because of the high molecular weight, they tend to stay in the vascular space for long time periods. (*) (IEC pp. 306–307)

38.

D. During fluid replacement therapy, it is important to monitor the patient's pulse, blood pressure, skin temperature, and color. Auscultate the chest frequently. Observe for signs of fluid overload, such as dyspnea, pulmonary congestion (edema), and altered mental status. (4-5.2) (IEC pp. 665–667)

39.

C. This patient is exhibiting signs of a transfusion reaction. This occurs from the administration of blood or blood products. Additional signs and symptoms include hypotension, fever, chills, tachycardia, flushing of the skin, headaches, loss of consciousness, vomiting, and shortness of breath. (4-5.2) (IEC p. 320)

40.

D. The two most important factors that affect flow rate are the length and diameter of the intravenous catheter. For the patient who requires fluid replacement, use the largest-diameter intravenous catheter practical and one of the shortest length. Use the shortest-length administration set as well. (4-5.2) (IEC pp. 312, 666)

41.

C. 0.9% sodium chloride is considered to be isotonic with the body, so a solution that is 3% sodium chloride is hypertonic. It will draw water into the vascular space. Finally, 0.45% is hypotonic and will result in water exiting from the vascular space. (4-5.2) (IEC pp. 306–307)

42.

C. The radial pulse and systolic blood pressure are used to guide fluid administration. The goal is to establish a radial pulse and/or a systolic blood pressure of 90 mm Hg. (4-5.2) (IEC pp. 665–667)

43.

A. When providing fluid replacement for blood loss, infuse at a wide-open rate at increments of 20 ml/kg. If the patient is still showing clinical signs of shock and has no radial pulse or the systolic blood pressure is less than 90 mm Hg, repeat the 20-ml/kg bolus and again reassess. (4-5.2) (IEC pp. 666–667)

44.

C. In a hypovolemic patient, the goal is intravenous cannulation, which will allow rapid fluid infusion if needed. The arrangement of a 16-gauge angio with a macrodrip administration set will allow the fastest flow rate. The 14-gauge response is an appropriate gauge for trauma, but the microdrip administration set would be prohibitive if infusing fluids rapidly. (4-5.2) (IEC pp. 312, 666)

45.

A. Starling's law of the heart discusses the increase in myocardial contraction when the muscle fibers are stretched by increases in preload. The enhanced recoil results in more forceful expulsion of a larger amount of blood. This increase in stroke volume will then translate into improved cardiac output and eventually into improved blood pressure. (*) (IEC p. 197)

46.

D. Human serum albumin is a hypertonic solution and will draw fluid into the intravascular space. Both lactated Ringer's and normal saline are isotonic solutions and will not cause a fluid shift. Packed cells will have no osmotic effect. (4-5.2) (IEC p. 306)

47.

B. When infusing fluid in a patient with internal hemorrhage that cannot be controlled, the goal of fluid resuscitation is to infuse only enough fluid to regain a radial pulse or increase the systolic blood pressure to 90 mm Hg. More aggressive fluid infusion may cause a more rapid blood loss and is contraindicated. (4-5.2) (IEC p. 667)

48.

A. Fluid can be infused at a rate of 20 ml/kg in a patient with blood loss where the bleeding is controlled. If the bleeding is controlled, the systolic blood pressure can be raised above 100 mm Hg. (4-5.2) (IEC pp. 665–667)

49.

D. The fluid can be infused most rapidly by using a 14-gauge catheter with a 10-drop macrodrip solution set. (4-5.2) (IEC pp. 312, 666)

50.

B. A pyrogenic reaction occurs from contaminated fluid, tubing, or catheters. It presents as a sudden onset of fever, chills, headache, nausea, and vomiting. On recognition, you should immediately stop and disconnect the IV line. Initiate another IV with a new solution, tubing, and catheter at a new site. (4-5.2) (IEC pp. 319–320)

Respiratory Emergencies

unit objectives

Questions in this unit relate to DOT objectives 5-1.1 to 5-1.8. The objectives are listed in the Appendix.

DIRECTIONS
Each of the questions or incomplete statements below is followed by suggested answers or completions. Select the **one answer** that is best in each case.

1. A patient who presents with orthopnea
   A. has difficulty in breathing when sitting straight up.
   B. has difficulty in breathing when lying flat.
   C. uses only the diaphragm.
   D. depends on hypoxic drive to breathe.

2. Coughing up blood from the respiratory tree is called
   A. hematemesis.
   B. hematoma.
   C. hemoptysis.
   D. hymenoptera.

3. Pulsus paradoxus occurs when
   A. the pulse increases during inspiration.
   B. the systolic blood pressure decreases 10 torr while breathing.
   C. the pulse rises and blood pressure drops when the patient sits up.
   D. none of the above

4. If your patient presents with carpopedal spasms, this is most likely the result of
   A. hyperventilation.
   B. severe respiratory acidosis.
   C. metabolic alkalosis.
   D. congestive heart failure.

5. Which of the following measures the maximum amount of air in lpm that your patient can expire?
   A. pulse oximeter
   B. Wright spirometer
   C. capnograph
   D. colormetric capnometer

Scenario
Questions 6–9 refer to the following scenario:

Your patient is a 59-year-old male who presents sitting at the kitchen table in moderate respiratory distress. His elbows are on the table in a tripod position, and he appears to be really working at breathing. Although this problem came on gradually today, his family states that he has had lung disease for a long time. He is a lifetime smoker and is on home oxygen at 2 lpm via nasal cannula. He takes Atrovent® (ipratropium bromide) inhaler, Theolair® (theophylline), and Proventil® (albuterol) inhaler. He appears very thin and barrel chested with a pink complexion. You immediately notice the pronounced accessory muscles in his neck and chest along with retractions. He labors to breathe, pursing his lips during exhalation. His vital signs are pulse 90, BP 140/80, respiratory rate 40, skin warm and pink, diffuse expiratory wheezes, and O_2 saturation 90%.

6. Your prehospital diagnosis is
   A. asthma.
   B. congestive heart failure.
   C. chronic bronchitis.
   D. emphysema.

7. This disease is characterized by
   A. alveolar wall destruction.
   B. hypermucous secretion.
   C. decreased left-ventricular function.
   D. allergic reaction.

8. His pink complexion is caused by
   A. decreased carbon dioxide levels.
   B. increased oxygen levels.
   C. increased red blood cell production.
   D. decreased tidal volume.

9. Immediate management of this patient includes
   A. continued oxygen at 2 lpm via nasal cannula.
   B. bronchodilation.
   C. IV fluid replacement with normal saline.
   D. all of the above

Scenario

Questions 10–14 refer to the following scenario:

Your patient is a 24-year-old male who presents in severe respiratory distress. His wife states that he has had increasing difficulty in breathing all morning but now is much worse. He has a history of asthma and takes two oral medications: Theo-Dur® (theophylline) and prednisone. He also takes two metered-dose inhalers: Ventolin® (albuterol) and Beclovent® (beclomethasone). On examination, you find an otherwise healthy person who speaks in words only. His vital signs are pulse 120 and strong, BP 140/80, respirations 40 and very labored, and skin pale. You auscultate inspiratory and expiratory wheezes and rhonchi bilaterally. He is hyperressonant to percussion.

10. Asthma is a disease characterized by
    A. airway edema.
    B. bronchospasm.
    C. hypermucous secretion.
    D. all of the above

11. Prednisone and beclomethasone are drugs that
    A. dilate the bronchioles directly.
    B. decrease inflammation.

C. stimulate the respiratory center.
D. block the allergic response.

12. Albuterol and theophylline are prescribed to
    A. dilate the bronchioles directly.
    B. decrease inflammation.
    C. inhibit the respiratory center.
    D. block the allergic response.

13. The hyperresonance is due to
    A. collapsed alveoli.
    B. associated pneumothorax.
    C. air trapped in the alveoli.
    D. decreased duration of the expiratory phase.

14. Prehospital management of this patient includes
    A. 100% oxygen.
    B. Proventil/Atrovent combination.
    C. IV access.
    D. all of the above

15. A patient who presents with shortness of breath, chest pain, fever, chills, general malaise, a productive yellow sputum streaked with blood, and rales and wheezes in the lower-right lobe probably has
    A. congestive heart failure.
    B. emphysema.
    C. an acute asthma attack.
    D. pneumonia.

16. The problem described in the previous question is a respiratory infection caused by a
    A. virus.
    B. bacterium.
    C. fungus.
    D. all of the above

Scenario

Questions 17–19 refer to the following scenario:

Your patient is a firefighter who took off his self-contained breathing apparatus (SCBA) while performing overhaul procedures in a house fire. He presents with a headache, irritability, loss of coordination, and confusion.

17. This patient is probably suffering from
    A. acute myocardial infarction.
    B. carbon monoxide poisoning.
    C. transient ischemic attack.
    D. stroke.

18. The pathophysiology of this problem includes
    A. CO binding on hemoglobin.
    B. cellular hypoxia.
    C. metabolic acidosis.
    D. all of the above

19. Management of this situation includes
    A. airway management.
    B. 100% oxygenation.
    C. transportation to a hyperbaric chamber.
    D. all of the above

Scenario

Questions 20–22 refer to the following scenario:

Your patient is a 45-year-old man who complains of sudden onset of upper-right-sided stabbing chest pain and shortness of breath. He has no other medical history except for being hospitalized with pneumonia 2 weeks ago and sent home to recuperate. Earlier this week, he had ex-perienced some lower-calf pain. He presents in moderate distress with the following vital signs: pulse 100, BP 140/80, respirations 28, skin warm and dry, and some expiratory wheezing in the area of chest pain.

20. Your prehospital diagnosis is
    A. acute asthma attack.
    B. acute myocardial infarction.
    C. acute pulmonary embolism.
    D. spontaneous pneumothorax.

21. This problem is characterized by
    A. an allergic reaction.
    B. coronary artery ischemia.
    C. a moving blood clot.
    D. a ruptured lung.

22. A predisposing factor of this condition is
    A. prolonged immobilization.
    B. atherosclerosis.
    C. a congenital defect.
    D. hyperreactive airways.

23. Your patient is a tall, thin male in his late 20s who presents with sudden onset of sharp pain in the upper-right chest and mild shortness of breath. He has no history and takes no medications but has smoked for 10 years. He has decreased lung sounds in the upper-right apex and some subcutaneous emphysema in the same area. He is tachycardic, diaphoretic, and pale. Your field diagnosis is
    A. spontaneous pneumothorax.
    B. traumatic asphyxia.
    C. ruptured aortic aneurysm.
    D. aortic valve stenosis.

Scenario

Questions 24–30 refer to the following scenario:

Your patient is a 79-year-old female who presents in moderate respiratory distress. She sits upright and can answer your questions only with short phrases. She describes having a recent cold and this worsening shortness of breath and cough. She denies any chest pain. She has a long history of breathing problems. She claims that she gets this every year at this time and that it lasts about 2 months. She also admits to smoking two packs of cigarettes each day for the past 50 years. Her vital signs are pulse 100 and regular, BP 150/80, respiratory rate 36 and labored, and skin cyanotic. You auscultate diffuse expiratory wheezes. She has a very productive cough, with her sputum being yellowish-brown and sticky. She has pitting pedal edema and ascites.

24. Your prehospital diagnosis should be
    A. acute asthma.
    B. emphysema.
    C. chronic bronchitis.
    D. acute pulmonary embolism.

25. The cause of this disease is
    A. allergies.
    B. venous stasis.
    C. years of toxic inhalation.
    D. none of the above

26. The pathophysiology of this disease involves
    A. the destruction of alveolar walls.
    B. increased mucus production.
    C. a traveling blood clot.
    D. hyperreactive airways.

27. This patient's smoking history is described as
    A. 50 pack years.
    B. 2 pack years.
    C. 100 pack years.
    D. none of the above.

28. Her sputum indicates
    A. respiratory infection.
    B. pulmonary edema.
    C. hematemesis.
    D. hemoptysis.

29. Her cyanosis is caused by
    A. hypocarbia.
    B. hypoxia.
    C. pulmonary hypertension.
    D. increased residual volume.

30. The base station physician orders you to administer albuterol via nebulizer in an attempt to
    A. decrease pulmonary edema.
    B. stop the allergic reaction.
    C. dilate the airways.
    D. increase cardiac contractions.

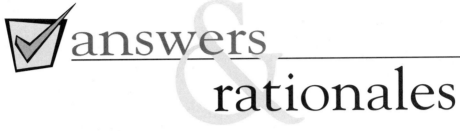

Following each rationale, you will find a reference to the corresponding objective in the DOT National Standard EMT-Intermediate curriculum. An asterisk denotes material that is supplemental to the DOT curriculum. Page numbers after a rationale indicate where the question topic may be discussed in the Brady text *Intermediate Emergency Care* (Bledsoe, Porter, Cherry).

1.

B. Orthopnea is the patient's sensation of difficulty in breathing while lying flat. It is a common complaint in patients with congestive heart failure. (5-1.4) (IEC p. 810)

2.

C. Hemoptysis is the coughing up of blood from the respiratory tree. Hemoptysis can be caused by tumors, pulmonary emboli, and many forms of blunt or penetrating chest trauma. (5-1.4) (IEC p. 810)

3.

B. Pulsus paradoxus occurs when there is a drop in the systolic blood pressure of 10 torr or more with each respiratory cycle. It is associated with chronic obstructive pulmonary disease and cardiac tamponade. As a rule, in the field, you should not take the time to look for pulsus paradoxus. (5-1.4) (IEC p. 813)

4.

A. A patient with carpopedal spasms presents with his fingers and toes in flexion. This is the result of transient shifts in blood calcium caused by changes in the serum CO_2 and pH levels from hyperventilating. Your main job in these cases is to find out **why** your patient was or is still hyperventilating. (5-1.4) (IEC p. 812)

5.

B. A Wright spirometer measures your patient's peak flow in lpm. It is useful in determining the degree of lower-airway resistance and measuring the efficacy of treatments. For example, if before treatment your asthmatic patient can blow only 45% of normal and after an albuterol treatment he can blow 75%, you can assume your treatments are working. (5-1.7) (IEC p. 814)

6.

D. The prehospital diagnosis of this patient should be emphysema. (5-1.8) (IEC p. 820)

7.

A. Emphysema results from destruction of the alveolar walls distal to the terminal bronchioles. This disease is caused by exposure to noxious substances, such as cigarette smoke, and results in the gradual destruction of the walls of the alveoli, decreasing the alveolar membrane surface area and lessening the area available for gas exchange. (5-1.8) (IEC p. 820)

8.

C. Patients with emphysema tend to be pink in color because of polycythemia and are referred to as "pink puffers." The polycythemia occurs as an excess of red blood cells is produced. (5-1.8) (IEC p. 821)

9.

B. Immediate management of this patient includes administering 100% oxygen via a nonrebreather mask and attempting to dilate the lower airways with albuterol, ipratropium, or a combination of both. (5-1.8) (IEC p. 823)

10.

D. Asthma is a disease characterized by lower-airway edema, bronchospasm, and hypermucous secretion. This is the classic pathophysiological triad of asthma. (5-1.8) (IEC p. 823)

11.

B. Prednisone and beclomethasone are drugs that decrease inflammation. These belong to a class known as corticosteroids. (5-1.8) (IEC p. 824)

12.

A. Albuterol (beta agonist) and theophylline (xanthine) are prescribed to directly dilate the bronchioles. (5-1.8) (IEC p. 824)

13.

C. The asthma patient may exhibit hyperresonance on percussion. This hyperresonance is due to the collapse of the bronchioles on exhalation, trapping air in the distal airways and alveoli. (5-1.8) (IEC p. 824)

14.

D. Prehospital management of this patient includes 100% oxygen, Proventil/Atrovent combination via nebulizer, IV access, ECG monitoring, and reassessment for deterioration or signs of status asthmaticus. (5-1.8) (IEC p. 825)

15.

D. A patient who presents with shortness of breath, chest pain, fever, chills, general malaise, a productive yellow sputum streaked with blood, and rales and wheezing in the lower-right lobe probably has pneumonia. Other clues include pleuritic chest pain, dull to percussion, and egophony. Pneumonia is an infection of the lungs and a common medical problem. (5-1.8) (IEC p. 827)

16.

D. Pneumonia is a common respiratory disease caused when an infectious agent invades the lungs. Pneumonia can be bacterial, viral, or fungal. It may involve part or all of the lung. (5-1.8) (IEC p. 827)

17.

B. A particular hazard for firefighters and rescue personnel is carbon monoxide poisoning, particularly during overhaul operations when some smoldering still occurs. A smoldering fire yields much carbon monoxide. (5-1.4) (IEC p. 830)

18.

D. Carbon monoxide is an odorless, tasteless, and colorless gas produced from the incomplete burning of fossil fuels. Carbon monoxide easily binds to the hemoglobin molecule. Once bound, receptor sites on the hemoglobin can no longer transport oxygen to the peripheral tissues. The result is hypoxia at the cellular level and ultimately metabolic acidosis. (*) (IEC p. 830)

19.

D. Management of any patient suspected of having carbon monoxide poisoning includes ensuring a patent airway, providing 100% oxygen, and transporting the patient rapidly to a hyperbaric chamber. Hyperbaric oxygen increases PaO_2 and promotes oxygen uptake on hemoglobin molecules not yet bound by carbon monoxide. (*) (IEC p. 830)

20.

C. This patient, who complains of sudden onset of upper-right-sided stabbing chest pain and shortness of breath following hospitalization and confinement to bed for a couple of weeks and of lower-leg pain, probably has suffered an acute pulmonary embolism. (5-1.8) (IEC p. 830)

21.

C. Pulmonary embolism is a blood clot or some other particle that lodges in a pulmonary artery. The condition is potentially life threatening because it can significantly decrease pulmonary blood flow, thus leading to hypoxemia. The problem occurs when a blood clot travels up the venous circulatory system and lodges in a pulmonary artery. (5-1.8) (IEC p. 831)

22.

A. Factors predisposing a patient to blood clots include prolonged immobilization, thrombophlebitis, the use of certain medications, and atrial fibrillation. (5-1.8) (IEC p. 831)

23.

A. A spontaneous pneumothorax occurs in the absence of trauma usually in tall, thin males between 20 and 40 years old. Risk factors include cigarette smoking. As with a pneumothorax, it is important to ensure adequate ventilation of the lungs while you monitor for a developing tension pneumothorax. (5-1.8) (IEC p. 832)

24.

C. Your patient presents with the classic signs and symptoms of chronic bronchitis. (5-1.8) (IEC p. 822)

25.

C. Following prolonged exposure to cigarette smoke, the number of mucus-secreting cells in the respiratory tree increases, producing a large quantity of sputum. (5-1.8) (IEC p. 822)

26.

B. The pathophysiology of chronic bronchitis involves increased mucus production. This increased mucus becomes a place for bacteria to grow, making the patient susceptible to frequent respiratory tract infections. (5-1.8) (IEC p. 822)

27.

C. Every patient suspected of having lung disease should be questioned about cigarette and tobacco use. This is generally reported in pack years. Multiply the number of cigarette packs smoked per day by the number of years smoked. This patient smoked two packs per day for 50 years, making her a 100-pack-years smoker (and a member of the Century Club). (5-1.8) (IEC p. 821)

28.

A. Yellow sputum indicates a lower respiratory infection typical of patients with exacerbations of chronic bronchitis. (5-1.8) (IEC p. 822)

29.

B. Patients with chronic bronchitis tend to be overweight and cyanotic. Because of this, they are referred to as "blue bloaters." This is due to the chronic hypoxia. (5-1.8) (IEC p. 822)

30.

C. Common first-line treatment for chronic bronchitis is to administer a sympathomimetic bronchodilator via nebulizer in an attempt to dilate the lower airways. These inhaled beta agonists include albuterol, metaproterenol, and isoetharine. Inhaled anticholinergics, such as ipratropium bromide, are also indicated. (5-1.8) (IEC p. 823)

Cardiovascular Emergencies

unit objectives

Questions in this unit relate to DOT objectives 5-2.1 to 5-2.39. The objectives are listed in the Appendix.

DIRECTIONS Each of the questions or incomplete statements below is followed by suggested answers or completions. Select the **one answer** that is best in each case.

1. The heart muscle is perfused by the
   A. coronary arteries.
   B. cerebral arteries.
   C. inferior vena cava.
   D. subclavian arteries.

2. The amount of blood ejected by the heart in one contraction is called
   A. preload.
   B. cardiac output.
   C. blood pressure.
   D. stroke volume.

3. Which of the following does not directly affect stroke volume?
   A. preload
   B. afterload
   C. heart rate
   D. contractile force

4. Up to a point, the greater the preload, the greater the
   A. contractile force.
   B. heart rate.
   C. afterload.
   D. blood pressure.

5. The resistance against which the heart must pump is called
   A. preload.
   B. afterload.
   C. Starling's effect.
   D. end-diastolic volume.

6. Another name for preload is
   A. afterload.
   B. end-diastolic volume.

   C. blood pressure.
   D. stroke volume.

7. A person with a stroke volume of 70 ml and a heart rate of 80 has a cardiac output of
   A. 5600 ml.
   B. 1500 ml.
   C. 560 ml.
   D. 150 ml.

8. Preload is dependent on
   A. arteriole vasoconstriction.
   B. venous return.
   C. stroke volume.
   D. ventricular strength.

9. A positive inotropic drug increases
   A. heart rate.
   B. conduction velocity.
   C. contractile force.
   D. refractoriness.

10. A negative chronotropic drug decreases
    A. heart rate.
    B. conduction velocity.
    C. contractile force.
    D. refractoriness.

11. Specialized structures designed to speed conduction from one muscle fiber to the next are the
    A. syncytial tissues.
    B. inotropic fibers.
    C. intercalated discs.
    D. autonomic cells.

12. The cells of the cardiac conductive system have
    A. automaticity.
    B. excitability.
    C. conductivity.
    D. all of the above

13. The normal intrinsic firing rate of the SA node is
    A. 20–40 beats per minute.
    B. 40–60 beats per minute.
    C. 60–100 beats per minute.
    D. none of the above

14. The normal intrinsic firing rate of the AV junction is
    A. 20–40 beats per minute.
    B. 40–60 beats per minute.
    C. 60–100 beats per minute.
    D. none of the above

15. The normal intrinsic firing rate of the Purkinje system is
    A. 20–40 beats per minute.
    B. 40–60 beats per minute.
    C. 60–100 beats per minute.
    D. none of the above

16. In Einthoven's triangle, lead 2 is characterized by
    A. right leg negative, left arm positive.
    B. left leg positive, right arm negative.
    C. right leg positive, left arm negative.
    D. left leg negative, right arm positive.

17. Which of the following can be obtained from a single-lead ECG reading?
    A. the presence of an infarct
    B. cardiac output
    C. chamber enlargement
    D. heart rate

18. The P wave represents
    A. atrial depolarization.
    B. ventricular depolarization.
    C. delay at the AV node.
    D. ventricular repolarization.

19. The T wave represents
    A. atrial depolarization.
    B. ventricular depolarization.
    C. delay at the AV node.
    D. ventricular repolarization.

20. The QRS complex represents
    A. atrial depolarization.
    B. ventricular depolarization.
    C. delay at the AV node.
    D. ventricular repolarization.

21. The P–R interval represents
    A. atrial depolarization.
    B. ventricular depolarization.
    C. delay at the AV node.
    D. ventricular repolarization.

22. Which of the following may produce artifact on the ECG?
    A. muscle tremors
    B. loose electrodes
    C. 60-Hz interference
    D. all of the above

23. The normal P–R interval is
    A. <0.12 second.
    B. 0.12–0.20 second.
    C. 0.04–0.1 second.
    D. none of the above

24. The normal QRS complex is
    A. <0.04 second.
    B. 0.12–0.20 second.
    C. 0.04–0.12 second.
    D. none of the above

25. Which of the following could cause a cardiac dysrhythmia?
    A. lateral wall myocardial infarction
    B. hyperkalemia
    C. hypoxia and acidosis
    D. all of the above

Scenario

Questions 26–28 refer to the following scenario:

Your patient is a 45-year-old male who experienced some chest discomfort while jogging. The pain is substernal and does not radiate. He has no previous medical history and takes no medications. The pain is somewhat relieved by rest. His BP is 150/88, pulse 96 and regular, respirations 18, and skin warm and pink. His lungs are clear bilaterally, and he has no other remarkable signs or symptoms. His ECG strip is shown in Figure 1.

26. This patient's probable diagnosis is
    A. stable angina.
    B. unstable angina.
    C. preinfarction angina.
    D. Prinzmetal's angina.

27. His ECG strip is
    A. sinus tachycardia.
    B. wandering atrial pacemaker.

C. premature atrial contractions.
D. normal sinus rhythm.

28. Initial prehospital management of this patient should include oxygen and
    A. morphine IV.
    B. nitroglycerin SL.
    C. epinephrine SC.
    D. atropine IV.

Scenario

Questions 29–32 refer to the following scenario:

Your patient is a 56-year-old female who complains of sudden onset of substernal chest pressure with no radiation while watching television. She denies any shortness of breath or nausea. She has a history of atherosclerotic heart disease and takes diltiazem. Her BP is 160/90, pulse 110, respirations 16, skin warm and dry, and lungs clear bilaterally. She has no other remarkable physical findings. Her ECG is shown in Figure 2.

29. This patient is probably experiencing
    A. stable angina.
    B. unstable angina.
    C. cardiogenic shock.
    D. Ludwig's angina.

FIGURE 1

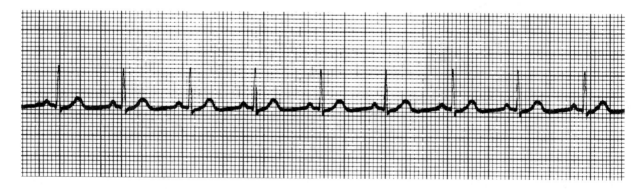

FIGURE 2

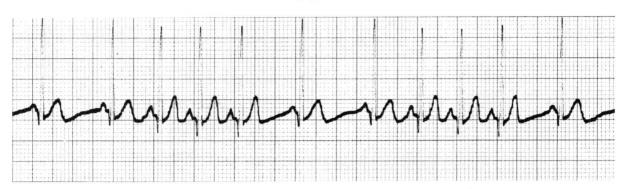

30. Her ECG strip is
    A. normal sinus rhythm.
    B. premature atrial contraction.
    C. wandering atrial pacemaker.
    D. sinus dysrhythmia.

31. The process by which fatty deposits collect within arterial walls is known as
    A. arteriosclerosis.
    B. atherosclerosis.
    C. arteriosclerotitis.
    D. atheritis.

32. Diltiazem is a drug in which class?
    A. nitrate
    B. beta blocker

C. calcium channel blocker
D. diuretic

Scenario

Questions 33–36 refer to the following scenario:

Your patient is a 65-year-old man who complains of sudden onset of substernal chest pain radiating to the neck and left shoulder. It began while eating 1 hour ago and has not subsided. He also complains of some shortness of breath, nausea, and dizziness. He has a history of coronary artery disease and hypertension. He takes Procardia XL once a day. His BP is 180/80, pulse 80 and irregular, respirations 26, lungs clear, and skin warm and dry. His ECG strip is shown in Figure 3.

FIGURE 3

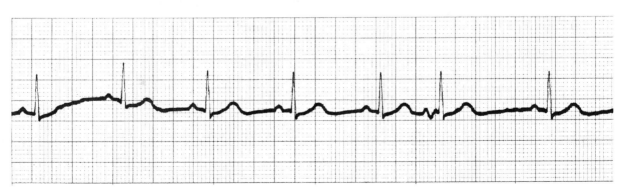

33. This patient is probably suffering from
    A. stable angina.
    B. unstable angina.
    C. acute myocardial infarction.
    D. cardiogenic shock.

34. His ECG strip is
    A. normal sinus rhythm.
    B. premature atrial contraction.
    C. wandering atrial pacemaker.
    D. sinus dysrhythmia.

35. Procardia XL is a drug in which class?
    A. nitrate
    B. beta blocker
    C. calcium channel blocker
    D. diuretic

36. Prehospital management of this patient includes
    A. high-flow oxygen.
    B. pain management.
    C. reassurance.
    D. all of the above

Scenario

Questions 37–40 refer to the following scenario:

Your patient is a 45-year-old female who complains of mild to moderate shortness of breath and some chest discomfort. She has a long history of cardiac problems and takes digoxin, Lasix, and Slow-K. Her BP is 180/80, pulse 94 and very irregular, respirations 20, and skin cool and pink. She has bilateral crackles (rales) in the lower lobes. She has no peripheral edema or JVD. Her ECG is shown in Figure 4.

37. Your diagnosis of this patient is
    A. right-heart failure.
    B. left-heart failure.
    C. cardiogenic shock.
    D. acute pulmonary edema.

38. Her medications suggest she has
    A. abnormal cardiac dysrhythmias.
    B. aortic valve problems.
    C. cor pulmonale.
    D. congestive heart failure.

FIGURE 4

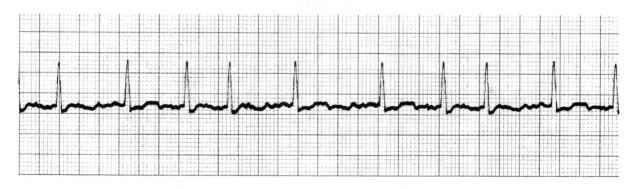

39. Her ECG is
    A. wandering atrial pacemaker.
    B. atrial flutter.
    C. atrial fibrillation.
    D. junctional rhythm.

40. Prehospital pharmacological management of this patient should include oxygen and
    A. nitroglycerin, furosemide, morphine.
    B. furosemide, albuterol, lidocaine.
    C. morphine, naloxone, furosemide.
    D. potassium, furosemide, morphine.

Scenario

Questions 41–44 refer to the following scenario:

Your patient is an 80-year-old male who presents in severe respiratory distress, sitting bolt upright, and gasping for each breath. He has a history of high blood pressure and breathing problems. He takes Inderal each day. His BP is 170/70, pulse 72 and irregular, respirations 40 and extremely labored, and skin warm and diaphoretic. On auscultation, you hear diffuse bilateral crackles and wheezing. He coughs up blood-tinged sputum. His ECG is shown in Figure 5.

41. This patient is experiencing
    A. acute pulmonary edema.
    B. cor pulmonale.
    C. cardiogenic shock.
    D. aortic aneurysm.

42. His ECG is
    A. wandering atrial pacemaker.
    B. atrial flutter.
    C. atrial fibrillation.
    D. junctional rhythm.

43. Inderal is a drug in which class?
    A. beta blocker
    B. nitrate
    C. calcium channel blocker
    D. cardiac glycoside

44. Which of the following is not a prehospital management goal for this patient?
    A. oxygenation
    B. preload increase
    C. diuresis
    D. coronary artery dilation

FIGURE 5

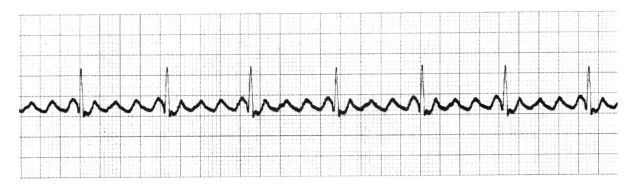

Scenario

Questions 45–49 refer to the following scenario:

Your patient is a 57-year-old woman who lies unconscious on her living room floor. Her husband claims she "just collapsed after clutching her chest." She has a previous medical history and takes Cardizem. Her BP is 70 palpated; pulse 140; respirations rate 20 and shallow; skin cool, pale, and clammy; lungs congested; and chemstrip 130. Her ECG strip is shown in Figure 6.

45. This patient is suffering from
    A. cardiogenic shock.
    B. acute pulmonary edema.
    C. right-heart failure.
    D. left-heart failure.

46. Her ECG is
    A. atrial fibrillation.
    B. paroxysmal supraventricular tachycardia.
    C. sinus tachycardia.
    D. atrial flutter.

47. The primary cause for this dysrhythmia is
    A. ectopic focus.
    B. reentry focus.

C. compensatory mechanism.
D. parasympathetic stimulation.

48. Cardizem is a drug in which class?
    A. nitrate
    B. cardiac glycoside
    C. beta blocker
    D. calcium channel blocker

49. Prehospital management of this patient includes all of the following **except**
    A. dopamine IV.
    B. oxygen.
    C. IV fluid challenge.
    D. positive pressure ventilation.

Scenario

Questions 50–52 refer to the following scenario:

Your patient is a 78-year-old male who collapsed in the bathroom while moving his bowels. He sits slumped on the toilet, moaning, pale, and extremely diaphoretic. He has no history of cardiac problems and takes no medications. His BP is 70 palpated, pulse 36, respirations 28 and shallow, lungs clear, and chemstrip 120. His ECG is shown in Figure 7.

FIGURE 6

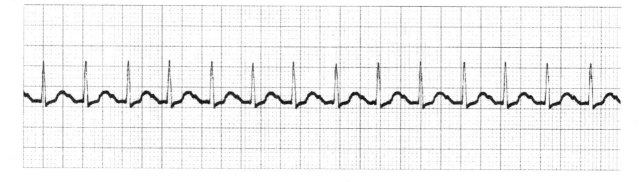

FIGURE 7

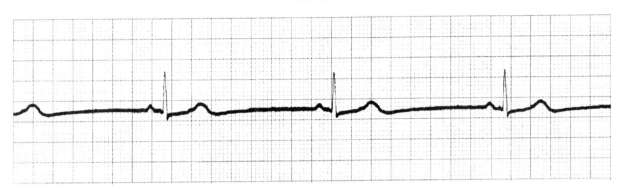

50. The most likely cause of this man's symptoms is
    A. hypoglycemia.
    B. decreased cardiac output.
    C. narcotic overdose.
    D. sympathetic overstimulation.

51. His ECG strip is
    A. junctional rhythm.
    B. sinus arrhythmia.
    C. sinus bradycardia.
    D. idioventricular rhythm.

52. The first prehospital treatment after oxygen is
    A. transcutaneous cardiac pacing.
    B. adenosine IV.
    C. epinephrine IV.
    D. atropine IV.

Scenario

Questions 53–55 refer to the following scenario:

Your patient is a 35-year-old female who developed heart palpitations while exercising. She complains of lightheadedness and some dizziness. She denies any chest pain. She has a history of Wolff-Parkinson-White syndrome and takes Pronestyl. Her BP is 140/70, pulse 190, respirations 18, skin warm and dry, and lungs clear bilaterally. Her ECG is shown in Figure 8.

FIGURE 8

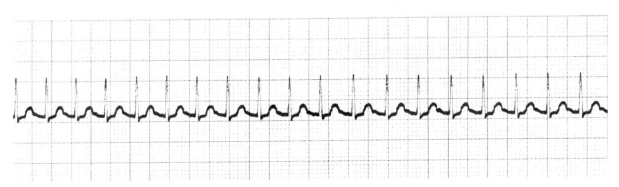

53. This patient's rhythm is
    A. sinus tachycardia.
    B. ventricular tachycardia.
    C. supraventricular tachycardia.
    D. atrial flutter.

54. The probable cause of this dysrhythmia is
    A. ectopic phenomena in the ventricle.
    B. reentry phenomena in the atria.
    C. compensatory mechanism.
    D. sympathetic stimulation.

55. The initial treatment of this patient includes oxygen and
    A. immediate cardioversion.
    B. immediate defibrillation.
    C. vagal maneuvers.
    D. verapamil IV.

Scenario

Questions 56–58 refer to the following scenario:

Your patient is a 67-year-old man who collapsed in the kitchen while cooking dinner. He presents on the floor, pale, clammy, and moaning, with vomit around his mouth. His wife states he has no history and takes no medications. His BP is 70/30, pulse 170 and weak, respirations 28 and shallow, lungs clear bilaterally, and chemstrip 120. His ECG is shown in Figure 9.

56. His ECG is
    A. ventricular tachycardia.
    B. SVT with aberrancy.
    C. ventricular fibrillation.
    D. idioventricular rhythm.

57. Initial management of this patient includes
    A. immediate synchronized cardioversion.
    B. aggressive airway management.
    C. diazepam IV.
    D. all of the above

58. Which of the following drugs may be ordered for this patient?
    A. atropine and epinephrine
    B. adenosine and verapamil
    C. naloxone and 50% dextrose
    D. lidocaine and procainamide

FIGURE 9

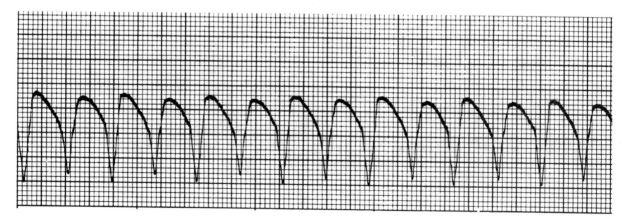

FIGURE 10

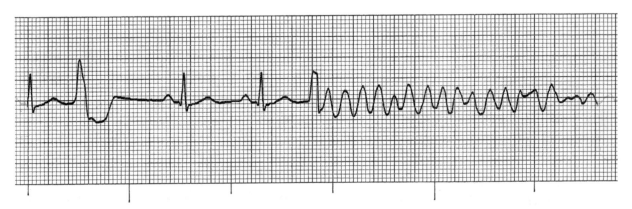

Scenario

Questions 59–62 refer to the following scenario:

Your patient is a 45-year-old male who complains of chest pain and shortness of breath. During your work-up, he suddenly loses consciousness and slumps over. His ECG changes are shown in Figure 10.

59. This patient's new ECG is
    A. ventricular fibrillation.
    B. ventricular tachycardia.
    C. asystole.
    D. idioventricular rhythm.

60. Your first move is to
    A. defibrillate at 200 joules.
    B. deliver a precordial thump.
    C. begin CPR.
    D. check your patient.

61. All of the following will decrease intrathoracic resistance during defibrillation **except**
    A. using electrode jelly.
    B. using proper paddle pressure.
    C. using proper paddle positioning.
    D. waiting 3–5 minutes between defibrillation attempts.

62. Pharmacological management of this patient includes oxygen and which of the following drugs?
    A. epinephrine, atropine
    B. epinephrine, lidocaine, amiodarone
    C. adenosine, verapamil, lidocaine
    D. epinephrine, isoproterenol, lidocaine

Scenario

Questions 63–66 refer to the following scenario:

Your patient is a 99-year-old male found in cardiac arrest by his family. CPR was begun immediately and is ongoing on your arrival. After a quick look, your patient is in the following rhythm shown in Figure 11. He is pulseless, apneic, and unconscious.

63. This patient's rhythm is
    A. supraventricular tachycardia.
    B. idioventricular rhythm.
    C. ventricular tachycardia.
    D. none of the above

FIGURE 11

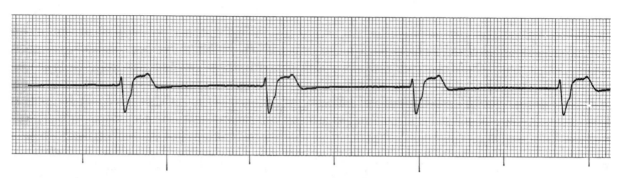

64. This patient's condition is described as
    A. AV dissociation.
    B. pulseless electrical activity.
    C. complete heart block.
    D. none of the above

65. Management of this patient includes all of the following **except**
    A. CPR and intubation.
    B. epinephrine and atropine IV.
    C. defibrillation and amiodarone.
    D. IV fluids.

66. Causes for this condition include
    A. hypovolemia.
    B. pericardial tamponade.
    C. hypoxia and acidosis.
    D. all of the above

Scenario

Questions 67 and 68 refer to the following scenario:

Your patient is a 65-year-old male complaining of malaise. He has no medical history and takes no medications. His BP is 120/70, pulse 60 and irregular, respirations 20, lungs clear, and skin warm and dry. His ECG is shown in Figure 12.

67. This patient's rhythm is
    A. second-degree AV block type 2.
    B. second-degree AV block type 1.
    C. third-degree AV block.
    D. first-degree AV block.

FIGURE 12

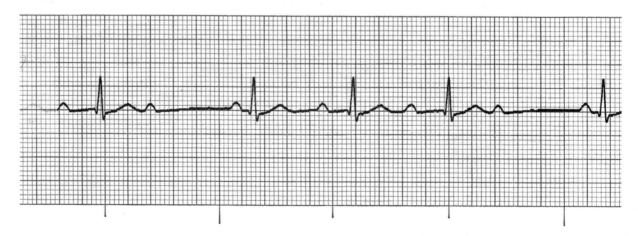

68. Prehospital management of this patient includes

   A. oxygen and monitoring only.

   B. oxygen, atropine IV.

   C. oxygen, transcutaneous pacing.

   D. oxygen, atropine, transcutaneous pacing.

Scenario

Questions 69 and 70 refer to the following scenario:

Your patient is an 89-year-old female who collapsed while shopping. No one is available to give you a history, and she responds to deep pain only. Her BP is 70/30, pulse 36, respirations 30 and shallow, skin pale and clammy, lungs clear bilaterally, and chemstrip 100. Her ECG is shown in Figure 13.

69. Her ECG is

   A. second-degree AV block type 2.

   B. junctional escape rhythm.

   C. third-degree AV block.

   D. ventricular escape rhythm.

70. Prehospital management of this patient includes

   A. CPR and intubation.

   B. atropine and transcutaneous pacing.

   C. lidocaine and bretylium.

   D. adenosine and verapamil.

FIGURE 13

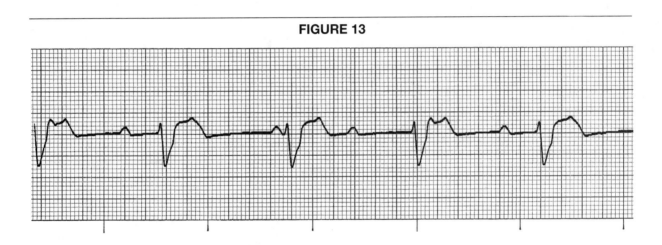

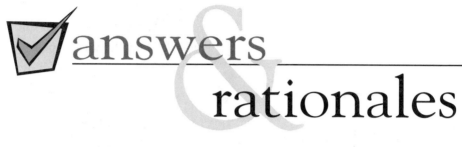

answers & rationales

Following each rationale, you will find a reference to the corresponding objective in the DOT National Standard EMT-Intermediate curriculum. An asterisk denotes material that is supplemental to the DOT curriculum. Page numbers after a rationale indicate where the question topic may be discussed in the Brady text *Intermediate Emergency Care* (Bledsoe, Porter, Cherry).

1.

A. The heart muscle itself is perfused by the coronary arteries. These vessels originate in the aorta just above the leaflets of the aortic valve and lie on the surface of the heart. (5-2.2) (IEC p. 839)

2.

D. Stroke volume is the amount of blood ejected by the heart in one contraction. Stroke volume is measured in milliliters. The average stroke volume is 60–100 ml, although this capacity can increase significantly in a healthy heart. (5-2.2) (IEC p. 840)

3.

C. Stroke volume is a reflection of three factors: preload, cardiac contractility, and afterload. (5-2.2) (IEC p. 840)

4.

A. The pressure in the ventricle at the end of diastole is referred to as preload. Preload influences the force of the next contraction. This is based on Starling's law of the heart,

which states that the more the myocardial muscle is stretched, up to a limit, the greater its force of contraction will be. (5-2.2) (IEC p. 840)

5.

B. The resistance against which the heart must pump is called afterload. In general, the greater the resistance or afterload, the less the stroke volume. An increase in peripheral vascular resistance will decrease stroke volume. Conversely, a decrease in peripheral vascular resistance, up to a point, will increase stroke volume. (5-2.2) (IEC p. 840)

6.

B. Another name for preload is end-diastolic volume. (5-2.2) (IEC p. 840)

7.

A. Cardiac output is defined as the volume of blood pumped by the heart in 1 minute. It is a calculation of stroke volume times heart rate. A person with a stroke volume of 70 ml and heart rate of 80 beats per minute has a cardiac output of 5600 ml. (5-2.2) (IEC p. 840)

8.

B. Preload represents the amount of blood or pressure in the ventricles prior to contraction. It is dependent on venous return from the body. (5-2.2) (IEC p. 840)

9.

C. The term inotropy refers to the strength of a muscular contraction of the heart. Therefore, a positive inotropic agent is one that increases the strength of a cardiac contraction. (5-2.28) (IEC p. 840)

10.

A. The term chronotrope refers to heart rate. A drug that is a negative chronotropic agent is one that suppresses the heart rate. (5-2.28) (IEC p. 840)

11.

C. Within the cardiac muscle fibers are special structures called intercalated disks. These disks connect cardiac muscle fibers and conduct electrical impulses quickly from one muscle fiber to the next. (5-2.2) (IEC p. 841)

12.

D. The cells of the cardiac conductive system have several important properties. First, they have excitability. They can respond to electrical stimulus. Second, they have conductivity. They can conduct an electrical impulse from one cell to another. Third, they have automaticity, the ability to self-depolarize without an impulse from an outside source. (5-2.2) (IEC p. 842)

13.

C. The normal intrinsic firing rate of the SA node is 60–100 beats per minute. (5-2.2) (IEC p. 843)

14.

B. The normal intrinsic firing rate of the AV junction is 40–60 beats per minute. (5-2.2) (IEC p. 843)

15.

A. The normal intrinsic firing rate of the Purkinje system is 20–40 beats per minute. (5-2.2) (IEC p. 843)

16.

B. According to Einthoven's triangle, lead 2 is characterized by left leg positive, right arm negative. (5-2.6) (IEC p. 844)

17.

D. Only a very limited amount of information can be obtained from a single-lead ECG reading. You can tell how fast the heart is beating, how regular the heartbeat is, and how long it takes to conduct the impulse through various parts of the heart. You cannot tell the presence or location of an infarct or a chamber enlargement or the quality or presence of pumping action. (5-2.7) (IEC p. 845)

18.

A. The P wave represents each atrial depolarization. (5-2.7) (IEC p. 846)

19.

D. The T wave represents ventricular repolarization. (5-2.7) (IEC p. 846)

20.

B. The QRS complex represents ventricular depolarization. (5-2.7) (IEC p. 846)

21.

C. The P–R interval represents delay at the AV node. The normal P–R interval is 0.12–0.20 second. (5-2.7) (IEC p. 851)

22.

D. Artifacts are deflections produced by factors other than the heart's electrical activity. Common causes of artifacts include muscle tremors, shivering, patient movement, loose electrodes, 60-Hz interference, and machine malfunction. (5-2.7) (IEC p. 843)

23.

B. The normal P–R interval is 0.12–0.20 second. (5-2.7) (IEC p. 851)

24.

C. The normal QRS complex is 0.04–0.12 second. (5-2.7) (IEC p. 851)

25.

D. Dysrhythmias are deviations from the normal electrical rhythm of the heart and can be caused by a number of situations: myocardial ischemia and infarction; electrolyte imbalances, such as hyperkalemia; and blood gas abnormalities, including hypoxia and an abnormal pH. (5-2.7) (IEC p. 855)

26.

A. Stable angina occurs during activity when the oxygen demands of the heart are increased. Angina can be of relatively short duration (3–5 minutes) or prolonged (lasting 15 minutes or more). The pain is often relieved by rest, nitroglycerine, or oxygen. (5-2.18) (IEC p. 924)

27.

D. Sinus rhythm is the standard heartbeat. It is distinguished by the following features: rate is 60–100 beats per minute, P–P and R–R rhythms are regular, and P waves are normal in shape, are upright, and appear only before each QRS complex. The P–R interval lasts 0.12–0.20 second and is constant. The QRS complex looks normal and has a duration of less than 0.12 second. (5-2.7) (IEC p. 846)

28.

B. Initial prehospital management of this patient should include oxygen and nitroglycerin sublingually. Nitroglycerin decreases myocardial work and dilates the coronary arteries. (5-2.22, 5-2.23) (IEC p. 924)

29.

B. Unstable angina occurs at rest. Because this condition often indicates severe atherosclerotic heart disease, it is also called preinfarction angina. (5-2.18) (IEC p. 923)

30.

D. Sinus dysrhythmia is often a normal finding and is sometimes related to the respiratory cycle and changes in intrathoracic pressure. It can also be caused by enhanced vagal tone. The identifying feature of sinus dysrhythmia is an irregular rhythm. In all other ways, it is identical to normal sinus rhythm. (5-2.7) (IEC p. 860)

31.

B. The major underlying factor in many cardiovascular emergencies is atherosclerosis. Atherosclerosis is a progressive, degenerative disease of the medium and large arteries. It results from the deposition of fats under the tunica intima layer of the involved vessels. (5-2.1) (IEC p. 922)

32.

C. Diltiazem (Cardizem) is a calcium channel blocker used increasingly for angina pectoris, dysrhythmias, hypertension, and other cardiovascular problems. It works by inhibiting calcium from entering the cells. (5-2.22) (IEC p. 924)

33.

C. Acute myocardial infarction is the death of a portion of the heart muscle from prolonged deprivation of arterial blood supply. It can also occur when the oxygen demand of the heart exceeds its supply for an extended period of time. It is most often associated with atherosclerotic heart disease. (5-2.18) (IEC p. 925)

34.

B. Premature atrial contractions (PACs) result from a single electrical impulse originating in the atria outside the SA node; in turn, this causes a premature depolarization of the heart before the next expected sinus beat. Identifying features of a PAC include an early beat with a normal-looking P wave and normal-looking QRS. (5-2.7) (IEC p. 865)

35.

C. Nifedipine (Procardia XL) is a calcium channel blocker. (5-2.22) (IEC p. 924)

36.

D. Prehospital management of a patient with acute myocardial infarction includes preventing pain and apprehension by reassuring the patient, administering high-flow oxygen, managing pain with nitroglycerine and morphine, and screening for the use of thrombolytics or angioplasty. (5-2.23) (IEC p. 927)

37.

B. Left-ventricular failure occurs when the left ventricle fails as an effective forward pump, causing back pressure of blood into the pulmonary circulation and often resulting in pulmonary edema. The patient with left-heart failure usually presents with bilateral rales in the lower lobes and shortness of breath. (5-2.26) (IEC p. 930)

38.

D. A patient with a history of congestive heart failure may take digoxin to increase cardiac output by increasing the force of contraction of the left ventricle. He may take a diuretic to decrease venous return and stimulate the kidneys to produce more urine and a potassium supplement, such as Slow-K, to replenish potassium lost through excessive diuresis. (*) (IEC p. 931)

39.

C. Atrial fibrillation is a dysrhythmia that results from multiple areas of reentry within the atria or from multiple ectopic foci bombarding an AV node. Identifying features of atrial fibrillation include a grossly irregular rhythm and no discernible P waves. (5-2.7) (IEC p. 870)

40.

A. The goals of prehospital management of a patient in left-ventricular failure include decreasing venous return to the heart, decreasing myocardial oxygen demands, and improving ventilation and oxygenation. Pharmacologically, we do this by administering nitroglycerin, furosemide, and morphine. (5-2.28) (IEC p. 932)

41.

A. Acute pulmonary edema is the most serious complication of left-ventricular failure when the lungs are literally bombarded with fluid. The fluid leaks out of the capillary beds into the interstitial spaces. (5-2.26) (IEC p. 932)

42.

B. Atrial flutter results from a rapid atrial reentry circuit and an AV node that cannot handle all impulses through to the ventricles. Identifying features of atrial flutter include the absence of P waves and the presence of flutter waves at a rate of 250–350 per minute. The flutter waves resemble a sawtooth or picket fence pattern. (5-2.7) (IEC p. 869)

43.

A. Beta blockers are frequently used to control dysrhythmias, high blood pressure, and angina. Many beta blockers, such as propranolol (Inderal), are nonselective, while others are selective for beta 1 or beta 2 receptors. (5-2.28) (IEC p. 931)

44.

B. Prehospital management of a patient in acute pulmonary edema includes decreasing the venous return of the heart, decreasing

myocardial oxygen demands, and improving ventilation and oxygenation. (5-2.39) (IEC p. 932)

45.

A. Cardiogenic shock is the most severe form of pump failure. It occurs when left-ventricular function is so compromised that the heart cannot meet the metabolic demands of the body and compensatory mechanisms are exhausted. (5-2.26) (IEC p. 935)

46.

C. Sinus tachycardia results from an increase in the rate of SA node discharge. Tachycardia is identical to normal sinus rhythm except that the rate is greater than 100. (5-2.7, 5-2.8) (IEC p. 859)

47.

C. Sinus tachycardia is often a benign process. In some cases, it is a compensatory mechanism for decreased stroke volume. (5-2.7) (IEC p. 860)

48.

D. Diltiazem (Cardizem) is a calcium channel blocker. Calcium channel blockers are used increasingly for angina, dysrhythmias, hypertension, and other cardiovascular problems. (*) (IEC p. 924)

49.

C. Prehospital management of the patient in cardiogenic shock is difficult. Even when the best technology is available, mortality rates approach 80–90%. Prehospital management should include rapid transport, high-flow oxygen, and a dopamine drip. (5-2.39) (IEC p. 936)

50.

B. The most common cause of this man's symptoms is decreased cardiac output from a decreased heart rate. Remember that cardiac output is rate times stroke volume. A decrease or increase in either component without compensation directly affects the cardiac output. (*) (IEC p. 856)

51.

C. Sinus bradycardia results from the slowing of the SA node. It can result from increased parasympathetic tone, SA node disease, or drug effects. (5-2.7, 5-2.8) (IEC p. 857)

52.

D. Treatment of sinus bradycardia is unnecessary unless hypotension or ventricular irritability is present. If treatment is required, administer 0.5 mg bolus of atropine sulfate. This can be repeated every 3–5 minutes until a satisfactory rate has been obtained or 0.04 mg/kg of the drug has been given. (5-2.39) (IEC p. 857)

53.

C. Supraventricular tachycardia occurs when rapid atrial depolarization overrides the SA node. It often occurs with a sudden onset and may last minutes to hours. (5-2.7) (IEC p. 865)

54.

B. Supraventricular tachycardia may be caused by increased automaticity of a single atrial focus or by reentry phenomena at the AV node. (5-2.7) (IEC p. 866)

55.

C. Initial treatment of a patient in supraventricular tachycardia with stable vital signs includes administering oxygen and performing vagal maneuvers, such as Valsalva or carotid sinus massage. (5-2.13) (IEC p. 867)

56.

A. Ventricular tachycardia is a rhythm that consists of three or more ventricular complexes in succession at a rate of 100 beats per minute or more. This rhythm overrides the normal pacemaker of the heart. (5-2.7, 5-2.8) (IEC p. 886)

57.

A. Initial management of this patient includes immediate synchronized cardioversion. (5-2.39) (IEC p. 887)

58.

D. Pharmacological management of this patient may include lidocaine, procainamide, or amiodarone. (5-2.13) (IEC p. 887)

59.

A. Ventricular fibrillation is a chaotic ventricular rhythm usually resulting from the presence of many reentry circuits within the ventricles. There is no ventricular depolarization or contraction. (5-2.7, 5-2.8) (IEC p. 889)

60.

D. The initial management of this patient is to check him clinically. Always correlate your patient's pulse with what you see on the ECG. In this case, a disconnected lead or faulty monitor could produce this ECG pattern. If you cannot detect a pulse, consider the rhythm ventricular fibrillation. (5-2.39) (IEC p. 889)

61.

D. Reducing intrathoracic resistance is an important factor in a successful defibrillation. Using electrode jelly, using proper paddle positioning and pressure, and delivering successive countershocks as quickly as possible will all decrease intrathoracic resistance. (*) (IEC p. 911)

62.

B. Pharmacological management of the patient with ventricular fibrillation includes oxygen, epinephrine, amiodarone, and lidocaine. (5-2.13) (IEC p. 889)

63.

B. Ventricular escape rhythm or idioventricular rhythm results when either impulses from the higher pacemakers fail to reach the ventricles or the rate of discharge of the higher pacemakers becomes less than that of the ventricles, normally 15–45 beats per minute. (5-2.7) (IEC p. 883)

64.

B. When a patient with a rhythm has no associated pulse, this is known as pulseless electrical activity. (5-2.7) (IEC p. 893)

65.

C. Management of a patient in idioventricular rhythm with pulseless electrical activity includes CPR; airway management and oxygenation, including intubation; epinephrine and atropine IV; and rapid IV fluid administration. (5-2.12) (IEC p. 895)

66.

D. Common causes for pulseless electrical activity include hypovolemia, hypoxia, acidosis, and cardiac tamponade. (*) (IEC p. 893)

67.

B. Second-degree AV block type 1 (Wenkebach phenomenon) is an intermittent block at the level of the AV node. It produces a characteristic cyclic pattern in which the P–R intervals become progressively longer until an impulse is blocked or not conducted through the AV node. This cycle is repetitive. An identifying feature of second-degree AV block type 1 is a P–R interval that progressively lengthens until a QRS complex is dropped. (5-2.7) (IEC p. 873)

68.

A. There is generally no treatment other than observation for patients in second-degree AV block type 1 with stable vital signs. (5-2.13) (IEC p. 874)

69.

C. Third-degree block, or complete heart block, is the absence of conduction between the atria and the ventricles, resulting from complete electrical block at or below the AV node. The atria and ventricles subsequently pace the heart independently of each other. (5-2.7) (IEC p. 876)

70.

B. Third-degree heart block can severely compromise cardiac output because of decreased heart rate and the loss of coordinated atrial kick. The prehospital management of this patient would include parasympathetic blockers, such as atropine, and transcutaneous external pacing. (5-2.13) (IEC p. 876)

UNIT

3 Diabetic Emergencies

unit objectives

Questions in this unit relate to DOT objectives 5-3.1 to 5-3.16. The objectives are listed in the Appendix.

DIRECTIONS
Each of the questions or incomplete statements below is followed by suggested answers or completions. Select the **one answer** that is best in each case.

1. Chemical substances released by a gland that control or affect other glands or body systems are called
   A. endocrines.
   B. hormones.
   C. polypeptides.
   D. ketones.

2. Which of the following statements is true regarding endocrine glands?
   A. They have ducts.
   B. They exert their effects locally.
   C. Salivary glands are endocrine.
   D. none of the above

3. The body's natural tendency to maintain a constant, stable, internal environment is known as
   A. homeostasis.
   B. hemostasis.
   C. metabolism.
   D. anabolism.

4. Low blood sugar reading is normally considered to be anything less than _____ in the healthy adult.
   A. 60 mg/dL
   B. 80 mg/dL
   C. 100 mg/dL
   D. 120 mg/dL

5. Which of the following hormones stimulates the liver to transform its glycogen stores into glucose for immediate use?
   A. prolactin
   B. glucagon

   C. insulin
   D. somatostatin

6. Which of the following hormones is **not** produced by the islets of Langerhans?
   A. glucagon
   B. somatostatin
   C. prolactin
   D. insulin

7. Insulin is necessary to
   A. facilitate transport of glucose into the cells.
   B. produce glucose from muscle tissue.
   C. enhance glycogen formation in the liver.
   D. promote gluconeogenesis.

8. Which of the following is **not** a characteristic of diabetes mellitus?
   A. ketone production
   B. excessive insulin production
   C. osmotic diuresis
   D. associated heart and kidney disease

9. Diabetic ketoacidosis is a direct result of
   A. the cells burning inefficient fuels.
   B. the pancreas secreting excessive insulin.
   C. the kidneys reabsorbing glucose.
   D. rapid, deep respirations.

10. Insulin shock is a direct result of
    A. insufficient insulin levels.
    B. insufficient blood glucose levels.
    C. hyperglycemia.
    D. not taking enough insulin.

11. Nonketotic hyperosmolar coma differs from DKA in that

    A. the pancreas produces some insulin.

    B. ketones are eliminated by the kidneys.

    C. osmotic diuresis does not occur.

    D. blood glucose levels do not rise greatly.

Scenario

Questions 12–20 refer to the following scenario:

Your patient is a 45-year-old male who lies unconscious in bed. His daughter states that he has a long history of diabetes and takes insulin daily. He lives alone and had not been seen for a few days. He has no other history. His heart rate is 100, BP 90/60, respirations 40 and deep with a fruity odor, lungs clear, skin warm and dry, and chemstrip 380. He had vomited twice prior to your arrival.

12. This patient is most likely experiencing

    A. hypoglycemia.

    B. insulin shock.

    C. hyperglycemia.

    D. nonketotic hyperosmolar coma.

13. His problem probably resulted from

    A. taking his insulin and not eating enough.

    B. not taking his insulin.

    C. taking his insulin and overeating.

    D. recent illness.

14. His hypotension and dehydrated look result from

    A. osmotic diuresis.

    B. overproduction of ketones.

    C. increased insulin levels.

    D. increased ADH release.

15. His respiratory pattern is known as

    A. Cheyne-Stokes.

    B. Kussmaul's.

    C. Graves'.

    D. Biot's.

16. This respiratory pattern occurs as the body attempts to

    A. increase insulin production.

    B. correct metabolic acidosis.

    C. decrease hypoxia from insulin shock.

    D. produce more ketonic acids.

17. The fruity breath results from _____ in the expired air.

    A. glucose

    B. insulin

    C. ketones

    D. glucagon

18. His chemstrip reads 380 because

    A. he cannot transport glucose into his cells.

    B. he cannot transform glycogen into glucose.

    C. he is hypoglycemic.

    D. he is in insulin shock.

19. Classic early signs of this disease include all of the following **except**

    A. polydipsia.

    B. polyuria.

    C. polyphagia.

    D. polyphasia.

20. Emergency prehospital treatment for this patient includes

    A. crystalloid fluid infusion.

    B. 50% dextrose IV.

    C. glucagon IM.

    D. naloxone IV.

Scenario

Questions 21–25 refer to the following scenario:

Your patient is a 39-year-old female who collapsed in a supermarket and lies unconscious on the floor. She is alone, and no one is available to provide you with a history. She has no medications in her purse, except for some Glucotabs. She is wearing a bracelet that states she is diabetic. Her heart rate is 110, BP 100/70, respirations 28 and shallow, skin cool and clammy, lungs clear, and chemstrip 40.

21. This patient is most likely experiencing
    A. hypoglycemia.
    B. insulin shock.
    C. hyperglycemia.
    D. A and B

22. This patient's condition could have resulted from any of the following **except**
    A. taking her insulin and not eating enough.
    B. not taking her insulin.
    C. too much exercise/activity.
    D. recent illness.

23. Her unconsciousness is due to
    A. cerebral hypoxia.
    B. cerebral hypoglycemia.
    C. ketoacidosis.
    D. osmotic diuresis.

24. Prehospital management of this patient includes
    A. insulin SC.
    B. 250 ml of lactated Ringer's.
    C. 50% dextrose IV.
    D. all of the above

25. If an accurate chemstrip cannot be obtained, management should include all of the following **except**
    A. thiamine IV.
    B. 50% dextrose IV.
    C. insulin SC.
    D. oral glucose.

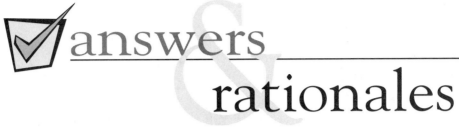
answers & rationales

Following each rationale, you will find a reference to the corresponding objective in the DOT National Standard EMT-Intermediate curriculum. An asterisk denotes material that is supplemental to the DOT curriculum. Page numbers after a rationale indicate where the question topic may be discussed in the Brady text *Intermediate Emergency Care* (Bledsoe, Porter, Cherry).

1.

B. Hormones are chemical substances released by glands that control or affect other glands or body systems. Endocrine glands secrete hormones directly into the bloodstream. Exocrine glands transport their hormones to target tissues via ducts. Emergencies are usually caused by the underproduction or overproduction of hormones. (*) (IEC p. 948)

2.

D. Endocrine glands are ductless and exert widespread effects because they release their hormones into the general circulation. Examples include the thyroid, pancreas, and gonads. (*) (IEC p. 948)

3.

A. Homeostasis is the body's natural tendency to maintain a constant, stable, internal environment. The endocrine system plays a major role in homeostasis by secreting hormones that regulate various body functions. (*) (IEC p. 949)

4.

B. Low blood sugar is anything less than 80 mg/dL in the healthy adult and constitutes documented hypoglycemia. (5-3.7) (IEC p. 951)

5.

B. Glucagon stimulates the liver to transform its glycogen stores into glucose for immediate use. It also stimulates the liver to manufacture glucose from other substances in a process called gluconeogenesis. Glucagon raises the blood level of glucose. (*) (IEC p. 950)

6.

C. The islets of Langerhans are specialized tissues within the pancreas that contain three types of hormone-secreting cells: alpha cells, beta cells, and delta cells. Alpha cells secrete glucagon, beta cells secrete insulin, and delta cells secrete somatostatin. (*) (IEC p. 951)

7.

A. Insulin is a hormone secreted by the beta cells of the islets of Langerhans. It is antagonistic to glucagon and causes the blood level of glucose to decrease. It combines with insulin receptors on the cell membrane and allows glucose to enter the cell. It is an absolute necessity for survival. (*) (IEC p. 951)

8.

B. Diabetes mellitus is a disease characterized by decreased insulin production by the beta cells of the islets of Langerhans of the pancreas. Insulin facilitates glucose transport into the cells. As the body cells become starved for glucose, they use other sources of energy, resulting in ketone production. Increased blood glucose levels cause an osmotic gradient, resulting in a water shift into the vascular compartment. This, in turn, causes glucose to be spilled into the urine, taking water with it. The diabetic is at risk for heart disease, kidney failure, and blindness. (5-3.1) (IEC p. 949)

9.

A. Diabetic ketoacidosis is a direct result of the cells using other sources of energy, such as fats. This inefficient fuel produces many by-products, such as ketones and other organic acids. If enough ketones are produced, metabolic acidosis and coma may ensue. (5-3.5) (IEC p. 953)

10.

B. Insulin shock (hypoglycemia) is a result of insufficient glucose to meet tissue demands. Usually this occurs as a result of taking injected insulin and not eating enough to feed the tissues. The insulin transports all available glucose into the cells, leaving very low blood levels. Untreated, the patient may sustain brain injury since the brain receives its energy from glucose metabolism. Hypoglycemia is a true emergency. (5-3.7) (IEC p. 956)

11.

A. Nonketotic hyperosmolar coma differs from diabetic coma. Patients suffering the former produced enough insulin to feed the cells but not enough to maintain normal blood glucose levels. Their glucose can reach extremely high levels, causing a tremendous osmotic gradient and dehydration. Ketones are not produced because glucose is burned as fuel in the cells. (5-3.11) (IEC p. 955)

12.

C. This patient is most likely experiencing diabetic ketoacidosis (DKA) or hyperglycemia. The history (positive for diabetes), onset (slow), chemstrip (high), respirations (rapid and deep), and skin condition (warm and dry) are all classic signs. (5-3.12) (IEC p. 953)

13.

B. Hyperglycemia most often results from not taking sufficient amounts of prescribed insulin. Without this messenger, glucose cannot enter the cells. (5-3.11) (IEC p. 953)

14.

A. Increased blood glucose levels cause an osmotic gradient. This gradient draws interstitial water into the intravascular compartment, resulting in glucose spillage into the urine. As water follows glucose, patients become dehydrated. If enough fluid is lost, hypotension and tachycardia follow. (5-3.11) (IEC p. 954)

15.

B. Kussmaul's respirations, characterized by rapid, deep breathing, represent the body's attempt to increase minute volume. (5-3.12) (IEC p. 954)

16.

B. Kussmaul's respirations are the body's attempt to compensate for the metabolic acidosis caused by excessive ketone production. As the buffer system changes metabolic acids (ketones) to respiratory acids (carbon dioxide), the respiratory system eliminates the excess by increasing minute volume ventilation. Minute volume is increased by breathing faster and deeper than normal. (5-3.11) (IEC p. 954)

17.

C. When ketones are eliminated through the respiratory tract, the patient will exhibit a fruity, or acetone, breath odor. (5-3.11) (IEC p. 954)

18.

A. Because this patient cannot transport glucose into his cells, blood levels rise dramatically. (5-3.11) (IEC p. 954)

19.

D. The early signs of diabetes include polyuria (frequent urination from osmotic diuresis), polydipsia (excessive thirst from the dehydration), and polyphagia (excessive hunger from the cells being starved of glucose). (5-3.12) (IEC p. 954)

20.

A. If blood glucose levels can be accurately determined to be high and the patient exhibits the signs and symptoms of DKA, a crystalloid infusion should be administered to reverse the dehydration and hypotension. A red top can be drawn to obtain baseline blood glucose levels. If allowed, insulin may be administered in the field. (5-3.16) (IEC p. 955)

21.

D. Your patient is most likely experiencing insulin shock (hypoglycemia). Her history (Medic-Alert bracelet and Glucotabs), level of consciousness (altered), and chemstrip (low) all strongly suggest hypoglycemia. An altered level of consciousness, low chemstrip, and improvement following dextrose therapy are known as Whipple's triad. (5-3.8) (IEC p. 956)

22.

B. Hypoglycemia may result from taking too much insulin, not eating enough, excessive exercise, or illness. (5-3.7) (IEC p. 956)

23.

B. This patient has no available glucose for brain metabolism. The brain is a very greedy organ, demanding a constant supply of oxygen and glucose. Withhold either from the brain for an extended period of time, and death may result. (5-3.7) (IEC p. 956)

24.

C. Prehospital treatment of this patient includes a rapid bolus of 25 g of 50% dextrose IV. A red top can be drawn to determine baseline blood glucose levels. (5-3.10) (IEC p. 956)

25.

C. If blood glucose levels cannot be determined, a rapid bolus of 25 g of 50% dextrose IV followed by 100 mg of thiamine IV should be administered. (5-3.10) (IEC p. 957)

UNIT
4

Allergic Reactions

unit objectives

Questions in this unit relate to DOT objectives 5-4.1 to 5-4.11. The objectives are listed in the Appendix.

DIRECTIONS

Each of the questions or incomplete statements below is followed by suggested answers or completions. Select the **one answer** that is best in each case.

1. Anaphylaxis is defined as
   A. an acute, generalized, misdirected immune reaction.
   B. an antigen/antibody reaction.
   C. a life-threatening emergency.
   D. all of the above

2. Any substance capable of producing an immune system response is a(n)
   A. antibody.
   B. antigen.
   C. receptor.
   D. idiosyncrasy.

3. The type of immune response that involves a chemical attack on the foreign substance by antibodies is known as _____ immunity.
   A. cellular
   B. anaphylactoid
   C. humoral
   D. anaphylactic

4. Antibodies are produced by specialized cells of the immune system called _____ cells.
   A. B
   B. G
   C. T
   D. E

5. During the primary response, _____ is/are released.
   A. IgA
   B. IgG
   C. IgM
   D. B and C

6. Which of the following types of immunity develops through vaccination?
   A. acquired
   B. natural
   C. naturally acquired
   D. induced active

7. The exposure of an individual to an antigen where antibodies are formed is referred to as
   A. hypersensitivity.
   B. sensitization.
   C. an allergic reaction.
   D. none of the above

8. The antibody responsible for producing allergic and anaphylactic responses is
   A. IgA.
   B. IgE.
   C. IgM.
   D. IgG.

9. Which of the following is true regarding vaccines?
   A. They stimulate antibody production.
   B. They contain antigenic proteins from a virus or bacterium.
   C. Some last a lifetime.
   D. all of the above

10. Which of the following is **not** considered a hymenopteran insect?
    A. fire ant
    B. spider
    C. wasp
    D. hornet

11. Histamine receptors are located in the
   A. airways.
   B. peripheral blood vessels.
   C. digestive tract.
   D. all of the above

12. Histamine causes all of the following physiological reactions **except**
   A. bronchodilation.
   B. increased peristalsis.
   C. increased capillary permeability.
   D. vasodilation.

13. The person with anaphylaxis may exhibit all of the following signs and symptoms **except**
   A. hypertension.
   B. stridor.
   C. urticaria.
   D. abdominal cramping.

14. Angioedema is best described as
   A. vasodilation and increased capillary permeability.
   B. third cranial nerve paralysis.
   C. generalized body hives.
   D. eczema of the neck.

15. In severe cases, the signs and symptoms of anaphylaxis begin _____ following exposure to the antigen.
   A. within 1 minute
   B. 5–10 minutes
   C. 10–20 minutes
   D. 1 hour

16. The anaphylactic shock patient should be managed with
   A. aggressive airway management.
   B. epinephrine and diphenhydramine.
   C. 100% oxygen.
   D. all of the above

17. Epinephrine causes all of the following **except**
   A. bronchodilation.
   B. peripheral blood vessel constriction.
   C. heart rate decrease.
   D. contractile force increase.

18. Diphenhydramine is given in anaphylaxis because it
   A. blocks histamine receptor sites.
   B. enhances the effects of epinephrine.
   C. renders the antigen inactive.
   D. produces permanent immunity.

19. When a foreign substance is introduced into the bloodstream, the body responds by manufacturing
   A. antibodies.
   B. antigens.
   C. histamine.
   D. allergens.

20. Sensitization refers to
   A. the process of creating antigens in response to antibodies.
   B. the release of chemical mediators into the bloodstream.
   C. the body's response to the released chemical mediators.
   D. the body's ability to attack a foreign substance on repeated exposure.

21. After being manufactured, antibodies can attach themselves to
   A. esinophils.
   B. basophils.
   C. neutrophils.
   D. monophils.

22. Antibodies are manufactured to eliminate or destroy _____, which may invade the body.
    A. immunoglobulins
    B. haptens
    C. basophils
    D. allergens

23. An anaphylactic reaction can best be described as an
    A. antibody–hapten reaction.
    B. allergy–antigen reaction.
    C. antigen–antibody reaction.
    D. antigen–allergen reaction.

24. The body system responsible for the anaphylactic reaction is the
    A. cardiovascular.
    B. immune.
    C. respiratory.
    D. integumentary.

25. What is the primary cause of death in a patient with a severe anaphylactic reaction?
    A. hypotension
    B. laryngeal edema
    C. tachycardia
    D. bronchospasm

26. Hypotension seen with a severe anaphylactic reaction is caused by
    A. peripheral shunting of blood.
    B. the antigen introduced into the bloodstream.
    C. vasoconstriction.
    D. a decrease in systemic vascular resistance.

27. Which of the following respiratory assessment findings is not consistent with anaphylaxis?
    A. bronchospasm
    B. decreased airway resistance
    C. increased mucus production
    D. bronchial edema

28. Increased vascular permeability and vasodilation secondary to anaphylaxis cause
    A. hypotension.
    B. bradycardia.
    C. tachypnea.
    D. hyperpnea.

29. Urticaria and pruritis associated with anaphylaxis are caused primarily by
    A. chemical mediator release from MAST cells.
    B. cellular changes from profound hypoxia.
    C. erythemic tissue.
    D. acidosis secondary to hypoperfusion.

30. One of the most prevalent chemical mediators associated with an anaphylactic reaction is
    A. phosphodiasterase.
    B. cyclic-AMP.
    C. histamine.
    D. glucagon.

31. An acute anaphylactic reaction could occur after the antigen was _____ into the body.
    A. injected
    B. ingested
    C. inhaled
    D. all of the above

32. Which of the following is **least** likely to cause anaphylaxis?
    A. wasp venom
    B. certain medications
    C. pollen
    D. food

33. Basophils are found primarily in
    A. connective tissue.
    B. the respiratory tree.
    C. vascular smooth muscle.
    D. circulating blood.

34. What are the hallmark integumentary signs indicative of an anaphylactic reaction?
    A. pruritis and urticaria
    B. rhinorrhea and edema
    C. erythema and lesions
    D. urticaria and rhinorrhea

35. You are assessing a 21-year-old male who was stung by a bee. The patient was initially complaining of hives, itching, wheezing, and tightness in his chest but now has a diminishing level of consciousness, is extremely cyanotic, and is hypotensive. Based on the given signs, he is experiencing which type of anaphylactic reaction?
    A. mild
    B. moderate
    C. severe
    D. fatal

36. Bronchoconstriction associated with an anaphylactic reaction is manifested as
    A. stridorous respirations.
    B. wheezing on auscultation.
    C. crackles on auscultation.
    D. rhonchi on auscultation.

37. Which of the following is an ominous sign of impending arrest in a severe anaphylactic reaction?
    A. tachycardia above 100 per minute
    B. cyanosis to the extremities
    C. absence of wheezing with diminished breath sounds on auscultation
    D. loss of radial pulses and a systolic blood pressure of 102 mm Hg

38. How is glottic edema, associated with an anaphylactic reaction, manifested in severe anaphylaxis?
    A. wheezing
    B. stridor
    C. hemoptysis
    D. pruritis

39. Respiratory stridor indicates
    A. bronchoconstriction.
    B. airway occlusion.
    C. massive vasodilation.
    D. hypoperfusion.

40. What vital signs are most consistent with severe anaphylaxis?
    A. BP 100/86, HR 68, RR 18
    B. BP 86/68, HR 130, RR 42
    C. BP 180/90, HR 140, RR 36
    D. BP 78/64, HR 98, RR 18

41. You have assessed and begun treatment on a 36-year-old male suffering an anaphylactic reaction. Initially, the patient was extremely dyspneic with coarse bilateral wheezing; was disoriented; had warm, dry, flushed skin; and was hypotensive. Currently, the patient is still hypotensive and disoriented, but now the breath sounds have diminished even further. Based on the presented findings, you conclude that
    A. the patient's status is probably improving.
    B. the patient's status is probably unchanged.
    C. the patient's status is probably deteriorating.
    D. you do not have enough information to tell.

42. As a general guideline, the _____ the onset of signs and symptoms of anaphylaxis after exposure, the _____ the severity of the reaction.
    A. quicker, milder
    B. slower, milder
    C. quicker, greater
    D. slower, greater

43. A severe anaphylactic reaction
    A. can occur with minutes after exposure.
    B. usually occurs within 10–15 minutes of exposure.
    C. usually develops over 30 minutes after exposure.
    D. takes at least an hour to develop after exposure.

44. Physical indications of histamine release in a sensitized patient can be evidenced by
    A. hypotension.
    B. bradycardia.
    C. hemataemesis.
    D. hypotonia.

45. An anaphylactic reaction is a function of which body system?
    A. cardiovascular
    B. respiratory
    C. central nervous system
    D. immune

46. Which immunoglobulin is responsible for initiating the anaphylactic reaction?
    A. IgE
    B. IgM
    C. IgA
    D. IgD

47. If the body has never been exposed to a specific antigen in an IgE reaction before, the response of the body to the first exposure
    A. is the same as the expected anaphylactic reaction.
    B. is more severe than the expected anaphylactic reaction.
    C. typically does not create an anaphylactic reaction.
    D. creates only a mild anaphylactic reaction.

48. Which of the following would not typically cause an anaphylactic reaction in an individual?
    A. aspirin
    B. X-ray contrast media
    C. antacids
    D. antibiotics

49. A patient is to receive epinephrine for an allergic reaction. All of the following statements about this administration are true **except**

   A. 1:1000 epinephrine should be used for IM administration.

   B. 1:10,000 epinephrine should be used for ET administration.

   C. 1:1000 epinephrine should be used for IV administration.

   D. 1:10,000 epinephrine should be used for IV administration.

50. Which of the following signs or symptoms is not a direct result of the chemical mediator release in anaphylaxis?

   A. tachycardia

   B. dyspnea

   C. low blood pressure

   D. itching and hives

51. You are conducting an initial assessment of a patient with a history of bee stings, to which he is allergic. Which of the following would best indicate that your patient is experiencing a severe reaction?

   A. urticaria

   B. unresponsiveness

   C. bilateral wheezing

   D. cool, clammy skin

52. Your immediate treatment during the initial assessment of a patient suffering a severe anaphylactic reaction would be

   A. administration of high-flow oxygen.

   B. spine stabilization.

   C. initiation of an IV line.

   D. administration of epinephrine.

53. Your anaphylactic patient needs tracheal intubation, and you note severe glottic edema. You should

   A. increase the rate of PPV.

   B. perform a needle cricothyrotomy.

   C. consider inserting a smaller-diameter endotracheal tube.

   D. force the tube in between the edematous tissue.

54. Which of the following clinical findings is **least** suggestive of a severe anaphylactic reaction?

   A. extreme anxiety

   B. hypotension

   C. bilateral wheezing on inspiration and expiration

   D. inspiratory stridor

55. In the severe anaphylactic reaction, it is imperative to try and maintain normal perfusion pressures. Which of the following will help with this goal?

   A. administration of IV fluids

   B. placing a constriction band between the injection site and the heart

   C. administration of epinephrine

   D. A and C

56. Nausea, vomiting, and diarrhea, when present in an anaphylactic reaction, are all associated with

   A. severe vasodilation.

   B. histamine release.

   C. bronchoconstriction.

   D. none of the above

57. What type of IV fluid is preferred in the treatment of an anaphylactic patient?

    A. isotonic colloid solution

    B. hypotonic crystalloid solution

    C. hypertonic colloid solution

    D. isotonic crystalloid solution

58. After starting an IV in your anaphylactic patient, you decide to administer a fluid bolus because of hypotension. The amount you will infuse is

    A. 10 ml/kg.

    B. 20 ml/kg.

    C. 30 ml/kg.

    D. 40 ml/kg.

59. Which IV setup will allow the fluid bolus to be administered the fastest?

    A. a 14-gauge with a microdrip administration set

    B. a 20-gauge with a macrodrip administration set

    C. a 16-gauge with a macrodrip administration set

    D. an 18-gauge with a microdrip administration set

60. Which of the following effects of epinephrine are **least** desirable when administering it to an anaphylactic shock patient?

    A. beta 1 effects

    B. beta 2 effects

    C. alpha effects

    D. all of the above

61. After administering epinephrine to an anaphylactic patient, which of the following would you expect to reverse?

    A. respiratory distress

    B. hypotension

C. altered mental status

D. all of the above

62. Which of the epinephrine dosages would be appropriate for a mild allergic reaction?

    A. 0.03 mg

    B. 3.0 mg

    C. 0.3 mg

    D. none of the above

63. Which of the epinephrine dosages would be appropriate for a severe allergic reaction?

    A. 0.03 mg

    B. 3.0 mg

    C. 0.3 mg

    D. none of the above

64. The major difference between administering epinephrine to a mild and severe allergic reaction is

    A. the route of administration.

    B. the dose of epinephrine to be administered.

    C. the concentration of epinephrine to be used.

    D. the repeat dose of epinephrine.

65. You have a patient who believes he is having an allergic reaction. The patient has a sudden onset of chest tightness, wheezing, stridor with dyspnea and a poor tidal volume, severe urticaria, erythema, and pruritis. Vitals are BP 88/palp, HR 118, and RR 36. Based on this presentation, the patient is having

    A. a severe allergic reaction.

    B. a mild allergic reaction.

    C. a subtle allergic reaction.

    D. no allergic reaction.

66. The route of antigen introduction into the body that produces the most rapid onset of a reaction is usually
    A. ingestion.
    B. inhalation.
    C. injection.
    D. absorption.

67. What is the number one cause of death in a patient with a severe anaphylactic reaction?
    A. urticaria
    B. glottic edema
    C. hypotension
    D. bronchoconstriction

68. All of the following options are appropriate for treating a severe hypotensive anaphylactic patient **except**
    A. tracheal intubation.
    B. administration of 0.5 mg of epinephrine IV.
    C. high-flow oxygen.
    D. IV therapy of normal saline at a KVO rate.

69. You arrive on the scene of a residence and find an 18-year-old female patient who is presenting with signs and symptoms consistent with a moderate anaphylactic reaction. During your history, you determine that the patient has taken Motrin for the first time ever and shortly began to experience the reaction. She reports no known allergies and states she has never taken Motrin or any other nonsteroidal anitinflammatory drug in the past. During your assessment, she is exhibiting all of the typical signs and symptoms of anaphylaxis. She denies exposure to any other substances. She is most likely suffering from
    A. an asthma attack that is presenting similar to an anaphylactic reaction.
    B. an anaphylactoid reaction.
    C. an IgE-mediated anaphylactic reaction.
    D. a nonhistamine reaction.

70. How would you treat the patient suffering from an anaphylactoid reaction?
    A. Only oxygen and intravenous therapy are recommended.
    B. Administer diphenhydramine and crystalloid solutions.
    C. Use beta 2 agonists only and oxygen therapy.
    D. Manage the condition the same as an anaphylactic reaction.

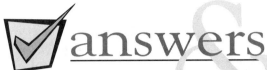

answers & rationales

Following each rationale, you will find a reference to the corresponding objective in the DOT National Standard EMT-Intermediate curriculum. An asterisk denotes material that is supplemental to the DOT curriculum. Page numbers after a rationale indicate where the question topic may be discussed in the Brady text *Intermediate Emergency Care* (Bledsoe, Porter, Cherry).

1.

D. Anaphylaxis is an acute, generalized, misdirected immune response to an antigen/antibody reaction that may be rapidly fatal even with prompt and appropriate emergency care. (5-4.2) (IEC p. 959)

2.

B. An antigen is any substance capable of producing an immune response. Among the many examples are bacteria, viruses, drug molecules, animal secretions or serum, and blood. (5-4.5) (IEC p. 960)

3.

C. Humoral immunity is a chemical attack on an invading substance by antibodies, also called immunoglobulins (Igs). (5-4.9) (IEC p. 960)

4.

A. Antibodies are produced by specialized cells of the immune system called B cells. There are five classes of antibodies: IgA, IgD, IgE, IgG, and IgM. (5-4.9) (IEC p. 960)

5.

D. During the primary response, IgG and IgM are released to help fight the antigen. (5-4.9) (IEC pp. 960–961)

6.

D. Immunity achieved through vaccination is known as induced active immunity. The vaccine is injected to stimulate development of antibodies to a specific antigen. This is also called artificially acquired immunity. An example is the immunity produced by the diphtheria/pertussis/tetanus (DPT) vaccine. (5-4.9) (IEC p. 961)

7.

B. The exposure of an individual to an antigen where IgE antibodies are formed is referred to as sensitization. This results in an immune response by which the person begins to develop antibodies. Subsequent exposure may produce an allergic reaction. (5-4.9) (IEC p. 962)

8.

B. The IgE (immunoglobulin E) antibody contributes to allergic and anaphylactic responses. (5-4.9) (IEC p. 962)

9.

D. A vaccine is an agent that, when injected, will produce an immune response. Most vaccines contain antigenic proteins from a virus or bacterium. Some vaccines, such as that for chicken pox, last a lifetime. Others, such as that for tetanus, must be repeated via boosters. (5-4.9) (IEC p. 961)

10.

B. Insect stings are the second most frequent cause of fatal anaphylactic reactions. Hymenopterans are insects that produce a unique venom that causes these severe reactions. These insects include fire ants, hornets, wasps, yellow jackets, and honey bees. (5-4.4) (IEC pp. 959–960)

11.

D. Histamine 1 receptors are located in the lower airways and peripheral blood vessels. Histamine 2 receptors are located in the stomach. (5-4.9) (IEC p. 963)

12.

A. Histamine causes bronchoconstriction, capillary leaking from increased permeability, peripheral vasodilation, increased gastric secretion, and increased movement of food through the digestive tract. (5-4.9) (IEC p. 963)

13.

A. Hypertension does not occur in true anaphylaxis. One of the cardinal effects is massive vasodilation, which results in hypotension. (5-4.7) (IEC pp. 964, 967)

14.

A. Vasodilation and increased capillary permeability cause swelling in the face and mucous membranes. This is called angioedema. (5-4.7) (IEC p. 963)

15.

A. The signs and symptoms of a severe anaphylactic reaction usually begin within 1 minute following exposure to the antigen. In a small percentage of patients, it can be delayed over 1 hour. The speed of onset usually predicts the severity of the response. (5-4.7) (IEC p. 963)

16.

D. The patient in anaphylactic shock should receive aggressive airway management and 100% oxygenation; IV fluid replacement; epinephrine SC, IM, or IV; antihistamines, such as diphenhydramine IV; corticosteroids, such as methylprednisolone, hydrocortisone, and dexamethasone; vasopressors, such as dopamine, norepinephrine, and epinephrine, as needed; and beta agonists, such as albuterol. (5-4.11) (IEC pp. 965–966)

17.

C. Epinephrine is the drug of choice for anaphylaxis because it reverses the effects of histamine by causing bronchodilation and peripheral vasoconstriction. This will reverse the angioedema that threatens the upper airway. It will also increase heart rate and strength of contractions. (5-4.8) (IEC pp. 965–966)

18.

A. Diphenhydramine is given in anaphylaxis because it competes with histamine at the receptor sites. By blocking the effects of histamine, you stop the life-threatening allergic response. (5-4.8) (IEC p. 966)

19.

A. The immune system will, when faced with a foreign substance, create antibodies to eliminate the invading substance. These invading substances, known as antigens or allergens, are components of the antigen/antibody reaction seen in acute anaphylactic reactions. (5-4.9) (IEC p. 960)

20.

D. Sensitization begins when the body is initially exposed to an antigen. This initiates the production of antibodies specific to that antigen. These antibodies allow the elimination of the antigen on repeated exposures. Chemical mediators are released along with the antibody/antigen reaction. This is what causes the clinical manifestation seen in an allergic reaction. (5-4.9) (IEC p. 962)

21.

B. Antibodies are created by plasma cells in response to exposure to an antigen (foreign substance). When manufactured, these antibodies attach themselves to MAST cells and basophils that house the chemical mediators. The other types of cells listed are types of white blood cells useful in fighting infections. (5-4.9) (IEC p. 963)

22.

D. Antibodies created by the immune system are designed to eliminate unwanted allergens that may invade the bloodstream. This is how the immune system helps to protect the body. Immunoglobulins are also structures created by the immune system to ward off invaders. Basophils are the white blood cells that the antibodies attach to. Haptens are a type or class of antibodies. (5-4.9) (IEC pp. 960–963)

23.

C. An anaphylactic reaction is also characterized as an antigen/antibody reaction. When an antigen (foreign substance) enters the bloodstream, antibodies specific to that antigen attack and eliminate it. An acute anaphylactic reaction occurs when there is an overwhelming antigen/antibody reaction. (5-4.2)

24.

B. The immune system is responsible for eliminating any foreign substance that gains access to the blood system. In an acute anaphylactic reaction, there is an inappropriate overwhelming response of the immune system. The chemical mediators released in such an emergency create the clinical signs and symptoms seen particularly in the cardiovascular, respiratory, and integumentary systems. It can also involve the gastrointestinal and nervous systems. (5-4.9) (IEC p. 960)

25.

B. The laryngeal edema resulting in occlusion of the airway develops rapidly and can be fatal within minutes if untreated. A severe allergic reaction can affect the cardiovascular and respiratory systems with fatal effects. In an acute reaction, the patient can display hypotension, tachycardia, stridor (from laryngeal edema), and bronchoconstriction. (5-4.9) (IEC pp. 964, 965)

26.

D. On introduction of the antigen in an allergic reaction, antibodies cause the release of chemical mediators from MAST cells and basophils, causing changes in the cardiovascular system. These changes include vasodilation or a decrease in systemic vascular resistance, peripheral pooling of blood, and increased capillary permeability. These changes cause the tachycardia and hypotension seen in acute reactions. (5-4.10) (IEC pp. 964–965)

27.

B. Chemical mediators released from MAST cells and basophils in an allergic reaction also affect the pulmonary system by causing profound bronchoconstriction, bronchial wall edema, and increased mucus production. This makes it harder for the person to breathe because of airway occlusion. This is known as an increase in airway resistance. (5-4.7) (IEC p. 964)

28.

A. The chemical mediators released in the anaphylactic reaction affect the cardiovascular system significantly. These changes often cause profound hypotension in the acute reaction. Tachycardia occurs as the body attempts to maintain a normal blood pressure by increasing cardiac output. Tachypnea (rapid breathing) may be seen due to hypoxia, but hyperpnea (deep breathing) is not likely due to the respiratory effects seen in anaphylactic reactions. (5-4.10) (IEC p. 964)

29.

A. Urticaria (hives) and pruritis (itching) are hallmark signs of an allergic reaction and are caused by the chemical mediators released from MAST cells and basophils. The skin may become reddened (erythemic) from the chemical mediators as well. Cellular changes due to hypoxia or acidosis do not play a role in the development of urticaria or pruritis but could be associated with cyanosis. (5-4.10) (IEC p. 964)

30.

C. Although numerous chemical mediators are released from MAST cells and basophils during an allergic reaction, histamine is one of the most prevalent. Histamine release has cardiovascular, respiratory, and integumentary manifestations. Phosphodiasterase is an intracellular enzyme and is not a component of an allergic reaction. Cyclic AMP is a second chemical messenger for cell transmission, and glucagon is a hormone that is involved with blood glucose levels. (5-4.9) (IEC p. 963)

31.

D. An acute reaction can occur from any mode of exposure—inhalation, absorption, or ingestion. In essence, if the antigen can gain access to the body, an allergic reaction can occur. (5-4.4) (IEC p. 963)

32.

C. Pollen is a common cause of asthmatic attacks and "hay fever" symptoms; however, it is not commonly associated with anaphylaxis. Wasp venom from stings, certain medications, and certain foods (nuts, shellfish) are commonly associated with anaphylaxis. Be aware, however, that almost any substance could create a reaction. (5-4.5) (IEC pp. 959–960)

33.

D. Basophils are a type of white blood cell that is important to the allergic reaction. Since it is a white blood cell, it is found within the bloodstream and circulates throughout the body. Basophils are immature mast cells. Once the basophil leaves the blood and enters connnective tissue, it becomes a MAST cell. MAST cells, also important to the allergic reaction, are stationary and are located within the walls of connective tissue, respiratory tree, and vascular smooth muscle. (5-4.9) (IEC pp. 103, 107)

34.

A. Hallmark integumentary signs seen in anaphylaxis include pruritis and urticaria. Rhinorrhea and erythema may also be present but are not considered as "hallmark" findings. (5-4.7) (IEC p. 964)

35.

C. The anaphylactic patient may present anywhere on the continuum of stable to severe, depending on his or her personal reaction to the antigen. However, alterations in the level of consciousness, hypotension, and stridorous respirations are considered as findings in a severe allergic reaction. (5-4.7) (IEC pp. 963–965, 967)

36.

B. Bronchoconstriction brought on by chemical mediator release, results in an increase in airway resistance and wheezing. Stridor may be present, but is from laryngeal edema. Rhonchi are secondary to mucous secretion in larger passages of the airway, not bronchoconstriction. Crackles, or rales, are from fluid in and around the alveolar sacs and are not common to allergic reactions. (5-4.10) (IEC p. 964)

37.

C. All of the clinical findings listed can be considered significant findings of a severe reaction; however absence of wheezing with minimal breath sounds upon auscultation is most likely indicative of poor air exchange due to bronchoconstriction. This patient is deteriorating to respiratory failure, and cardiac arrest may follow shortly thereafter. (5-4.7) (IEC pp. 964, 965, 967)

38.

B. Glottic edema from fluid shifting out of the cells due to an increase in capillary permeability creates a narrowing of the glottic opening. As the person inhales against the narrowed opening, it creates stridor. Stridor is a high pitched inspiratory noise indicative of at least 75 percent glottic closure. Wheezing is from bronchoconstriction, while pruritis is the perception of itching. Hemoptysis is coughing up blood. (5-4.10) (IEC p. 967)

39.

B. Inspiratory stridor is indicative of glottic closure caused by the swelling of the glottic tissues from the anaphylaxis and airway occlusion. This indicates a severe reaction and the patient may require advanced airway interventions. Vasodilation causes a drop in systemic vascular resistance and hypotension. (5-4.10) (IEC p. 967)

40.

B. The blood pressure of 86/68, respiratory rate of 42, and heart rate of 130 would be most likely. Vital signs in the severe allergic reaction will be the result of the body's response to the chemical mediator release. Generally, the patient will be hypotensive, tachycardic, and tachypneic. (5-4.7) (IEC pp. 964–965, 967)

41.

C. Diminishing breath sounds are most likely due to respiratory failure, not improvement. Given the seriousness of the patient initially and the lack of response to initial treatment, the patient's status is most likely deteriorating. With appropriate management, the anaphylactic patient's status should improve in the prehospital environment. (5-4.10) (IEC p. 964)

42.

C. The quicker the onset of the anaphylactic reaction, especially after an injection mechanism, the more likely the overall reaction will be more severe. (5-4.10) (IEC p. 963)

43.

A. The most severe of reactions can occur within minutes of the exposure, but a severe anaphylactic reaction can occur hours after exposure to the antigen. However, bee stings and intravenous medications (injection mechanisms) are most commonly associated with a rapid onset and serious manifestations. (5-4.10) (IEC p. 963)

44.

A. Hypotension from an increase in capillary permeability, a decrease in systemic vascular resistance, and peripheral pooling of blood are the results of histamine release in anaphylaxis. Bradycardia is unlikely since the normal feedback mechanism is tachycardia. Hemataemesis (vomiting blood) is not a common finding, and hypotonia is secondary to profound hypoxemia and hypoperfusion and is not directly due to the histamine release. (5-4.10) (IEC pp. 964–965)

45.

D. Anaphylaxis is an overwhelming response by the immune system to an antigen to which it has been sensitized. It is the immune system that creates the emergency, and its effects are seen primarily in the respiratory, cardiovascular, and central nervous systems. (5-4.9) (IEC p. 960)

46.

A. IgE is the one antibody that contributes to allergic and anaphylactic responses. There are five classes of human antibodies, also called immunoglobulins. They include IgM, IgG, IgA, IgE, and IgD. These all play a role in the immune response. (5-4.9) (IEC p. 962)

47.

C. The first time an antigen enters the body in an IgE-mediated reaction, there is usually not an anaphylactic reaction until sensitization occurs. After the person is sensitized, the body is primed for a reaction. An anaphylactoid reaction is a non-IgE-mediated reaction and can produce a severe and life-threatening reaction on the first exposure to an anaphylactoid reaction substance. (5-4.9) (IEC p. 962)

48.

C. Of the listed possibilities, the only one that has not been commonly cited as a probable antigen is antacids. All of the others have been found to create allergic reactions with exposure. Gathering a good history about allergic reactions is very important. Patient needs may make it necessary to alter your protocols. (5-4.5) (IEC p. 960)

49.

C. When administering epinephrine for anaphylaxis, there are four things to consider. First, is the reaction severe or mild? This determines the route of administration. Second, what is the desired dose? In either case, it is 0.3–0.5 mg. Third, what concentration of epinephrine should be used? This depends on route and severity. A 1:1000 dilution of epinephrine must be used for IM or SQ adminstration. In a severe reaction, a 1:10,000 dilution can be administered either IV (preferred) or endotracheally. Subcutaneous administration of epinephrine should not be used in the presence of hypotension because of the impaired absorption rate. A deep intramuscular injection should be used as an alternative to intravenous or tracheal routes when hypotension is present. (5-4.8) (IEC p. 966)

50.

A. Tachycardia is a reflex mechanism for hypoxia and hypotension that accompanies anaphylaxis and is a common manifestation of a mild or severe reaction. Dyspnea is caused by the bronchoconstriction and airway edema, and low blood pressure is a result of severe peripheral vasodilation and increased capillary permeability. The itching and hives are from histamine release and capillary dilation. (5-4.10)

51.

B. During the initial assessment, you are looking for significantly life-threatening conditions to the airway, breathing, and circulation. If you are assessing a patient thought to be having an anaphylactic reaction and he or she presents as unresponsive, this is a grave sign of severe hypoxemia and cerebral hypoperfusion. The other findings may well be present but may also be seen with a milder reaction. (5-4.10) (IEC pp. 964, 967)

52.

A. During the initial assessment, you treat life threats as they are discovered. Airway, ventilation, and oxygenation are the priorities in the patient management. After the oxygenation, you would initiate an IV and give epinephrine according to need. Immobilization is necessary only if you suspect spinal injury. (5-4.11) (IEC p. 963)

53.

C. If possible, try using a smaller-diameter tube that may fit in the edematous glottic opening. Any airway is better than none, as PPV will be totally ineffective if the glottic opening completely swells shut. Forcing a tube through is damaging. Performing a needle cricothyrotomy is beyond the scope of an EMT-Intermediate. (5-4.11) (IEC p. 965)

54.

A. Extreme anxiety may be present in a patient who has been exposed to an antigen to which he knows he is allergic. The person may be aware that he can have a severe reaction and may be scared. Additionally, the release of catecholamines early in the anaphylactic process may precipitate anxiety. The other findings are more suggestive of a moderate to severe reaction. (5-4.10) (IEC pp. 964, 967)

55.

D. Administration of intravenous fluids will increase intravascular volume, which might raise perfusion pressures. The concentration of epinephrine will cause vasoconstriction and increase perfusion pressure by raising SVR. (5-4.11) (IEC pp. 965–966)

56.

B. Histamine release can cause the patient to experience nausea, vomiting, and diarrhea. This effect is enhanced by the increased capillary permeability as more fluid enters the intestinal tract. Vasodilation and bronchoconstriction occur as a result of histamine as well, but they do not cause the GI distress. (5-4.10) (IEC p. 963)

57.

D. Fluids such as normal saline and lactated Ringer's are isotonic crystalloid solutions that will immediately increase intravascular volume in the anaphylactic patient. (5-4.11) (IEC p. 965)

58.

B. Whenever you have a fluid-depleted patient, the standard bolus amount is 20 ml/kg infused at a wide-open rate. Following this, reassess your patient to see if you need to repeat the bolus. (5-4.11) (IEC p. 666)

59.

C. When infusing a large amount of fluid in a short amount of time, use a setup that utilizes a large-bore angiocatheter (14 or 16 gauge) and a macrodrip administration set. Also, if possible, use the shortest catheter possible, like an inch and a quarter. These steps will reduce the resistance to flow as much as possible. (5-4.11) (IEC pp. 308, 666)

60.

A. Beta 1 stimulation is the least desirable in an anaphylactic reaction. This causes an increase in cardiac activity that will then require more perfusion and oxygenation. Beta 2 causes smooth-muscle relaxation of the bronchioles, and alpha causes peripheral vasoconstriction. (5-4.8)

61.

D. Because of the effects of epinephrine administration, you can expect to see all the above findings. Respiratory distress should diminish because of beta 2 stimulation, the blood pressure should normalize from vasoconstriction, and the orientation should improve with enhanced oxygenation and perfusion to the CNS. (5-4.8) (IEC pp. 965–966)

62.

C. Epinephrine for a mild allergic reaction is 0.3–0.5 mg of a 1:1000 solution administered SQ or IM. Subcutaneous administration in cases of anaphylaxis associated with hypotension is not a desirable route since the rate of absorption will be impaired and the efficacy of the epinephrine will be lessened. (5-4.8) (IEC p. 966)

63.

C. Epinephrine for a severe allergic reaction is 0.3–0.5 mg of a 1:10,000 solution administered IV push or via the ET tube. (5-4.8) (IEC p. 966)

64.

A. The most significant difference is the route of administration. The route of administration will determine the concentration. For SQ or IM, 1:1000 is used. For a severe reaction, you use 1:10,000 IV or ET. The dose remains the same regardless of the route or severity of the reaction. (5-4.8) (IEC p. 966)

65.

A. These clinical findings are most consistent with a severe allergic reaction. The major clinical findings that demonstrate a severe reaction are hypotension, stridor, severe wheezing, and an altered mental status. The skin findings are also found with a mild reaction but persist through a severe reaction. (5-4.7) (IEC p. 967)

66.

C. Injection of an antigen typically produces the most rapid onset of signs and symptoms associated with an anaphylactic reaction. Injection places the antigen within the body where it may be immediately absorbed and transported. (5-4.4) (IEC pp. 959–960, 963)

67.

B. The number one cause of death in any severe anaphylactic reaction is glottic edema causing an airway obstruction. That is why airway maintenance is so important and the presence of inspiratory stridor a significant finding. Severe bronchoconstriction and hypotension can also be fatal, but its presentation is not as rapid as the glottic edema. (5-4.10) (IEC p. 967)

68.

D. The IV at a KVO rate is inappropriate. The IV should be a 20-ml/kg bolus run at a wide-open rate. Treatment of a severe allergic reaction must occur rapidly if the patient is to have a successful recovery. The cornerstones of treatment are reversal of the bronchoconstriction, oxygenation, correcting vasodilation, and restoring intravascular volume. (5-4.11) (IEC pp. 666, 965–967)

69.

B. The patient is experiencing an anaphylactoid reaction. Anaphylactoid reactions present the same, clinically, as anaphylactic reactions; however, a patient suffering an anaphylactoid reaction does not need to be sensitized in order to experience the reaction. First-time exposure to medications and other substances could trigger the breakdown of the mast cells and basophils with a subsequent chemical mediator release. IgE antibodies are not required to be produced or attached onto the mast cells and basophils in order for the reaction to occur. (5-4.11)

70.

D. Since the anaphylactoid reaction results in the same chemical mediators being released from the mast cells and basophils, the same physiologic response of the organs and cells will occur as in an anaphylactic reaction. Thus, the patient should be treated the same as if suffering an anaphylactic reaction. (5-4.11)

Poisoning/Overdose Emergencies

unit objectives

Questions in this unit relate to DOT objectives 5-5.1 to 5-5.14. The objectives are listed in the Appendix.

DIRECTIONS Each of the questions or incomplete statements below is followed by suggested answers or completions. Select the **one answer** that is best in each case.

1. The most common route of entry for toxic exposure is
   A. inhalation.
   B. ingestion.
   C. surface absorption.
   D. injection.

2. Toxic gases, such as methyl chloride, chlorine, and carbon monoxide, enter the bloodstream through the
   A. blood-brain barrier.
   B. skin.
   C. alveolar-capillary membrane.
   D. intestinal tract.

3. Which of the following is an advantage of having a poison control center?
   A. It is staffed by poison control specialists.
   B. It is available 24 hours a day.
   C. It offers the most current information.
   D. all of the above

4. The poison antidote that works by adsorbing large amounts of poisonous molecules in the stomach is
   A. syrup of ipecac.
   B. naloxone.
   C. activated charcoal.
   D. amyl nitrite.

5. Which of the following describes the pathophysiology of cyanide poisoning?
   A. Cyanide binds with hemoglobin, preventing oxygen transport.
   B. Cyanide paralyzes the central nervous system.
   C. Cyanide prevents cellular use of oxygen.
   D. Cyanide can only be inhaled.

6. A cyanide antidote kit should contain
   A. amyl nitrite ampules.
   B. sodium nitrate solution.
   C. a sodium thiosulfate solution.
   D. all of the above

Scenario

Questions 7 and 8 refer to the following scenario:

Your patient is a 26-year-old male who was barbecuing in his garage with the overhead door half closed. His wife called 911 because he began acting strangely and vomited. You find him walking around the house disoriented, complaining of a severe headache and nausea.

7. This man is most likely suffering from
   A. carbon monoxide poisoning.
   B. acute methanol intoxication.
   C. cyanide poisoning.
   D. organophosphate poisoning.

8. Management of this patient includes
   A. removal from the toxic environment.
   B. oxygen administration.
   C. transport to a hyperbaric chamber.
   D. all of the above

9. Which of the following statements is true regarding caustic agents?
   A. Strong acids tend to cause deeper burns than strong alkalis.
   B. Eschar is the result of coagulation from an alkali burn.
   C. Strong alkalis produce liquefaction necrosis.
   D. Strong alkaline agents tend to pass quickly through the esophagus.

Scenario

Questions 10 and 11 refer to the following scenario:

Your patient is a 56-year-old man who presents on the floor with an altered mental status. He is confused and is hallucinating. His heart rate is 180, and he is hypotensive. He shows torsade de pointes on the monitor. You learn that he has no cardiac history, but he is being treated for clinical depression.

10. You suspect he may have taken an overdose of what type of medication?
    A. beta blockers
    B. calcium channel blockers
    C. tricyclics
    D. benzodiazepines

11. The most important part of your field management of this patient is to
    A. administer flumazenil.
    B. administer thiamine.
    C. monitor for cardiac dysrhythmias.
    D. induce emesis.

12. Prozac, Paxil, and Zoloft all belong to a class of drugs known as
    A. monoamine oxidase inhibitors (MAOIs).
    B. selective serotonin reuptake inhibitors (SSRIs).
    C. tricyclic antidepressants (TCAs).
    D. phenothiazines.

13. Your patient takes lithium. He most likely is being treated for
    A. manic-depressive disorder.
    B. obsessive-compulsive disorder.
    C. hallucinations.
    D. chronic pain.

14. A lethal type of food poisoning caused by improper food storage methods is
    A. Clostridium botulinum.
    B. Salmonella.
    C. E. coli.
    D. scomboid.

15. For which of the following bites or stings is there no antivenin?
    A. black widow spiders
    B. scorpions
    C. pit vipers
    D. brown recluse spiders

Scenario

Questions 16–18 refer to the following scenario:

Your patient is a 25-year-old rock climber who was bitten by a rattlesnake and walked to call for help (1 mile). She presents on the ground complaining of weakness, dizziness, and pain at the injection site. She has fang marks on her left leg with oozing. She is nauseated and has vomited twice. Her BP is 80/50; pulse 120 and weak; and skin cool, pale, and clammy to the touch.

16. Rattlesnakes are members of what class of snakes?
    A. *hymenoptera*
    B. pit vipers
    C. elapidae
    D. coral

17. Which of the following statements is true regarding rattlesnakes?
    A. Their bites can result in death within 30 minutes.
    B. Their bites seldom cause systemic reactions.
    C. All rattlesnakes have rattles.
    D. All rattlesnake bites inject poisonous venom.

18. Management of a rattlesnake bite includes all of the following **except**

    A. applying a constricting band proximal to the wound.

    B. keeping the patient calm.

    C. applying ice and compression and elevating the wound.

    D. immobilizing the extremity.

19. Your patient is a 63-year-old homeless male who is a habitual ambulance customer. This evening you find him slumped against a tree in the park, seemingly unconscious. He is alive but responds neither to voice nor to deep pain. Next to him you find a jar labeled "wood alcohol." His BP is 150/90, pulse 90, and respirations 40. He lies in a pool of vomit and reeks of alcohol. This patient is most likely suffering from

    A. alcohol intoxication.

    B. acute methanol poisoning.

    C. cyanide poisoning.

    D. none of the above

20. Your patient is a 35-year-old chronic alcoholic who calls you 2 days after leaving the detox unit. He presents with general weakness, tremors of the hands, and sweating and is very anxious. He complains of nausea and vomiting and inability to sleep. His skin is cool and clammy, BP 140/70, pulse 90, and respirations 20. He claims he sees pink elephants behind you and generally acts very strangely. This patient is most likely suffering from

    A. acute psychosis.

    B. delusions.

    C. acute alcohol withdrawal.

    D. ethylene glycol poisoning.

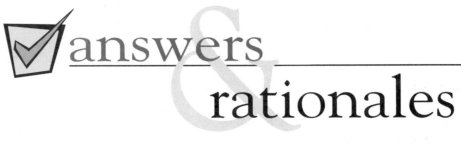

answers & rationales

Following each rationale, you will find a reference to the corresponding objective in the DOT National Standard EMT-Intermediate curriculum. An asterisk denotes material that is supplemental to the DOT curriculum. Page numbers after a rationale indicate where the question topic may be discussed in the Brady text *Intermediate Emergency Care* (Bledsoe, Porter, Cherry).

1.

B. Ingestion is the most common route of entry for toxic exposure. Frequently ingested poisons include household products, petroleum-based agents (gasoline and paint), cleaning agents (alkalis and soaps), cosmetics, prescribed drugs, plants, and foods. (5-5.3) (IEC p. 971)

2.

C. Inhalation of a poison results in rapid absorption of the toxic agent through the alveolar-capillary membrane. Commonly inhaled poisons include toxic gases; carbon monoxide; ammonia; chlorine; freon; toxic vapors, fumes, or aerosols; carbon tetrachloride; methyl chloride; teargas; mustard gas; and nitrous oxide. (5-5.3) (IEC p. 972)

3.

D. Poison control centers have been set up across the United States and Canada to assist in the treatment of poison victims and to provide information on new products and new treatment recommendations. Centers are usually staffed by physicians, pharmacists, nurses, or poison control specialists trained in toxicology and are available to callers 24 hours a day. (5-5.4) (IEC p. 971)

4.

C. Activated charcoal promotes gastrointestinal decontamination via its large surface area, which can adsorb molecules from the offending poison. (5-5.8) (IEC p. 974)

5.

C. Cyanide inflicts its damage by inhibiting cytochrome oxidase, an enzyme vital to cellular use of oxygen. Once cyanide enters the body, it acts as a cellular asphyxiant. (*) (IEC p. 978)

6.

D. A cyanide antidote kit should contain amyl nitrite ampules, a sodium nitrite solution, and a sodium thiosulfate solution. (5-5.8) (IEC p. 981)

7.

A. Carbon monoxide is an odorless, tasteless gas that is often the by-product of incomplete combustion. It has more than 200 times the affinity of oxygen to bind with hemoglobin, producing carboxyhemoglobin. Once this molecule has bound with hemoglobin, it is very resistant to removal and causes hypoxia. (5-5.9) (IEC p. 981)

8.

D. Management of carbon monoxide poisoning includes removing the patient from the toxic environment, administering high concentrations of oxygen, and transporting the victim as soon as possible to a hyperbaric chamber. (5-5.9) (IEC p. 982)

9.

C. Strong alkaline agents cause injury by inducing liquefaction necrosis, which allows deeper penetration and more extensive burns. Strong acids, on the other hand, produce coagulation, which acts as a protective barrier to further burns. (*) (IEC p. 983)

10.

C. Tricyclic antidepressants were once used to treat depression but are on the decline because of their narrow therapeutic index and the availability of safer drugs. However, they are still prescribed. Signs of tricyclic toxicity include an altered mental status, hallucinations, hypotension, and cardiac dysrhythmias, such as torsade de pointes. A severe overdose of tricyclics can result in PEA (pulseless electrical activity). (5-5.14) (IEC p. 985)

11.

C. Field management of a tricyclic overdose requires standard toxicological therapy, such as managing the ABCs and determining the need for GI decontamination. In addition, sodium bicarbonate may be required. But it is crucial that you perform cardiac monitoring because dysrhythmias are the most common cause of death. (5-5.14) (IEC p. 985)

12.

B. Paxil, Zoloft, and Prozac belong to a new class of drugs known as selective serotonin reuptake inhibitors (SSRIs). They are prescribed for clinical depression. While the true mechanism of action is unclear, they prevent the reuptake of serotonin, making it more available for the brain. (*) (IEC p. 986)

13.

A. Even though its mechanism of action is unclear, lithium remains the drug of choice for treating manic-depressive disorder. (*) (IEC p. 987)

14.

A. *Clostridium botulinum*, the world's most toxic poison, occurs in cases of improper food storage methods, such as canning. (*) (IEC p. 990)

15.

D. Since there is no antivenin for a brown recluse spider bite, treatment is mostly supportive. While antivenin exists and is available for the bites and stings of scorpions, black widow spiders, and pit vipers, all these may produce severe reactions themselves. (*) (IEC p. 993)

16.

B. Rattlesnakes are members of the pit viper class. Pit vipers are so named because of the distinctive pit between the eye and the nostril on each side of the head. (*) (IEC p. 996)

17.

A. A severe bite of a pit viper, such as a rattlesnake, can result in death from shock within 30 minutes. (5-5.6) (IEC p. 996)

18.

C. Management of a rattlesnake bite includes applying a constrictive band proximal to the wound on the extremity, keeping the patient calm, and immobilizing the extremity. (5-5.9) (IEC p. 997)

19.

B. Methanol, which is used in a variety of automotive products and cooking fuel, is toxic when ingested. Consumption of as little as 4 cc of methanol has produced blindness, while 15 cc has caused death. It is used occasionally by chronic alcoholics trying to get intoxicated. (5-5.9) (IEC p. 1003)

20.

C. The alcoholic may suffer a withdrawal reaction from either abrupt discontinuence of ingestion after prolonged use or a rapid fall in the blood alcohol level after acute intoxication. Withdrawal symptoms can occur several hours after sudden abstinence and can last up to 5–7 days. (*) (IEC pp. 1004–1006)

UNIT

6 Neurological Emergencies

unit objectives

Questions in this unit relate to DOT objectives 5-6.1 to 5-6.8. The objectives are listed in the Appendix.

DIRECTIONS
Each of the questions or incomplete statements below is followed by suggested answers or completions. Select the **one answer** that is best in each case.

1. The central nervous system consists of the
   A. sympathetic and parasympathetic branches.
   B. cranial nerves and peripheral nerves.
   C. axial and appendicular skeleton.
   D. brain and spinal cord.

2. Which of the following is an early sign of increased intracranial pressure?
   A. dilated, nonreactive pupils
   B. dilated, reactive pupils
   C. unilaterally dilated pupil
   D. none of the above

Match the following respiratory patterns with their respective descriptions:

3. _____ Cheyne-Stokes
4. _____ central neurogenic
5. _____ ataxic
6. _____ apneustic
7. _____ diaphragmatic

   A. prolonged inspiration
   B. no intercostal movement
   C. increase/decrease/apnea
   D. rapid, deep breathing; hyperventilation
   E. ineffective muscular coordination

8. Which of the following is true?
   A. Carbon dioxide is a potent vasodilator.
   B. Hyperventilation can decrease intracranial pressure.
   C. At a $PaCO_2$ of approximately 25 mm Hg, the cerebral blood vessels constrict.
   D. all of the above

9. A patient who responds to questions but is disoriented is categorized
   A. A.
   B. V.
   C. P.
   D. U.

10. Decorticate posturing is characterized by
    A. arms extended, legs extended.
    B. arms flexed, legs extended.
    C. arms extended, legs flexed.
    D. arms flexed, legs flexed.

11. A common mnemonic for remembering the causes for coma is
    A. PQRST.
    B. AEIOU–TIPS.
    C. SLUDGE.
    D. ABCDE.

12. Inadequate thiamine intake may result in all of the following **except**
    A. Wernicke's syndrome.
    B. Kernig's sign.
    C. Korsakoff's psychosis.
    D. encephalopathy.

Scenario

Questions 13–17 refer to the following scenario:

Your patient is a 75-year-old female who presents at home slumped to one side of the couch. She appears awake but disoriented. Per her family, she has a long history of hypertension and one stroke. Her respiratory rate is 18, pulse 90 and regular, BP

170/90, and pupils equal and reactive. Her left side is obviously weakened, she slurs her speech, and she has facial drooping. According to her family, all these signs are new.

13. Strokes are caused by
    A. hemorrhage of cerebral blood vessels.
    B. thrombus formation.
    C. embolism.
    D. all of the above

14. Transient ischemic attacks are defined as
    A. minor strokes.
    B. temporary strokes.
    C. strokes caused by hypoxia.
    D. none of the above

15. Patients with strokes commonly present with
    A. bilateral paralysis or paresthesia.
    B. polyuria, polydipsia, polyphagia.
    C. hemiparesis or hemiplegia.
    D. all of the above

16. Hemiplegia means
    A. weakness to the legs.
    B. inability to speak.
    C. unilateral paralysis.
    D. numbness.

17. Management of this patient should include
    A. blood glucose determination.
    B. 100% oxygen administration.
    C. cardiac monitoring.
    D. all of the above

Scenario

Questions 18–25 refer to the following scenario:

Your patient is a 56-year-old homeless man who, per bystanders, experienced a seizure. He presents to you on the street, comatose, and smelling of alcohol and urine, with vomit and blood around his mouth. Further examination finds him responsive to deep pain with purposeful movement, breathing at 20 per minute, heart rate 90 and regular, BP 140/70, and pupils equal but sluggish to react. As you prepare to examine him further, he seizes once again, full grand mal.

18. The most common cause of seizures is
    A. hypoglycemia.
    B. hypoxia.
    C. drug overdose.
    D. epilepsy.

Match the following types of seizures with their respective descriptions:

19. _____ grand mal
20. _____ petit mal
21. _____ jacksonian
22. _____ psychomotor
23. _____ pseudoseizure

    A. brief loss of consciousness
    B. dysfunction to one area of body
    C. tonic/clonic extremity movement
    D. involves temporal lobe with aura
    E. can be interrupted, no postictal period

24. Status epilepticus is defined as
    A. a seizure due to epilepsy.
    B. a seizure that does not stop following diazepam therapy.
    C. two or more seizures without a lucid interval.
    D. all of the above

25. Which of the following is **not** recommended in the management of this patient?
    A. IV D$_5$W
    B. blood glucose determination
    C. diazepam IV push
    D. 100% oxygen administration

26. Your patient suffered a sudden loss of consciousness and was unresponsive for approximately 5 minutes. Your differential field diagnosis includes all of the following **except**
    A. syncope.
    B. seizure.
    C. TIA.
    D. cardiac dysrhythmia.

27. Which of the following is a cause of syncope?
    A. idiopathic reasons
    B. cardiovascular conditions
    C. hypoglycemia
    D. all of the above

28. Your patient is a 30-year-old woman who complains of recurring right-sided headaches. She describes them as intense and throbbing. She also complains of photophobia, nausea, and vomiting. She claims she can feel it coming on through some auditory signals. Her neck is supple. Your probable field diagnosis is
    A. cluster headache.
    B. migraine headache.
    C. tension headache.
    D. organic headache.

29. Which of the following statements is true regarding back pain?
    A. Fifteen percent of lower-back pain is due to sciatica.
    B. The cause of most lower-back pain is unknown.
    C. Sciatica never causes motor or sensory deficits.
    D. Men report 50% more lower-back pain than women.

30. Which is the most common cause of a herniated disc?
    A. degeneration
    B. trauma
    C. improper lifting
    D. none of the above

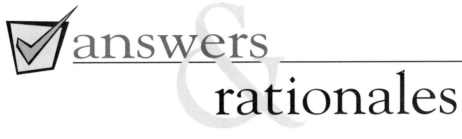

answers & rationales

Following each rationale, you will find a reference to the corresponding objective in the DOT National Standard EMT-Intermediate curriculum. An asterisk denotes material that is supplemental to the DOT curriculum. Page numbers after a rationale indicate where the question topic may be discussed in the Brady text *Intermediate Emergency Care* (Bledsoe, Porter, Cherry).

1.

D. The central nervous system consists of the brain and spinal cord. (*) (IEC p. 1009)

2.

C. A unilaterally dilated pupil that remains reactive to light may be the earliest sign of increasing intracranial pressure. The patient who presents with or develops the unilaterally dilated pupil is in the immediate transport category. (5-6.2) (IEC p. 1012)

Matching (5-6.2) (IEC p. 1013)

3.	C	Cheyne-Stokes
4.	D	central neurogenic
5.	E	ataxic
6.	A	apneustic
7.	B	diaphragmatic

8.

D. The blood level of carbon dioxide has a critical effect on cerebral blood vessels. The normal blood $PaCO_2$ is 40 mm Hg. Increasing the $PaCO_2$ causes cerebral vasodilation, while decreasing it results in cerebral vasoconstriction. If the patient is poorly ventilated, the $PaCO_2$ will increase, causing even further vasodilation with a subsequent increase in intracranial pressure. Hyperventilation can decrease the $PaCO_2$ to nearly 25 mm Hg, effectively causing vasoconstriction of the cerebral vessels. This will help minimize brain swelling. Therefore, hyperventilate any patient suspected of having increased intracranial pressure at a rate of 24 breaths per minute or more. (5-6.1) (IEC p. 1014)

9.

A. A patient who responds to questions but is disoriented is categorized A for alert. He is alert but disoriented. To be oriented, he must know who he is, where he is, and the approximate time. (5-6.7) (IEC p. 1010)

10.

B. Decorticate posturing is characterized by flexion of the arms and extension of the legs. Decerebrate posturing is characterized by arm and leg extension. Both signify deep cerebral or brain-stem injury. (5-6.2) (IEC p. 1014)

11.

B. Unconsciousness or coma is a state in which the patient cannot be aroused even by powerful external stimuli. There generally are only two mechanisms capable of producing alterations in mental status: structural lesions and toxic-metabolic states. Within these two general categories, there are many causes of altered mental status. The mnemonic AEIOU–TIPS is an easy way to remember some of them. (5-6.7) (IEC p. 1018)

A — acidosis, alcohol

E — epilepsy

I — infection

O — overdose

U — uremia (kidney failure)

T — trauma, tumor, toxin

I — insulin

P — psychosis, poison

S — stroke, seizure

12.

B. Thiamine deficiency may cause Wernicke's syndrome (an acute and reversible encephalopathy) or Korsakoff's psychosis. (5-6.1) (IEC p. 1019)

13.

D. A stroke or CVA is a term that describes injury or death of brain tissue, usually due to interruption of cerebral blood flow from either ischemic or hemorrhagic lesions. This may be caused by hemorrhage in the brain

tissue, an embolus in the cerebral blood vessels, or thrombus formation that occludes arterial supply to the brain. (5-6.1) (IEC p. 1020)

14.

B. Transient ischemic attacks or TIAs are temporary strokes. These are usually caused by emboli that temporarily interfere with the blood supply to the brain, producing symptoms of neurologic deficit. These symptoms may last for only a few minutes or for several hours. (5-6.5) (IEC p. 1023)

15.

C. Patients with strokes commonly present with hemiplegia or hemiparesis, unilateral facial droop, speech disturbances, confusion and agitation, eating disturbances, uncoordinated fine motor movements, vision problems, inappropriate behavior with excessive laughing or crying, or coma. (5-6.4) (IEC p. 1022)

16.

C. Hemiplegia means paralysis of one side of the body. (5-6.4) (IEC p. 1022)

17.

D. Management of a patient with stroke symptoms should include blood glucose determination and administration of 50% dextrose if the patient is hypoglycemic, administration of 100% oxygen, and cardiac monitoring. Of utmost importance are ascertaining the time of onset of symptoms and rapidly transporting the patient to a stroke center if still within the 3-hour window for administering fibrinolytic therapy. (5-6.4) (IEC p. 1024)

18.

D. A seizure is a temporary alteration in behavior due to massive electrical discharge of one or more groups of neurons in the brain. The most common cause is idiopathic epilepsy. (5-6.1) (IEC p. 1025)

Matching (5-6.6) (IEC p. 1026)

19.	C	grand mal
20.	A	petit mal
21.	B	jacksonian
22.	D	psychomotor
23.	E	pseudoseizure

24.

C. Status epilepticus is a series of two or more generalized motor seizures without an intervening return of consciousness. The most common cause in adults is failure to take prescribed anticonvulsive medications. (5-6.6) (IEC p. 1028)

25.

A. Managing the patient in status epilepticus includes aggressive airway management, oxygenation, IV access with normal saline or lactated Ringer's, determination of blood glucose level and administration of 50% dextrose if the patient is hypoglycemic, and administration of a diazepam IV push. (5-6.6) (IEC p. 1029)

26.

A. Syncope is, by definition, a transient loss of consciousness due to inadequate blood flow to the brain. Syncope involves rapid recovery of consciousness. If your patient does not regain consciousness within a few moments, it is not syncope but something more serious. (5-6.7) (IEC p. 1029)

27.

D. Syncope can be caused by cardiovascular conditions, such as dysrhythmias (e.g., bradycardia, tachycardia) or mechanical problems; noncardiovascular disease, such as metabolic (e.g., hypoglycemia), neurological (e.g., transient ischemic attack) or psychiatric (e.g., anxiety) conditions; or idiopathic (unknown) reasons. (5-6.7) (IEC p. 1029)

28.

B. Migraine headaches afflict approximately 17 million people. They are characterized by an intense, throbbing, unilateral headache accompanied by photophobia, nausea, and vomiting. Often patients experience a visual or auditory aura just prior to the headache. (5-6.7) (IEC p. 1030)

29.

B. Most back pain is idiopathic. That is, the cause may be difficult or impossible to diagnose. This makes the treatment of many cases of lower-back pain frustrating and sometimes unsuccessful. (5-6.1) (IEC p. 1032)

30.

C. This is probably the most important question and answer in this book for a prehospital provider. Improper lifting is the most common cause of disc herniation. Through adequate exercise and proper mechanics, you can avoid this career-ending injury. (5-6.1) (IEC p. 1032)

Nontraumatic Abdominal Emergencies

unit objectives

Questions in this unit relate to DOT objectives 5-7.1 to 5-7.4. The objectives are listed in the Appendix.

DIRECTIONS Each of the questions or incomplete statements below is followed by suggested answers or completions. Select the **one answer** that is best in each case.

1. Poorly localized, dull pain that originates in the walls of hollow organs is known as _____ pain.
   A. somatic
   B. referred
   C. visceral
   D. peritoneal

2. Sharp, localized pain that originates in the walls of the body, such as skeletal muscles, is known as _____ pain.
   A. somatic
   B. referred
   C. visceral
   D. peritoneal

3. Pain that originates in a region other than where it is felt is known as _____ pain.
   A. somatic
   B. referred
   C. visceral
   D. peritoneal

4. Signs of GI bleeding include
   A. nausea and vomiting.
   B. hematemesis.
   C. melena.
   D. all of the above

5. Which of the following contributes to the formation of a peptic ulcer?
   A. ibuprofen
   B. smoking
   C. *H. pylori*
   D. all of the above

Match the following types of bowel diseases with their respective characteristics:

6. _____ hernia
7. _____ intussusception
8. _____ volvulus
9. _____ Crohn's disease
10. _____ ulcerative colitis
11. _____ adhesions
12. _____ diverticulosis

   A. destruction of the mucosal layer of bowel
   B. out-pouchings of mucosa and submucosa
   C. bowel protruding through the abdominal muscle wall
   D. inflammatory disease of small bowel
   E. part of the intestine slips into the part just distal to itself
   F. twisting of the intestine on itself
   G. union of separate tissues by fibrous band

13. Your patient presents with severe lower-right abdominal pain at McBurney's point. It began as a vague discomfort around the umbilicus. He also complains of anorexia, nausea, vomiting, and fever and has pronounced rebound tenderness. He may be suffering from
   A. gastritis.
   B. acute appendicitis.
   C. cholecystitis.
   D. pylonephritis.

14. An epigastric pain condition characterized by inflammation of the gallbladder is known as
    A. pylonephritis.
    B. cholecystitis.
    C. gastritis.
    D. hepatitis.

15. A positive Murphy's sign indicates
    A. gastritis.
    B. cholecystitis.
    C. hepatitis.
    D. pylonephritis.

16. Classic signs of acute renal failure include
    A. hot, flushed skin.
    B. peripheral edema.
    C. bradycardia.
    D. polyuria.

17. Which of the following statements is true regarding chronic kidney failure?
    A. End-stage renal failure occurs when 50% of nephrons are destroyed.
    B. Anuria is always present in end-stage renal failure.

C. Most cases are caused by diabetes and hypertension.
    D. Metabolic instability occurs even in the early stages.

18. Your patient in chronic renal failure may present with
    A. ascites.
    B. rales in the lung bases.
    C. jugular venous distention.
    D. all of the above

19. Which of the following presentations is most suggestive of a kidney stone?
    A. quiet patient in fetal position
    B. distended abdomen, supine with knees drawn up
    C. gross hematuria, severe peritonitis
    D. squirming, uncomfortable patient

20. Your nontrauma patient presents with percussion tenderness at the costovertebral angle. Your most likely field diagnosis is
    A. nephrolithiasis.
    B. pylonephritis.
    C. cystitis.
    D. lower UTI.

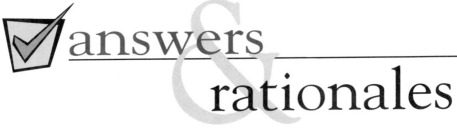

Following each rationale, you will find a reference to the corresponding objective in the DOT National Standard EMT-Intermediate curriculum. An asterisk denotes material that is supplemental to the DOT curriculum. Page numbers after a rationale indicate where the question topic may be discussed in the Brady text *Intermediate Emergency Care* (Bledsoe, Porter, Cherry).

1.

C. Dull, poorly localized pain that originates in the walls of hollow organs, such as the gallbladder and intestines, is known as visceral pain. Many hollow organs cause visceral pain as they become distended, inflamed, or ischemic. For example, the pain of appendicitis often presents as vague periumbilical pain. (5-7.2) (IEC p. 1036)

2.

A. Sharp, localized pain that originates in the walls of the body, such as skeletal muscles, is known as somatic pain. It travels along definite neural routes determined by dermatomes or tissue blocks developed during the embryonic stage. Bacterial and chemical irritation can cause somatic pain. As the appendix ruptures, it sends its chemical contents into the abdominal cavity, causing irritation and localized pain. (5-7.2) (IEC p. 1037)

3.

B. Pain that originates in a region other than where it is felt is known as referred pain. Many neural pathways from various organs pass through areas where the organ was formed during the embryonic stage. For example, splenic injuries and myocardial ischemia often cause left-shoulder pain. (5-7.2) (IEC p. 1037)

4.

D. Because blood severely irritates the GI system, patients can present with nausea and vomiting, hematemesis (bloody vomit), and melena (bloody stool). The blood may be bright red (new, fresh), dark brown (old, partially digested), or black and tarry in the stool. (5-7.2) (IEC p. 1041)

5.

D. Peptic ulcers are commonly caused by nonsteroidal anti-inflammatory drugs, such as ibuprofen and aspirin; acid-stimulating products, such as alcohol and nicotine; and the *H. pylori* bacterium. All contribute to the erosion of the protective mucosal lining in the stomach. When this lining is gone, hydrochloric acid used in the digestive process is allowed to erode the stomach lining. (5-7.1) (IEC p. 1040)

Matching (5-7.1) (IEC p. 1042)

6. C hernia
7. E intussusception
8. F volvulus
9. D Crohn's disease
10. A ulcerative colitis
11. G adhesions
12. B diverticulosis

13.

B. Appendicitis is the inflammation of the appendix. The patient suffering from appendicitis will usually complain of lower-right-quadrant abdominal pain, nausea, vomiting, fever, and anorexia. The peritoneum will generally become inflamed, and rebound tenderness will be present. (5-7.2) (IEC p. 1038)

14.

B. Inflammation of the gallbladder is called cholecystitis. It usually occurs when gallstones lodge in the cystic duct that drains the gallbladder. (5-7.2) (IEC p. 1038)

15.

B. Murphy's sign pain is caused when an inflamed gallbladder is palpated by pressing under the right costal margin. (5-7.2) (IEC p. 1039)

16.

B. Classic signs of acute renal failure include cool, clammy, pale skin; oliguria; peripheral edema; and, if in circulatory collapse, tachycardic, hypotensive, with an altered mental status. (5-7.2) (IEC p. 1044)

17.

C. End-stage renal failure occurs when 80% of nephrons are destroyed. Anuria is not necessarily present in end-stage renal failure. Most cases are caused by diabetes and hypertension. Metabolic instability occurs in end-stage failure. At this stage, only dialysis or a transplant will keep the patient alive. (5-7.1) (IEC p. 1044)

18.

D. The patient in chronic renal failure may present with severe dyspnea, neck vein distention, ascites, and rales at the lung bases. (5-7.2) (IEC p. 1046)

19.

D. Because of extreme pain and an inability to get into a position of comfort, a patient who is passing a kidney stone usually squirms continuously. (5-7.2) (IEC p. 1047)

20.

B. Tenderness to percussion at the costovertebral angle (Lloyd's sign) is a classic sign of pylonephritis (kidney infection). (5-7.3) (IEC p. 1049)

UNIT

8

Environmental Emergencies

unit objectives

Questions in this unit relate to DOT objectives 5-8.1 to 5-8.40. The objectives are listed in the Appendix.

DIRECTIONS
Each of the questions or incomplete statements below is followed by suggested answers or completions. Select the **one answer** that is best in each case.

1. Heat loss in the form of infrared rays is known as
   A. radiation.
   B. convection.
   C. conduction.
   D. evaporation.

2. Heat flows from the skin to the air because of
   A. radiation.
   B. convection.
   C. conduction.
   D. evaporation.

3. Heat is carried away from the body by air currents in a process known as
   A. radiation.
   B. convection.
   C. conduction.
   D. evaporation.

4. When the body becomes too hot, which of the following happens?
   A. peripheral vasodilation
   B. decreased cardiac output
   C. decreased respiratory rate
   D. increased thermogenesis

5. When the body becomes too cold, which of the following does **not** happen?
   A. sympathetic stimulation
   B. piloerection
   C. vasodilation
   D. thermogenesis

6. Heat cramps are caused by
   A. a rapid change in extracellular osmolarity.
   B. potassium and water losses.

C. increased thermogenesis (shivering).
D. decreased perfusion of abdominal muscles.

7. Heat exhaustion is caused by
   A. increased sodium and water losses.
   B. a rapid, dangerous elevation of body temperature.
   C. peripheral vasoconstriction.
   D. increased circulating blood volume.

8. Prehospital management of the heat stroke patient includes all of the following **except**
   A. rapid cooling.
   B. oxygen administration.
   C. dopamine IV.
   D. IV access.

9. Prehospital management of the frostbite victim includes all of the following **except**
   A. immersing the frozen part in 102–104°F water.
   B. gently massaging the frozen part.
   C. elevating the thawed part.
   D. covering the thawed part with loose sterile dressings.

10. The primary cause of death from drowning is
    A. acid-base abnormality.
    B. asphyxia.
    C. pulmonary edema.
    D. hemodilution.

11. Which of the following is a result of the mammalian diving reflex?

    A. tachypnea

    B. bradycardia

    C. vasodilation

    D. all of the above

12. Prehospital management of the near-drowning victim includes all of the following **except**

    A. C-spine management and oxygenation.

    B. the Heimlich maneuver.

    C. defibrillation as indicated.

    D. CPR as indicated.

Match the following terms of basic nuclear physics with their respective definitions:

    13. _____ protons

    14. _____ neutrons

    15. _____ electrons

    16. _____ isotopes

    17. _____ alpha particles

    18. _____ gamma rays

    A. unstable atoms emitting ionizing radiation

    B. positively charged particles present in all elements

    C. particles lacking an electrical charge

    D. negatively charged minute particles

    E. low-energy particles, easily blocked by clothing

    F. dangerous, high-energy particles, requiring lead shielding

19. According to Boyle's law, 1 L of air at sea level will be compressed to _____ at a depth of 33 feet of water.

    A. 1000 ml

    B. 500 ml

    C. 333 ml

    D. 250 ml

20. According to Henry's law, at 33 feet below the surface, the quantity of nitrogen and oxygen dissolved in the tissues will be _____ that at sea level.

    A. one-half

    B. three times

    C. two times

    D. four times

21. A person experiencing sinus headache pain, dizziness, and hearing loss after diving too fast may be suffering from

    A. barotrauma.

    B. eustachian tube rupture.

    C. middle ear infection.

    D. all of the above

22. A diver who appears to be intoxicated and takes unnecessary risks may be experiencing

    A. carbon monoxide poisoning.

    B. barotrauma.

    C. the bends.

    D. nitrogen narcosis.

23. A diver who holds his breath during ascent may experience

    A. air embolism.

    B. pneumothorax.

    C. alveoli rupture.

    D. all of the above

24. A diver who ascends without allowing time for gradual recompression may experience

    A. air embolism.

    B. pneumomediastinum.

    C. eustachian tube rupture.

    D. the bends.

Scenario

Questions 25 and 26 refer to the following scenario:

Your patient is a 23-year-old construction worker who collapsed on the job. The temperature is 88°F with 78% humidity. He presents on the ground with skin that is hot, wet, and red. He has no medical history according to his coworkers, and there is no Medic-Alert identification. His BP is 90/60, pulse 120, respirations 30 and shallow, lungs clear, chemstrip 100, and axillary temperature 107°F.

25. This patient is most likely suffering from
    A. heat cramps.
    B. heat exhaustion.
    C. heat stroke.
    D. heat prostration.

26. Immediate prehospital management of this patient includes all of the following **except**
    A. rapid cooling.
    B. oxygenation.
    C. IV fluids.
    D. vasopressors.

Scenario

Questions 27–30 refer to the following scenario:

Your patient is a 38-year-old female who got lost in the woods on a hiking trip. She spent the night in a small cave with overnight temperatures dropping to the mid-20s. It had rained earlier in the day, and she had no time to dry off before settling in the cave. She was found by searchers at around 10:00

A.M. the next day. She presents awake but confused and disoriented. She appears very stiff, and her movements are uncoordinated. Her BP is 100/60, pulse 80, respirations slow and shallow, skin cool and pale, chemstrip 120, and axillary temperature 86°F.

27. This person is suffering from
    A. mild hypothermia.
    B. mild hyperthermia.
    C. severe hypothermia.
    D. hyperpyrexia.

28. In severe hypothermia, the patient's ECG may show the presence of
    A. delta waves.
    B. J waves.
    C. coving.
    D. ST segment depression.

29. Since the nearest hospital is 1 hour by car, which of the following statements is true regarding the prehospital management of this patient?
    A. Rewarming should not be attempted.
    B. Heated oxygen should not be administered.
    C. External heat should never be applied.
    D. The patient must be handled gently.

30. If the patient loses consciousness and arrests, prehospital management should include all of the following **except**
    A. CPR.
    B. defibrillation.
    C. medication administration.
    D. heated and humidified oxygen.

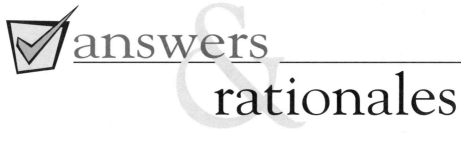

answers & rationales

Following each rationale, you will find a reference to the corresponding objective in the DOT National Standard EMT-Intermediate curriculum. An asterisk denotes material that is supplemental to the DOT curriculum. Page numbers after a rationale indicate where the question topic may be discussed in the Brady text *Intermediate Emergency Care* (Bledsoe, Porter, Cherry).

1.

A. Heat loss in the form of infrared rays is called radiation. All objects not at absolute zero temperature will radiate heat. (*) (IEC p. 1058)

2.

C. Direct contact of the body surface with another, cooler object causes the body to lose heat by conduction. Heat flows from higher-temperature matter to lower-temperature matter. If the ambient air temperature is cooler than the skin temperature, then heat will flow from the skin to the air. (*) (IEC p. 1057)

3.

B. Heat loss to air currents passing over the body is called convection. (*) (IEC p. 1058)

4.

A. When the body becomes too hot, it attempts to eliminate body heat through five mechanisms: vasodilation, perspiration, decreased heat production, increased cardiac output, and increased respiratory rate. (5-8.8) (IEC p. 1058)

5.

C. When the body becomes too cold, it attempts to preserve heat by engaging the following mechanisms: vasoconstriction, piloerection, increased heat production by shivering, and sympathetic stimulation. (5-8.9) (IEC p. 1058)

6.

A. Heat cramps are caused primarily by a rapid change in extracellular fluid osmolarity, resulting from sodium and water losses. This causes intermittent painful contractions of various skeletal muscles. (5-8.11) (IEC p. 1061)

7.

A. Heat exhaustion results from excessive water and salt losses due to sweating. Deficiencies in water and sodium combine to cause electrolyte volume and vasomotor regulatory disturbances. (5-8.11) (IEC p. 1061)

8.

C. Prehospital management of the heat stroke patient includes rapid cooling, oxygen administration, IV access, ECG monitoring, and core temperature monitoring. Vasopressors and anticholinergic drugs should be avoided. (5-8.21) (IEC p. 1063)

9.

B. Prehospital management of the frostbite victim includes immersing the frozen part in water heated to 102–104°F, elevating the thawed part, and covering the thawed part with loose sterile dressings. (*) (IEC p. 1071)

10.

B. Deaths due to drowning and near drowning are primarily caused by asphyxia from airway obstruction in the lungs secondary to the aspirated water or laryngospasm. (*) (IEC p. 1072)

11.

B. When a person dives into cold water, he or she reacts to the submersion of the face. This is known as the mammalian diving reflex. As a result of this reflex, breathing is inhibited, the heart rate becomes slower, and vasoconstriction develops in the tissues. (*) (IEC p. 1073)

12.

B. Prehospital management of the near-drowning victim includes C-spine management, oxygenation, defibrillation, and CPR as indicated. (5-8.36) (IEC p. 1074)

Matching (*) (IEC p. 1085)

13. B protons
14. C neutrons

15. D electrons
16. A isotopes
17. E alpha particles
18. F gamma rays

19.

B. Air is compressible. Boyle's law states that for every 33 feet below the surface you dive, the pressure of gas in your lungs doubles, while the volume decreases by one-half. One liter of air at the surface, therefore, is compressed to 500 ml at 33 feet below the surface. (*) (IEC p. 1075)

20.

C. Henry's law states that the amount of gas dissolved in a given volume of fluid is proportional to the pressure of the gas with which it is in equilibrium. Since the body is made up primarily of liquid, gases that are inhaled will be dissolved in the body in proportion to the partial pressure of each breath. The body uses oxygen, but it does not use nitrogen. Therefore, the primary gas dissolved in the body is nitrogen because it is inert and not used by the body. At 33 feet below the surface, the quantity of oxygen and nitrogen dissolved in the tissues will be two times that at sea level. (*) (IEC p. 1076)

21.

A. Barotrauma, commonly called "the squeeze," becomes a concern during descent. If the diver cannot equilibrate the pressure between the nasopharynx and the middle ear through the eustachian tube, he can experience middle-ear pain. (5-8.38) (IEC p. 1077)

22.

D. Major diving emergencies while at the bottom of the dive involve nitrogen narcosis, commonly called "raptures of the deep." This is due to nitrogen's effect on cerebral function. (5-8.38) (IEC p. 1077)

23.

D. The most serious barotrauma can occur if a diver holds his breath during ascent. As a diver ascends, the air in the lungs, which has been compressed, expands. If it is not exhaled, the alveoli may rupture. If this occurs, the result may be structural damage to the lung and air embolism. This may also produce mediastinal and subcutaneous emphysema or pneumothorax. (5-8.37) (IEC p. 1077)

24.

D. A diver who ascends without allowing time for gradual recompression may experience "the bends." This is a condition that develops in divers subjected to a rapid reduction of air pressure after ascending to the surface following exposure to compressed air. Nitrogen bubbles enter the tissue spaces in small blood vessels. Bubbles produced by rapid decompression are thought to obstruct blood flow and lead to local ischemia, subjecting tissues to anoxia stress. (5-8.37) (IEC p. 1077)

25.

C. This patient is most likely suffering from heat stroke. Heat stroke occurs when the body's hypothalamic temperature regulation is lost, causing uncompensated hyperthermia, which, in turn, causes cell death and physiologic collapse. (5-8.21) (IEC p. 1062)

26.

D. Immediate prehospital management of the heat stroke patient includes cooling the patient rapidly, administering oxygen, establishing IVs, and monitoring the ECG and core temperature. Vasopressors and anticholinergic drugs are contraindicated since they may inhibit sweating. (5-8.21) (IEC p. 1063)

27.

C. With a core temperature of less than 90°F, this patient is suffering from severe hypothermia. (5-8.30) (IEC p. 1066)

28.

B. The typical hypothermic ECG shows the presence of J waves, also called Osborne waves. (5-8.28) (IEC p. 1066)

29.

D. Rewarming of this patient should be attempted since transportation to the hospital will take more than 15 minutes. External application of heat by warm blankets is a safe and effective means of rewarming the hypothermic patient. Another excellent means of rewarming the hypothermic patient is by administering heated and humidified oxygen. Of course, the hypothermic patient should be moved gently. (5-8.30) (IEC p. 1068)

30.

C. Prehospital management of the hypothermic cardiac arrest includes CPR, defibrillation, and administration of heated and humidified oxygen. (5-8.30) (IEC p. 1070)

9 Behavioral Emergencies

unit objectives

Questions in this unit relate to DOT objectives 5-9.1 to 5-9.12. The objectives are listed in the Appendix.

DIRECTIONS Each of the questions or incomplete statements below is followed by suggested answers or completions. Select the **one answer** that is best in each case.

1. Which of the following interviewing techniques is considered appropriate for the behavioral emergency patient?
   A. using a formal checklist of questions
   B. never allowing the patient to lead the interview
   C. pressing the patient for specific answers
   D. communicating honestly and firmly

2. During long periods of silence, you should
   A. press the patient to keep talking.
   B. keep talking yourself.
   C. stay calm and relaxed.
   D. leave the patient alone.

3. If the behavioral emergency patient believes that there are large pink elephants in the room, you should
   A. tell him you see them too.
   B. understand they are real for him.
   C. tell him there are no pink elephants.
   D. tell him he has an obvious psychiatric problem.

4. If the distraught patient says he wants to "end it all," you should
   A. let him.
   B. try to stop him from talking about it.
   C. tell him everything will be all right.
   D. try to get him to talk more about it.

5. Your first priority in any behavioral emergency is
   A. your safety.
   B. the patient's safety.
   C. the underlying reason for the patient's behavioral problem.
   D. the patient's life-threatening injuries.

6. The patient who believes he is Jimmy Hoffa and is being chased by mobsters is probably suffering from
   A. manic depression.
   B. paranoid schizophrenia.
   C. acute anxiety.
   D. none of the above

7. A mood disorder characterized by feelings of helplessness and hopelessness is
   A. anxiety.
   B. depression.
   C. mania.
   D. schizophrenia.

8. Which of the following organic causes can mimic depression?
   A. hyperthyroidism
   B. hypothyroidism
   C. Cushing's disease
   D. Graves' disease

9. A patient with bipolar disorder usually suffers from
   A. frequent hallucinations.
   B. wide mood swings.
   C. delusional behavior.
   D. altered disorganization.

10. Lithium (Lithobid) is often prescribed for _____ patients.
    A. schizophrenic
    B. suicidal
    C. organic brain syndrome
    D. manic-depressive

11. Which of the following statements best describes somatoform disorders?

    A. Patients are preoccupied with physical symptoms.

    B. Patients exaggerate common physical symptoms as serious illness.

    C. Patients complain of pain unexplained by a physical ailment.

    D. all of the above

12. Munchausen syndrome is a type of _____ disorder.

    A. factitious

    B. somatoform

    C. hypochondriasis

    D. dissociative

13. Psychogenic amnesia, multiple personality disorder, depersonalization, and fugue state are all examples of _____ disorder.

    A. factitious

    B. somatoform

    C. hypochondriasis

    D. dissociative

Match the following types of personality disorders with their respective characteristics:

14. _____ paranoid

15. _____ schizoid

16. _____ schizotypal

17. _____ antisocial

18. _____ depersonalizing

19. _____ histrionic

20. _____ narcissistic

21. _____ avoidant

22. _____ dependent

23. _____ obsessive-compulsive

24. _____ kleptomanic

25. _____ pyromanic

26. _____ trichotillomanic

27. _____ bulimic

28. _____ anorexic

    A. voluntary refusal to eat

    B. social inhibition, inadequacy

    C. distrust and suspicion

    D. impulse to pull out one's hair

    E. disregard for rights of others

    F. recurrent episodes of binge eating/abnormal elimination

    G. feeling detached from oneself

    H. impulse to steal objects not for immediate use

    I. excessive emotions and attention seeking

    J. detachment from social relationships

    K. acute discomfort in close relationships

    L. impulse to set fires

    M. preoccupation with orderliness, perfectionism, control

    N. submissive and clinging behavior

    O. need for admiration, lack of empathy

29. Which of the following is a major suicide risk factor?

    A. previous attempts

    B. depression

    C. widowed spouses

    D. all of the above

30. Headache, palpitations, insomnia, and hyperventilation may be signs of

    A. depression.

    B. schizophrenia.

    C. anxiety.

    D. extrapyramidal symptoms.

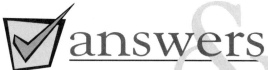

answers & rationales

Following each rationale, you will find a reference to the corresponding objective in the DOT National Standard EMT-Intermediate curriculum. An asterisk denotes material that is supplemental to the DOT curriculum. Page numbers after a rationale indicate where the question topic may be discussed in the Brady text *Intermediate Emergency Care* (Bledsoe, Porter, Cherry).

1.

D. Certain interviewing techniques are appropriate for the behavioral patient. These include communicating self-confidence as well as honesty, firmness, and a reasonable attitude about issues important to the patient and the situation. (5-9.5) (IEC p. 1093)

2.

C. A EMT-Intermediate should not be afraid of long silent periods during the interview. During this time, the EMT-Intermediate should remain relaxed and attentive. (5-9.5) (IEC p. 1093)

3.

B. Some behavioral patients have delusions. Avoid being judgmental. When a patient exhibits delusional behavior, understand that this behavior is reality for this patient. (5-9.5) (IEC p. 1094)

4.

D. If your patient expresses suicidal thoughts, stay calm and do not appear uncomfortable. Instead, try to get him to talk more about it and be frank. Ask him if he has ever tried to kill himself or if he has a plan, the means, and the opportunity. (5-9.5) (IEC p. 1094)

5.

A. Your top priority in any behavioral emergency is your own personal safety. (5-9.3) (IEC p. 1092)

6.

B. The patient suffering from paranoid schizophrenia often feels that someone, such as the FBI or CIA, is after him. Such paranoia often results from the patient's feeling of self-importance. Some paranoid schizophrenics become delusional and believe that they are famous figures, such as Jesus Christ or Napoleon. (5-9.2) (IEC p. 1097)

7.

B. Depression is a common psychiatric disorder. It is characterized by feelings of helplessness and hopelessness. (5-9.2) (IEC p. 1099)

8.

B. Certain conditions such as substance abuse, medications, organic brain syndrome, hypothyroidism, and chronic steroid use may mimic depression. (5-9.2) (IEC p. 1099)

9.

B. Bipolar disorder, also called manic-depressive disorder, is a condition characterized by tremendous mood swings from euphoria to debilitating depression. (5-9.2) (IEC p. 1099)

10.

D. Lithium is a drug often prescribed for patients with manic-depressive disorder, also known as bipolar disorder. (*) (IEC p. 1100)

11.

D. Somatoform disorders are characterized by physical symptoms that have no apparent physiological cause. There are many forms of this disorder. Patients may be preoccupied with physical symptoms. They may exaggerate common physical symptoms as serious illness or complain of pain unexplained by a physical ailment. (5-9.2) (IEC p. 1101)

12.

A. Munchausen syndrome is the severe form of factitious disorder. A factitious disorder is characterized by three criteria: an intentional production of physical signs or symptoms, motivation to assume the "sick role," and external incentives for the behavior. (5-9.2) (IEC p. 1101)

13.

D. Psychogenic amnesia, multiple personality disorder, depersonalization, and fugue state are all examples of dissociative disorder, in which the patient attempts to avoid stress by separating from his core personality. (5-9.2) (IEC p. 1101)

Matching (5-9.2) (IEC p. 1102)

14.	C	paranoid
15.	J	schizoid
16.	K	schizotypal
17.	E	antisocial
18.	G	depersonalizing
19.	I	histrionic
20.	O	narcissistic
21.	B	avoidant
22.	N	dependent
23.	M	obsessive-compulsive
24.	H	kleptomanic
25.	L	pyromanic
26.	D	trichotillomanic
27.	F	bulimic
28.	A	anorexic

29.

D. Some major suicidal risk factors include previous attempts, history of depression, and widowed spouses. (5-9.6) (IEC p. 1104)

30.

C. Headache, palpitations, insomnia, and hyperventilation may be signs of an acute anxiety attack. Anxiety is a normal response to stress. However, it can build up to such a point that it overwhelms the patient, who then feels helpless and becomes unable to function normally. (5-9.2) (IEC p. 1098)

UNIT

10

Gynecological Emergencies

unit objectives

Questions in this unit relate to DOT objectives 5-10.1 to 5-10.6. The objectives are listed in the Appendix.

DIRECTIONS Each of the questions or incomplete statements below is followed by suggested answers or completions. Select the **one answer** that is best in each case.

1. Fertilization normally occurs in the
   A. ovaries.
   B. fallopian tubes.
   C. uterus.
   D. vagina.

2. The uterine lining that sloughs off during the menstrual period is the
   A. perineum.
   B. endometrium.
   C. myometrium.
   D. perimetrium.

3. The function of the ovaries is to produce
   A. estrogen.
   B. progesterone.
   C. eggs for reproduction.
   D. all of the above

4. A fertilized egg normally implants on the
   A. uterine wall.
   B. cervix.
   C. perineum.
   D. urethra.

5. The area surrounding the vagina that sometimes tears during childbirth is the
   A. perineum.
   B. endometrium.
   C. urethra.
   D. cervix.

6. A woman's gravidity refers to her number of
   A. pregnancies.
   B. viable deliveries.
   C. abortions.
   D. cesarean sections.

7. A woman's parity refers to her number of
   A. pregnancies.
   B. viable deliveries.
   C. abortions.
   D. cesarean sections.

8. The beginning of menses is called
   A. menopause.
   B. menarche.
   C. ovulation.
   D. menstruation.

9. Physical examination of the gynecological patient includes all of the following **except**
   A. palpating for masses.
   B. inspecting for distention and guarding.
   C. asking about tenderness.
   D. performing an internal vaginal exam.

10. Common complications of pelvic inflammatory disease include
    A. sepsis.
    B. future ectopic pregnancies.
    C. pelvic organ adhesions.
    D. all of the above

11. The most common site for ectopic pregnancies is
    A. the uterus.
    B. a fallopian tube.
    C. the cervix.
    D. the abdomen.

12. Prehospital management of female gynecological trauma includes
   A. vaginal packing.
   B. IV D$_5$W run wide open.
   C. direct pressure on the external genitalia.
   D. none of the above

13. Which of the following statements is true regarding sexual assault?
   A. Most victims are female.
   B. EMT-Intermediates should not question the victim about the incident in the field.
   C. EMT-Intermediates should not perform physical examination of the genitalia.
   D. all of the above

14. Which of the following statements is true regarding the preserving of evidence in sexual assault cases?
   A. Place all clothing items in the same bag.
   B. Use plastic bags for blood-soaked articles.
   C. Do not allow the patient to clean her fingernails.
   D. Clean the patient's wounds.

15. Your female patient who complains of lower-abdominal pain while walking and during sexual intercourse, fever, and vaginal discharge may be suffering from
   A. ovarian cyst.
   B. mittelschmerz.
   C. epididymitis.
   D. pelvic inflammatory disease.

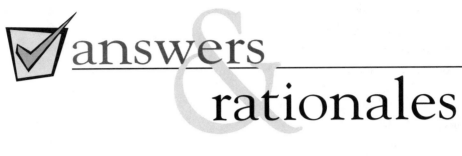

Following each rationale, you will find a reference to the corresponding objective in the DOT National Standard EMT-Intermediate curriculum. An asterisk denotes material that is supplemental to the DOT curriculum. Page numbers after a rationale indicate where the question topic may be discussed in the Brady text *Intermediate Emergency Care* (Bledsoe, Porter, Cherry).

1.

B. The fallopian tubes are hollow tubes that transport the egg from the ovary to the uterus. Fertilization usually occurs in a fallopian tube. (5-10.1) (IEC p. 227)

2.

B. The endometrium is the lining of the uterus. Each month, under the influence of estrogen and progesterone, the endometrium builds up in preparation for a fertilized ovum. If fertilization does not occur, the lining simply sloughs off. The sloughing off of the uterine lining is referred to as the menstrual period. (5-10.1) (IEC p. 227)

3.

D. The ovaries are the female gonads. They produce estrogen, progesterone, and eggs for reproduction. (5-10.1) (IEC p. 227)

4.

A. The uterus is a small, pear-shaped organ that connects with the vagina. The fertilized egg normally implants on the uterine wall. (5-10.1) (IEC p. 225)

5.

A. The perineum is the area surrounding the vagina and anus. This area is sometimes torn during childbirth. (5-10.1) (IEC p. 225)

6.

A. A woman's gravidity refers to her number of pregnancies. A nulligravida has never been pregnant. A primigravida is pregnant for the first time. A multigravida has been pregnant more than once.

Common Obstetrical Terminology

Term	Meaning
antepartum	the time interval prior to delivery of the fetus
postpartum	the time interval after delivery of the fetus
prenatal	the time interval prior to birth, synonymous with antepartum

natal	literally means birth
gravidity	the number of times a woman has been pregnant
primigravida	a woman who is pregnant for the first time
multigravida	a woman who has been pregnant more than once
nulligravida	a woman who has not been pregnant
parity	the number of times a woman has delivered a viable fetus
primipara	a woman who has delivered her first child
multipara	a woman who has delivered more than one baby
nullipara	a woman who has yet to deliver her first child
grand multipara	a woman who has delivered at least seven babies

The gravidity and parity of a woman are expressed in the following convention: G_4P_2. "G" refers to the gravidity, and "P" refers to the parity. (5-10.2) (IEC p. 1113)

7.

B. A woman's parity refers to her number of viable deliveries. A nullipara has never delivered a viable infant. A primipara has delivered one child. A multipara has delivered many babies. (5-10.2) (IEC p. 1113)

8.

B. The female undergoes a monthly hormonal cycle that prepares the uterus to receive a fertilized egg. A girl's menses or menstrual period usually begins when she is between 12 and 14 years old. The beginning of the menses is called menarche. (5-10.1) (IEC p. 228)

9.

D. Physical examination of the gynecological patient should be limited to taking a good history and palpating for masses, distention, and guarding. Never perform an internal vaginal exam in the field. (5-10.2) (IEC p. 1114)

10.

D. Pelvic inflammatory disease (PID) is an infection of the female reproductive tract. Common complications of PID include sepsis, pelvic organ adhesions, and future ectopic pregnancies. (5-10.5) (IEC p. 1115)

11.

B. Ectopic pregnancy is the implantation of a growing fetus in a place where it does not belong. The most common site is within a fallopian tube. (5-10.5) (IEC p. 1117)

12.

C. Prehospital management of female gynecological trauma includes managing a laceration by direct pressure on the external genitalia, maintaining intravascular blood volume by starting an IV of lactated Ringer's, and treating for shock. Never pack the vagina with any material or dressing regardless of the severity of the bleeding. (5-10.4) (IEC p. 1118)

13.

D. Sexual assault is one of the fastest-growing crimes in the United States. Most victims are female and know their assailants. The victim should not be questioned about the incident in the field since it is not important from the standpoint of prehospital care to determine whether penetration took place. A medic should never perform a physical examination of the genitalia in a possible sexual abuse case. (5-10.6) (IEC p. 1118)

14.

C. There are certain things an EMT-Intermediate can do to preserve physical evidence in a sexual assault case: Do not use plastic bags for blood-stained articles; bag each item separately if it must be bagged; handle clothing as little as possible, if at all; do not allow the patient to comb her hair or clean her fingernails; do not allow her to change her clothes, bathe, or douche before the medical exam; and do not clean wounds, if at all possible. (5-10.6) (IEC p. 1119)

15.

D. Pelvic inflammatory disease is an infection of the female reproductive organs. It is usually sexually transmitted. The patient presents with fever, chills, lower-abdominal pain, and vaginal bleeding or discharge. In addition, the patient may complain of pain on walking or pain with intercourse. (5-10.5) (IEC p. 1116)

UNIT

1

Obstetrical Emergencies

unit objectives

Questions in this unit relate to DOT objectives 6-1.1 to 6-1.20. The objectives are listed in the Appendix.

DIRECTIONS Each of the questions or incomplete statements below is followed by suggested answers or completions. Select the **one answer** that is best in each case.

1. The EDC refers to the
   A. date of conception.
   B. due date.
   C. date the mother will be admitted to the hospital.
   D. date of implantation.

2. Which of the following statements is true regarding vital sign changes in the pregnant woman?
   A. The blood pressure rises, and the pulse rate falls.
   B. The blood pressure falls, and the pulse rate rises.
   C. The blood pressure and the pulse rate rise.
   D. The blood pressure and the pulse rate fall.

3. The bulging of the baby's head past the opening of the vagina is called
   A. effacement.
   B. primipara.
   C. prolapsing.
   D. crowning.

4. The first stage of labor begins with the
   A. crowning of the infant's head.
   B. dilation of the cervix.
   C. delivery of the baby.
   D. onset of uterine contractions.

5. The second stage of labor begins with the
   A. crowning of the infant's head.
   B. dilation of the cervix.
   C. delivery of the baby.
   D. onset of uterine contractions.

6. The third stage of labor begins with the
   A. crowning of the infant's head.
   B. dilation of the cervix.
   C. delivery of the baby.
   D. onset of uterine contractions.

7. Complete dilation of the cervix is considered to be
   A. 5 cm.
   B. 10 cm.
   C. 15 cm.
   D. 20 cm.

8. Management of a patient with postpartum hemorrhage includes all of the following **except**
   A. fundal massage.
   B. pitocin IV.
   C. PASG.
   D. vaginal packing.

9. Which of the following distinguishes eclampsia from preeclampsia?
   A. vaginal bleeding
   B. visual disturbances
   C. grand mal seizures
   D. peripheral edema

10. Magnesium IV may be ordered for which of the following situations?
    A. lower-abdominal pain
    B. postpartum hemorrhage
    C. eclamptic seizures
    D. preterm labor pains

Scenario

Questions 11–13 refer to the following scenario:

Your patient is a 19-year-old woman who presents with severe lower-abdominal pain and vaginal bleeding. She claims she is not pregnant but has not had her period for at least 7 weeks. She also complains of weakness, nausea, and vomiting. She admits to being sexually active with multiple partners. She was seen in the ED for several cases of PID in the past 2 years. Her BP is 90/60, pulse 110, respirations 24, and skin cool and clammy.

11. You should suspect
    A. abruptio placenta.
    B. placenta previa.
    C. PID.
    D. ruptured ectopic pregnancy.

12. Her problem was caused by
    A. the premature separation of the placenta from the uterine wall.
    B. the uterus covering the cervical opening.
    C. an inflamed appendix.
    D. implantation of the fertilized ovum in a fallopian tube.

13. Management of this patient includes all of the following **except**
    A. IV fluids.
    B. vaginal packing.
    C. PASG.
    D. high-flow oxygen.

Scenario

Questions 14–17 refer to the following scenario:

Your patient is a 26-year-old 30-weeks-pregnant patient who complains of severe, tearing abdominal pain and some minor vaginal bleeding. On palpation, her abdomen is very tender, and her uterus seems to be tightly contracted. Fetal heart tones are absent. She is multigravida but nullipara.

14. You should suspect
    A. abruptio placenta.
    B. placenta previa.
    C. miscarriage.
    D. ectopic pregnancy.

15. Her problem was caused by
    A. the premature separation of the placenta from the uterine wall.
    B. the uterus covering the cervical opening.
    C. a spontaneous abortion.
    D. implantation of the fertilized ovum in a fallopian tube.

16. This patient's pregnancy history includes
    A. one pregnancy and one birth.
    B. many pregnancies and one birth.
    C. one pregnancy and no births.
    D. many pregnancies and no births.

17. Management of this patient includes all of the following **except**
    A. IV fluids.
    B. vaginal packing.
    C. PASG.
    D. high-flow oxygen.

Scenario

Questions 18–20 refer to the following scenario:

Your patient is a 30-year-old multigravida in her thirtieth week. She presents with bright red vaginal bleeding but denies any abdominal pain. Her uterus is soft and feels "out of place." Her problem began following sexual intercourse with her husband.

18. You should suspect
    A. abruptio placenta.
    B. placenta previa.
    C. miscarriage.
    D. ectopic pregnancy.

19. Her problem was caused by
    A. the premature separation of the placenta from the uterine wall.
    B. the uterus covering the cervical opening.
    C. a spontaneous abortion.
    D. implantation of the fertilized ovum in a fallopian tube.

20. Management of this patient includes all of the following **except**
    A. IV fluids.
    B. vaginal exam.
    C. PASG.
    D. high-flow oxygen.

21. Which of the following statements is true regarding the pregnant trauma patient?
    A. Overt signs of shock are seen early.
    B. The earlier the pregnancy, the greater the likelihood for fetal injury.
    C. The mother's body will shunt blood to the fetus following acute blood loss.
    D. none of the above

22. The proper treatment for a normovolemic patient with supine-hypotensive syndrome is
    A. Trendelenburg positioning.
    B. left lateral recumbent positioning.
    C. furosemide 40 mg IV.
    D. dopamine 5 mcg/kg/min IV.

23. Which of the following statements is true regarding gestational diabetes?
    A. It normally occurs in the first trimester.
    B. Prehospital management of diabetic emergencies is the same as in the nonpregnant patient.
    C. The younger the mother, the higher the incidence.
    D. all of the above

24. The difference between Braxton-Hicks contractions and true labor is
    A. cervical changes.
    B. intensity of pain.
    C. presence of blood discharge.
    D. none of the above

25. Airway maintenance of the infant during a breech birth is accomplished by
    A. inserting an endotracheal tube.
    B. using a meconium aspirator.
    C. using a nasopharyngeal airway.
    D. inserting two fingers into the vagina.

26. If the umbilical cord is prolapsed, you should
    A. push it back into the vagina.
    B. attempt to deliver the baby.
    C. pull on the cord.
    D. transport immediately.

27. If the baby presents with thick meconium staining around the mouth and nose, you should

   A. intubate and suction the trachea after initial ventilation.

   B. intubate and suction the trachea before initial ventilation.

   C. suction the oropharynx with a bulb syringe and ventilate.

   D. use a high-pressure demand valve to ventilate.

28. A few days following delivery of the baby, the mother complains of sudden onset of sharp chest pain and severe shortness of breath. The most likely cause of her condition is

   A. acute myocardial infarction.

   B. uterine rupture.

   C. uterine inversion.

   D. pulmonary embolism.

29. For which of the following complications of delivery should you **not** attempt to deliver the baby in the field?

   A. shoulder dystocia

   B. cephalopelvic disproportion

   C. precipitous delivery

   D. multiple births

30. A baby whose body is pink, whose extremities are blue, who has a pulse rate of 88, and who is crying strongly and actively moving receives an APGAR score of

   A. 4.

   B. 6.

   C. 8.

   D. 10.

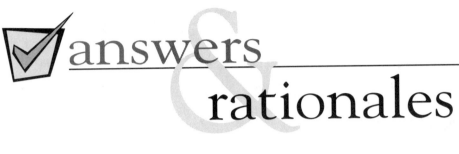

answers & rationales

Following each rationale, you will find a reference to the corresponding objective in the DOT National Standard EMT-Intermediate curriculum. An asterisk denotes material that is supplemental to the DOT curriculum. Page numbers after a rationale indicate where the question topic may be discussed in the Brady text *Intermediate Emergency Care* (Bledsoe, Porter, Cherry).

1.

B. The estimated date of confinement (EDC) is the mother's due date. (6-1.3) (IEC p. 1126)

2.

B. Because of normal changes occurring in the cardiovascular system of the pregnant woman, her blood pressure tends to be lower and her pulse rate tends to be faster during pregnancy. (6-1.3) (IEC p. 1124)

3.

D. Crowning is the bulging of the fetal head past the opening of the vagina during a contraction. It is an indication of an impending delivery. (6-1.8) (IEC p. 1130)

4.

D. The first stage of labor begins with the onset of uterine contractions and ends with the complete dilation of the cervix. It lasts approximately 8 hours in nulliparous women and 5 hours in multiparous women. (6-1.4) (IEC p. 1140)

5.

B. The second stage of labor begins with the complete dilation of the cervix and ends with the delivery of the fetus. In nulliparous patients, the second stage lasts approximately 50 minutes, and in multiparous women, it lasts approximately 20 minutes. (6-1.4) (IEC p. 1106)

6.

C. The third stage of labor begins with the delivery of the fetus and ends with the delivery of the placenta. The delivery of the placenta usually occurs within 30 minutes after birth. (6-1.4) (IEC p. 1141)

7.

B. Complete dilation of the cervix is considered to be 10 cm. (6-1.4) (IEC p. 1140)

8.

D. Postpartum hemorrhage is the loss of 500 ml or more of blood in the first 24 hours following delivery. Prehospital management of the postpartum hemorrhage patient includes administering oxygen and beginning external fundal massage, administering large-bore IVs of normal saline or lactated Ringer's, and applying antishock trousers. Never pack the vagina. (6-1.15) (IEC p. 1151)

9.

C. Eclampsia is the most serious manifestation of hypertensive disorders of pregnancy. It is characterized by grand mal seizure activity. (6-1.6) (IEC p. 1136)

10.

C. Magnesium sulfate may be ordered for eclamptic seizures. (6-1.17) (IEC p. 1137)

11.

D. Ectopic pregnancy is difficult to diagnose in the field. However, any woman of childbearing age who presents with lower-abdominal pain, vaginal bleeding, and a late menstrual period should be suspected of having a ruptured ectopic pregnancy. (6-1.6) (IEC p. 1133)

12.

D. Ectopic pregnancy is the implantation of a fertilized ovum outside of the uterus, most commonly in a fallopian tube. The ovum, however, can implant anywhere else in the abdominal cavity. (6-1.6) (IEC p. 1133)

13.

B. Management of the patient with a suspected ruptured ectopic pregnancy includes treatment for shock, IV fluids, pneumatic antishock garment, and high-flow oxygen. (6-1.17) (IEC p. 1133)

14.

A. Any pregnant patient in her third trimester who complains of tearing abdominal pain and vaginal bleeding should be suspected of having an abruptio placenta. (6-1.6) (IEC p. 1134)

15.

A. Abruptio placenta is the premature separation of the placenta from the wall of the uterus. The separation can be either partial or complete. (6-1.6) (IEC p. 1134)

16.

D. This patient is multigravida and nullipara. Gravida refers to her number of pregnancies (many). Her parity refers to her number of viable births (none). (6-1.3) (IEC p. 1128)

17.

B. Management of this patient includes IV fluids, pneumatic antishock garment (legs only), and high-flow oxygen, generally treating for shock. (6-1.17) (IEC p. 1135)

18.

B. This patient probably has placenta previa. Her history of third-trimester pregnancy, multigravida, and bleeding following intercourse is consistent with this diagnosis. (6-1.6) (IEC p. 1133)

19.

B. Placenta previa is the attachment of the placenta very low in the uterus so that it partially or completely covers the internal cervical opening. (6-1.6) (IEC p. 1133)

20.

B. Treatment for this patient is aimed at treating for shock: IV fluids, pneumatic antishock garment, and high-flow oxygen. (6-1.17) (IEC p. 1134)

21.

D. During pregnancy, overt signs of shock are late and often inconsistent. The later the pregnancy, the larger the gravid uterus and the greater the likelihood of fetal injury. The mother's body will shunt blood away from the fetus following acute blood loss. (6-1.6) (IEC p. 1131)

22.

B. Supine-hypotensive syndrome usually occurs late in pregnancy when the large uterus compresses the inferior vena cava when the mother lies in a supine position. If she is normovolemic and shows no signs of dehydration, place her in the left lateral position or elevate her right hip to decompress the vena cava. This is known as caval decompression. (6-1.9) (IEC p. 1137)

23.

B. Gestational diabetes usually occurs in the last 20 weeks of pregnancy, when placental hormones cause an increased resistance to insulin and a decreased glucose tolerance. Prehospital management of a diabetic emergency (hypoglycemia or hyperglycemia) is the same as with the nonpregnant patient. (6-1.17) (IEC p. 1138)

24.

A. In true labor contractions, the cervix effaces (thins and shortens). During Braxton-Hicks contractions, also known as false labor, there are no cervical changes. (6-1.4) (IEC p. 1138)

25.

D. During a breech birth, the baby's face may be pressed against the vaginal wall as he attempts to take a breath. In this case, you must insert two fingers in a "V" shape into the vagina and push the vaginal wall away from the infant's nose. (6-1.16) (IEC p. 1147)

26.

D. If the umbilical cord is prolapsed, you should not try to push it back into the vagina, attempt to deliver the baby, or pull on the cord. Simply place the mother in Trendelelburg or knee-chest position, administer high-flow oxygen, apply a moist dressing to the presenting part, and transport immediately. (6-1.16) (IEC p. 1148)

27.

B. Meconium is a sign of fetal distress. The thicker and darker it is, the worse it is and the higher the infant mortality rate is. If the meconium is thin and watery, merely suction it with a bulb syringe and allow the infant to breathe as you normally would. If it is thick and dark (some describe it as axle grease), you must remove as much of it as possible before the infant aspirates it into the lungs. Immediately intubate the infant and suction the trachea prior to allowing ventilation. (6-1.19) (IEC p. 1151)

28.

D. Pulmonary embolism is the presence of a blood clot in the pulmonary vasculature system. It is most often caused by a thrombus that developed during pregnancy and appears to occur more frequently following cesarean section than vaginal delivery. (6-1.6) (IEC p. 1153)

29.

B. Cephalopelvic disproportion occurs when the infant's head is too big to pass through the maternal pelvis easily. There may be strong contractions, but generally labor does not progress. The usual management of this condition is cesarean section. Administer oxygen, establish IV access, and transport the mother immediately to the hospital. (6-1.16) (IEC p. 1150)

30.

C. The APGAR score table is as follows: (6-2.8) (IEC p. 1146)

Element	0	1	2
Appearance	Body and extremities blue, pale	Body pink, extremities blue	Completely pink
Pulse rate	Absent	<100	>100
Grimace	No response	Grimace	Cough, cry, sneeze
Activity	Limp	Some flexion	Active
Respiratory effort	Absent	Slow and irregular	Strong cry

Neonatal Resuscitation

unit objectives

Questions in this unit relate to DOT objectives 6-2.1 to 6-2.39. The objectives are listed in the Appendix.

DIRECTIONS

Each of the questions or incomplete statements below is followed by suggested answers or completions. Select the **one answer** that is best in each case.

1. Which of the following is considered an antepartum risk factor for possible complications in newborns?

   A. more than one fetus

   B. mother's age is >35

   C. postterm gestation

   D. all of the above

Match the following congenital anomalies with their respective descriptions:

2. _____ meningomyelocele

3. _____ omphalocele

4. _____ choanal atresia

5. _____ cleft palate

6. _____ Pierre Robin syndrome

   A. spinal cord herniation

   B. small jaw/large tongue/no gag

   C. nasopharyngeal blockage

   D. fissure in roof of mouth

   E. umbilical herniation

7. Which of the following is recommended immediately following delivery of the infant?

   A. Position the baby, head down, at the level of the vagina.

   B. Suction the mouth and then the nose.

   C. Dry the baby off.

   D. all of the above

8. Which of the following is recommended practice regarding the umbilical cord?

   A. Milk the cord toward the baby.

   B. Milk the cord toward the mother.

   C. Clamp and cut the cord shortly after delivery.

   D. Disregard the cord until the placenta delivers.

9. The normal respiratory rate of the neonate should be _____ breaths per minute.

   A. 10–20

   B. 20–40

   C. 30–60

   D. 60–100

10. A pulse rate of less than 100 beats per minute in the newborn infant

    A. is normal after 2–3 minutes postpartum.

    B. indicates an infant in distress.

    C. requires immediate atropine administration.

    D. requires aggressive fluid therapy.

11. Which of the following statements is true regarding the APGAR score?

    A. It should be calculated at 1 and 5 minutes after delivery.

    B. An infant with a score of 3 requires immediate resuscitation.

    C. Scores in the 7–10 range indicate a normal infant.

    D. all of the above

12. The presence of meconium at birth requires immediate

    A. bag-valve-mask ventilation.

    B. suctioning of the trachea.

    C. stimulation of the baby to breathe.

    D. cardiopulmonary resuscitation.

13. Which of the following statements is true regarding neonatal suctioning?
    A. Normal suctioning should be performed by bulb syringe or Delee trap.
    B. Suctioning should last no longer than 10 seconds.
    C. Meconium should be suctioned through an endotracheal tube.
    D. all of the above

14. Which of the following is **not** part of the first step of the inverted pyramid?
    A. oxygen administration
    B. tactile stimulation
    C. drying and warming
    D. positioning

15. An infant's best indicator of distress is the
    A. respiratory effort.
    B. heart rate.
    C. cardiac rhythm.
    D. blood pressure.

16. If the infant presents with cyanosis after performing step 1 of the inverted pyramid, you should
    A. administer blow-by oxygen.
    B. perform bag-valve-mask ventilation.
    C. begin CPR.
    D. insert an endotracheal tube.

17. If the heart rate is less than 100 or the infant is still cyanotic after performing step 2, you should
    A. administer blow-by oxygen.
    B. perform bag-valve-mask ventilation.
    C. begin CPR.
    D. insert an endotracheal tube.

18. If the infant's heart rate is less than 80 after performing steps 1–3, you should
    A. administer atropine.
    B. perform chest compression.
    C. insert an endotracheal tube.
    D. administer epinephrine.

19. The infant's heart rate can best be checked by
    A. auscultating the heart at the apex.
    B. feeling the umbilical cord.
    C. palpating the brachial pulse.
    D. all of the above

20. Which of the following is true regarding neonatal resuscitation?
    A. Pop-off valves on bag-valve devices should be disengaged.
    B. Cuffed ET tubes should be used on all neonates.
    C. Chest compression should be performed on the midsternum.
    D. all of the above

21. The umbilicus contains
    A. two arteries and two veins.
    B. two arteries and one vein.
    C. one artery and two veins.
    D. one artery and one vein.

22. Mothers taking narcotics have been known to produce infants with
    A. low birth weight.
    B. withdrawal symptoms and tremors.
    C. respiratory depression.
    D. all of the above

Scenario

Questions 23–25 refer to the following scenario:

Your newborn infant presents with respiratory distress and cyanosis; unresponsiveness to ventilations; a small, flat abdomen; heart sounds displaced to the right; and bowel sounds in the chest.

23. Your suspected field diagnosis is
    A. spontaneous pneumothorax.
    B. herniated diaphragm.
    C. pericardial tamponade.
    D. phrenic nerve paralysis.

24. Proper positioning of this patient is
    A. Trendelenburg.
    B. left lateral recumbent.
    C. supine with head and chest elevated.
    D. prone.

25. Which of the following treatments is **contraindicated** for this patient?
    A. oxygen administration
    B. bag-valve-mask ventilation
    C. orogastric tube insertion and gastric suctioning
    D. endotracheal intubation

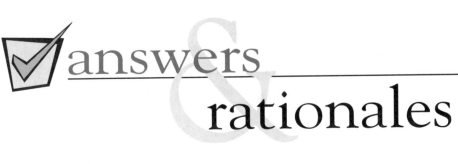

answers & rationales

Following each rationale, you will find a reference to the corresponding objective in the DOT National Standard EMT-Intermediate curriculum. An asterisk denotes material that is supplemental to the DOT curriculum. Page numbers after a rationale indicate where the question topic may be discussed in the Brady text *Intermediate Emergency Care* (Bledsoe, Porter, Cherry).

1.

D. Approximately 6% of field deliveries require neonatal life support. Antepartum (before birth) risk factors that indicate the possibility of complications in newborns include multiple gestation, inadequate prenatal care, mother younger than 16 or older than 35, history of perinatal morbidity or mortality, postterm gestation (baby overdue), drugs or medications, and toxemia/hypertension/diabetes during pregnancy. (6-2.3) (IEC p. 1156)

Matching (*) (IEC p. 1158)

2. A meningomyelocele
3. E omphalocele
4. C choanal atresia
5. D cleft palate
6. B Pierre Robin syndrome

7.

D. Routine care of the newborn infant is the first step of the inverted pyramid. This step includes drying and warming the baby; positioning the baby, head down, at the level of the vagina; suctioning the mouth and then the nose; and performing tactile stimulation if necessary. (6-2.6) (IEC p. 1162)

8.

C. After you have stabilized the neonate's airway and prevented heat loss, clamp and cut the umbilical cord. Apply the umbilical clamps within 30–45 seconds after birth. Place the first clamp approximately 10 cm from the neonate; place the second clamp approximately 5 cm distal from the first clamp; then cut the cord between the two clamps. After the cord is cut, inspect it periodically to make sure there is no additional bleeding. (6-2.6) (IEC p. 1161)

9.

C. The normal respiratory rate of the neonate should be 30–60 breaths per minute. (6-2.9) (IEC p. 1158)

10.

B. The heart rate is the critical component of neonatal resuscitation. A pulse rate of less than 100 beats per minute in the newborn indicates an infant in distress. (6-2.26) (IEC p. 1158)

11.

D. As soon as possible, assign the neonate an APGAR score. Do this at 1 and 5 minutes after birth. A score of 7–10 indicates an active and vigorous neonate that requires only routine care. Neonates with APGAR scores of less than 4 are severely distressed and require immediate resuscitation. (6-2.7) (IEC p. 1158)

12.

B. The presence of fetal meconium at birth indicates the possibility of fetal respiratory distress. Aspiration of meconium can cause severe lung inflammation and pneumonia in the neonate. If you spot meconium during delivery, do not induce respiratory effort until you have removed the meconium from the trachea by suctioning under direct visualization with the laryngoscope. This is a true emergency. (6-2.23) (IEC p. 1159)

13.

D. Normal suctioning of the neonate should be performed by bulb syringe or Delee trap and should last no longer than 10 seconds. Meconium should be suctioned through an endotracheal tube. (6-2.6, 6-2.23) (IEC p. 1159)

14.

A. As stated in question 1, the first step of the inverted pyramid includes drying and warming the infant; positioning the baby, head down, at the level of the vagina; suctioning the mouth and nose; and providing tactile stimulation when necessary. (6-2.6) (IEC p. 1162)

15.

B. An infant's best indicator of stress is the heart rate. If the heart rate is greater than 100 beats per minute and spontaneous respirations are present, continue assessing the baby. If the heart rate is less than 100 beats per minute, begin positive pressure ventilation immediately. If the heart rate is less than 60 beats per minute or between 60 and 80 beats per minute after 30 seconds of positive pressure ventilation and supplemental oxygen, begin chest compression. (6-2.5) (IEC p. 1167)

16.

A. If the infant presents with cyanosis after performing step 1 of the inverted pyramid, you should then move to step 2 and administer blow-by oxygen. (6-2.14, 6-2.31) (IEC p. 1167)

17.

B. If the heart rate is less than 100 or the infant is still cyanotic after performing step 2, immediately move to step 3 and perform bag-valve-mask ventilation. (6-2.9, 6-2.31) (IEC p. 1168)

18.

B. If the infant's heart rate is less than 80 after performing steps 1, 2, and 3, move to step 4 and perform chest compression. Encircle the neonate's chest and place both of your thumbs on the lower third of the sternum. Compress the sternum one-third to one-half of the chest's total height at a rate of at least 100 per minute. (6-2.11, 6-2.31) (IEC p. 1168)

19.

D. The infant's heart rate can best be checked by auscultating the heart at the apex, feeling for pulsation at the umbilical cord, or palpating the brachial pulse. (6-2.5, 6-2.26) (IEC p. 1167)

20.

A. When performing bag-valve-mask ventilation on the neonate, the pop-off valve, if present, should be disengaged. This will prevent underinflation of the infant's lungs. (6-2.10) (IEC p. 1186)

21.

B. The umbilicus contains three vessels—two arteries and one vein. The vein is easy to locate, as it is larger and has a thinner wall. Accessing the umbilical vein for resuscitation is a relatively easy process. (*) (IEC p. 1170)

22.

D. Maternal abuse of narcotics can produce infants with low birth weight, withdrawal symptoms and tremors, and respiratory depression. Unless the mother is a narcotic addict, administer naloxone to reverse any respiratory depression if the mother used within four hours of delivery. For the child of a narcotic addict, provide ventilation instead to avoid infant narcotic withdrawal. (6-2.3) (IEC p. 1170)

23.

B. Diaphragmatic hernias occur very rarely, in approximately 1 in 2200 births. When they do occur, the mortality is 50% for an infant presenting with respiratory distress in the first 18–24 hours. Signs and symptoms include respiratory distress and cyanosis unresponsive to ventilations; a small, flat abdomen; heart sounds displaced to the right; and bowel sounds in the chest. (*) (IEC p. 1174)

24.

C. Proper positioning of an infant with a herniated diaphragm is supine with the head and chest higher than the abdomen. (*) (IEC p. 1174)

25.

B. Do not use bag-valve-mask ventilation with an infant suspected of having a herniated diaphragm, as it may worsen the condition by causing gastric distention. If necessary, deliver positive pressure ventilation directly to the lungs through an endotracheal tube. (*) (IEC p. 1174)

3 Pediatrics

unit objectives

Questions in this unit relate to DOT objectives 6-3.1 to 6-3.106. The objectives are listed in the Appendix.

DIRECTIONS Each of the questions or incomplete statements below is followed by suggested answers or completions. Select the **one answer** that is best in each case.

1. A sunken anterior fontanel may indicate
   A. increased intracranial pressure.
   B. meningitis.
   C. epidural hematoma.
   D. dehydration.

2. Your 2-year-old patient requires head and neck immobilization on a backboard. Which of the following techniques will most likely maintain the child's head in the neutral position?
   A. padding underneath the head
   B. padding underneath the back and shoulders
   C. no padding
   D. padding underneath the head, back, and shoulders

3. The most common cause of cardiac arrest in infants and young children is
   A. respiratory arrest.
   B. circulatory collapse.
   C. cardiac dysrhythmia.
   D. drug overdose.

4. Usually the first sign of respiratory distress in infants is
   A. bradycardia.
   B. tachycardia.
   C. bradypnea.
   D. tachypnea.

5. Bradycardia in a distressed infant or young child is usually
   A. an ominous sign of impending cardiac arrest.
   B. transient.

C. a normal response to effective treatment.
D. the first sign of circulatory collapse.

6. Which of the following signs may signify impending cardiac arrest in a child?
   A. respiratory rate over 60
   B. pulse rate 170
   C. pulse rate 70 in a 5-year-old
   D. none of the above

7. Your patient is a 6-month-old girl who appears to have a complete upper-airway obstruction. Which of the following foreign body removal techniques is recommended?
   A. abdominal thrusts
   B. Heimlich maneuver
   C. back blows
   D. blind finger sweeps

8. Pop-off valves should be functional when ventilating the pediatric patient
   A. to avoid overinflation of the lungs.
   B. to avoid causing a pneumothorax.
   C. to avoid barotrauma to the lungs.
   D. none of the above

9. Which of the following is an approved method for estimating the correct ET tube size in an infant or young child?
   A. diameter of the patient's ring finger
   B. diameter of the patient's nasal opening
   C. patient's age in years $\times 4 + 16$
   D. all of the above

10. The commonly accepted age limit for attempting an intraosseous infusion is
    A. 3 years old.
    B. 6 years old.
    C. 8 years old.
    D. none of the above

11. Verifying proper placement of an intraosseous needle includes
    A. noting a lack of resistance.
    B. observing the needle standing upright.
    C. achieving free flow of the infusion without infiltration.
    D. all of the above

12. The initial dose for defibrillation in the pediatric patient is
    A. 1 J/kg.
    B. 2 J/kg.
    C. 4 J/kg.
    D. 200 J.

13. A 3-year-old child who burns both legs and arms has burned approximately _____ % of his entire body surface area.
    A. 54
    B. 46
    C. 72
    D. 36

14. Which of the following children may be at a higher risk for child abuse?
    A. child with disabilities
    B. twin child
    C. premature child
    D. all of the above

15. Which of the following is a classic characteristic of a child abuser?
    A. parent who spends majority of time with child
    B. parent who was abused as child

C. parent who is experiencing financial or marital stress
    D. all of the above

16. Which of the following statements regarding febrile seizures is true?
    A. They usually occur between the ages of 6 months and 1 year.
    B. They are caused by extremely high temperatures.
    C. They are caused by a sudden increase in temperature.
    D. The patient usually does not need to be transported.

Scenario

Questions 17–19 refer to the following scenario:

Your patient is a 2-month-old who presents lethargic and febrile. His mother says that he has been ill with upper respiratory congestion for 2 days. He has not eaten well, and he generally appears to be very ill. His anterior fontanels are sunken; he is tachycardic and tachypneic, with a 4-second capillary refill.

17. You should suspect _____ until proven otherwise.
    A. Reye's syndrome
    B. Down syndrome
    C. meningitis
    D. bronchiolitis

18. His vital signs indicate that this patient
    A. is in respiratory failure.
    B. is in shock.
    C. has increased intracranial pressure.
    D. none of the above

19. Prehospital management should include oxygen and
    A. IV mannitol.
    B. 20 ml/kg IV fluid challenge.
    C. IV antibiotics.
    D. the pneumatic antishock garment.

Scenario

Questions 20–22 refer to the following scenario:

Your patient is a 3-year-old who presents with a sudden onset of severe difficulty in breathing. She has not been ill and had been playing with friends at the time of onset. She presents afebrile with inspiratory stridor, a weak cough, and ashen skin.

20. You should suspect
    A. foreign body obstruction.
    B. croup.
    C. epiglottitis.
    D. asthma.

21. Initial prehospital management of this patient includes
    A. back blows.
    B. abdominal thrusts.
    C. leaving the patient alone.
    D. encouraging the patient to cough.

22. Further management of this patient may include
    A. direct laryngoscopy.
    B. removal with Magill forceps.
    C. cricothyrotomy.
    D. all of the above

Scenario

Questions 23–25 refer to the following scenario:

Your patient is a 5-year-old who presents sitting forward using all accessory muscles to breathe. He has inspiratory stridor, retractions, and a sore throat, and he drools. He is febrile and has been ill for almost a week prior to this incident.

23. In this patient, you should suspect
    A. foreign body obstruction.
    B. croup.
    C. epiglottitis.
    D. asthma.

24. Initial prehospital management of this patient includes
    A. racemic epinephrine.
    B. direct laryngoscopy.
    C. Heimlich maneuver.
    D. none of the above

25. If the patient totally occludes his airway, you should immediately
    A. deliver five abdominal thrusts.
    B. perform bag-valve-mask ventilation.
    C. inject 0.03 mg/kg epinephrine 1:1000 SC.
    D. none of the above

Scenario

Questions 26–28 refer to the following scenario:

Your patient is an 8-month-old child who presents with difficulty in breathing. She has diffuse expiratory wheezing and retractions and uses accessory muscles to move air. She is tachypneic and tachycardic. She is warm and has been ill since yesterday.

26. In this patient, you should suspect
    A. asthma.
    B. bronchitis.
    C. bronchiolitis.
    D. croup.

27. Signs that this patient is in imminent respiratory arrest include
    A. slowing of the respiratory rate.
    B. decrease in the respiratory effort.
    C. decrease in breath sounds.
    D. all of the above

28. Prehospital management of this patient should include
    A. administering oxygen.
    B. administering albuterol via nebulizer.
    C. sitting the child upright.
    D. all of the above

Scenario

Questions 29 and 30 refer to the following scenario:

Your patient is a 4-year-old who presents listless and appears very ill. She has a decreased level of consciousness and responds only to loud voices. Her mother says she has had diarrhea for 2 days and has not been able to keep food or drink down. She has tenting, dry mucous membranes, tachycardia, and delayed capillary refill.

29. From this patient's presentation, you should suspect
    A. respiratory failure.
    B. severe dehydration.
    C. pulmonary edema.
    D. respiratory infection.

30. Prehospital management should include oxygen and
    A. 20 ml/kg IV fluid challenge.
    B. 40 mg furosemide IV.
    C. IV antibiotics.
    D. albuterol via nebulizer.

Scenario

Questions 31 and 32 refer to the following scenario:

Your patient is a 6-year-old boy who presents with a rapid heart rate (260 beats per minute) and complains of palpitations. He is alert and oriented, his skin is warm and dry, he has no respiratory distress, and his blood pressure is 106/88. The ECG shows a narrow-complex tachycardia.

31. You suspect his problem is caused by
    A. dehydration.
    B. airway compromise.
    C. cardiac dysrhythmia.
    D. any of the above

32. Proper initial field management of this patient includes all of the following **except**
    A. oxygen administration.
    B. adenosine administration.
    C. synchronized cardioversion.
    D. fluid challenge.

33. Which of the following analgesics is **not** recommended for children?
    A. morphine
    B. fentanyl
    C. meperidine
    D. nalbuphine

34. The leading cause of poisoning in toddlers and preschoolers is
    A. cardiac medications.
    B. cleaning supplies.
    C. iron-containing vitamins.
    D. aspirin.

35. The most common type of burn injury suffered in the home by children is
    A. electrical.
    B. chemical.
    C. scald.
    D. direct fire.

36. Prehospital fluid resuscitation of children should be accomplished with
    A. 10 ml/kg IV colloid.
    B. 10 ml/kg IV crystalloid.
    C. 20 ml/kg IV 0.45% sodium chloride.
    D. 20 ml/kg IV lactated Ringer's.

37. Which of the following is the correct initial dose of epinephrine for a child in asystolic cardiac arrest?
    A. 0.1 mg/kg IV of 1:1000
    B. 0.01 mg/kg IV of 1:1000
    C. 0.1 mg/kg ET of 1:10,000
    D. 0.01 mg/kg IO of 1:10,000

38. Which of the following prehospital treatments is **not** indicated for a patient with croup?
    A. administering cool mist oxygen
    B. administering racemic epinephrine
    C. starting an IV
    D. sitting on mother's lap during transport

39. Epiglottitis has become a rare childhood disease because of
    A. better parental care at home.
    B. the *H. flu* vaccine.
    C. the advent of non–aspirin-containing analgesics.
    D. more tonsillectomies being performed.

40. An EMT-Intermediate should never attempt to visualize the oropharynx of a child suspected of having
    A. croup.
    B. epiglottitis.
    C. laryngotracheobronchitis.
    D. all of the above

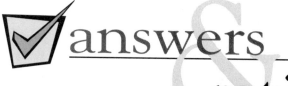answers

rationales

Following each rationale, you will find a reference to the corresponding objective in the DOT National Standard EMT-Intermediate curriculum. An asterisk denotes material that is supplemental to the DOT curriculum. Page numbers after a rationale indicate where the question topic may be discussed in the Brady text *Intermediate Emergency Care* (Bledsoe, Porter, Cherry).

1.

D. The anterior fontanel should be inspected in all infants. It should be level with the surface of the skull or slightly sunken, and it may pulsate. With dehydration, the anterior fontanel may often fall below the level of the skull and appear sunken. (6-3.7) (IEC p. 1192)

2.

B. As a rule, for children under the age of 3, padding underneath the back and shoulders will be necessary to maintain a neutral position because of the large occiput. (6-3.89) (IEC p. 1192)

3.

A. The most common causes of cardiac arrest in infants and young children are airway and respiratory problems. (6-3.68) (IEC p. 1196)

4.

D. In general, the first manifestation of respiratory distress in infants and young children is tachypnea. (6-3.21) (IEC p. 1198)

5.

A. Bradycardia in a distressed infant or young child is an ominous sign of impending cardiac arrest. Bradycardia is age dependent, so it is important to know the normal heart rate for each age-group. (6-3.68) (IEC p. 1198)

6.

A. Recognizing and preventing cardiac arrest in the pediatric patient is the key. Vital signs that place a pediatric patient at risk for cardiopulmonary arrest include a respiratory rate >60, heart rate >180, and heart rate <80 (under 5 years) and <60 (over 5 years). (6-3.68) (IEC p. 1200)

7.

C. For children less than 1 year old, back blows and chest thrusts are the only techniques recommended for removal of a foreign body. (6-3.32) (IEC p. 1205)

8.

D. Pediatric bag-valve-masks should not contain pressure pop-off valves. If one exists, it should be disengaged. The reason is that higher pressures may be needed to ventilate the pediatric patient. (6-3.13) (IEC p. 1208)

9.

B. Approved techniques for estimating the correct ET tube size for infants and young children include the diameter of the patient's little finger, the diameter of the nasal opening, and the patient's age in years + 16 divided by 4. Of course, you can always refer to a chart for the recommended size for your patient's age and size. (6-3.14) (IEC p. 1210)

10.

B. Indications for intraosseous infusion include an unresponsive child less than 6 years of age in shock or cardiac arrest, after unsuccessful attempts at peripheral IV insertion. In children over the age of 6, the bones become more solid. (6-3.4) (IEC p. 1215)

11.

D. Placement of the needle into the marrow cavity can be determined by noting a lack of resistance if the needle passes through the bony cortex. Other indications include the needle standing upright without support, the ability to aspirate bone marrow into a syringe, and the free flow of the infusion without infiltration into the subcutaneous tissues. (6-3.86) (IEC p. 1215)

12.

B. The initial dose for defibrillation in pediatric patients is 2 J/kg. Perform all subsequent defibrillation attempts at 4 J/kg. (6-3.71) (IEC p. 1217)

13.

B. Estimation of the burn surface is slightly different for children. When using the rule of nines to calculate the percentage of burns in infants and small children, each leg is worth 14%, while the head is worth 18%. For this patient, who burned both legs and arms, the body surface area adds up to 46%. (*) (IEC p. 1250)

14.

D. There are several characteristics common to abused children. Often they are seen as special and different from others. Also, premature infants or twins, children less than 5 years of age, children with disabilities, uncommunicative children, boys, and children of the wrong sex are at higher risk. (6-3.98) (IEC p. 1251)

15.

D. The child abuser can come from any geographic, religious, ethnic, occupational, educational, or socioeconomic group. However, people who abuse children tend to share certain characteristics. The abuser is usually a parent or someone in the role of a parent. When the mother spends most time with the child, she is the parent most frequently identified as the abuser. Most child abusers were abused as children. Common crises (financial stress, marital or relationship stress, and physical illness in a parent or child) may precipitate abuse. (6-3.98) (IEC p. 1251)

16.

C. Febrile seizures occur as a result of a sudden increase in body temperature. They seem related to the rate at which the body temperature increases, not to the degree of fever. (6-3.73) (IEC p. 1236)

17.

C. Documented fever in a child less than 3 months of age is considered meningitis until proven otherwise. (*) (IEC p. 1237)

18.

B. The patient's vital signs, sunken anterior fontanels, tachycardia, tachypnea, and delayed capillary refill all indicate shock. (6-3.53) (IEC p. 1228)

19.

B. Prehospital management of this patient should include oxygen and a fluid challenge of 20 ml/kg of IV crystalloid (normal saline, lactated Ringer's). (6-3.54) (IEC p. 1230)

20.

A. Any afebrile child who presents with a sudden onset of stridor without previous history of illness should be suspected as having a foreign body obstruction. (6-3.31) (IEC p. 1224)

21.

B. Initial prehospital management of this patient includes delivering five abdominal thrusts. (6-3.32) (IEC p. 1225)

22.

D. Further management of this patient may include direct laryngoscopy and removal of the foreign body with Magill forceps. (6-3.32) (IEC p. 1225)

23.

C. Your 5-year-old patient who sits forward, drooling and presenting with stridor, fever, and illness, should be suspected of having epiglottitis. (6-3.35) (IEC p. 1222)

24.

D. Initial prehospital management of this patient includes placing the child in a position of comfort and administering humidified oxygen by face mask or blow-by. Direct visualization of the larynx may cause laryngospasm and is contraindicated. (6-3.36) (IEC p. 1223)

25.

B. If the patient totally closes his airway (usually from laryngospasm), immediately perform bag-valve-mask ventilation. (6-3.36) (IEC p. 1223)

26.

C. In this patient, who is less than 1 year old, presenting with wheezing and difficulty breathing, you should suspect bronchiolitis. (6-3.39) (IEC p. 1226)

27.

D. Signs that a pediatric patient is in imminent respiratory arrest include a slowing of the respiratory rate, a decrease in the respiratory effort, and a decrease in breath sounds. (6-3.21, 6-3.39) (IEC p. 1220)

28.

D. Prehospital management of this patient should include oxygen administration, sitting the child upright, and administering albuterol via nebulizer. (6-3.40) (IEC p. 1227)

29.

B. This child who presents with dry mucous membranes, poor skin turgor, tachycardia, and delayed capillary refill is suspected of having severe dehydration. (*) (IEC p. 1228)

30.

A. Prehospital management of this patient should include oxygen and 20 ml/kg of IV crystalloid (normal saline, lactated Ringer's). (*) (IEC p. 1230)

31.

C. A heart rate of 260 indicates a cardiac dysrhythmia rather than any other cause, such as dehydration or hypoxia. The narrow complex suggests supraventricular tachycardia. (6-3.62) (IEC p. 1232)

32.

C. For this stable patient in probable supraventricular tachycardia, proper field management includes oxygen therapy, IV–KVO, and adenosine administration (0.1–0.2 mg/kg IV) to convert the rhythm. If the patient becomes unstable, deliver synchronized cardioversion (0.5–1 J/kg). (6-3.63) (IEC p. 1233)

33.

D. Unless there is a contraindication, children should receive pain management. Natural analgesics, such as morphine, meperidine, and fentanyl, are effective. Synthetic analgesics, such as nalbuphine and butorphanol, should be avoided because their effects on children are unpredictable. (*) (IEC p. 1247)

34.

C. Iron-containing vitamin supplements are the leading cause of poisoning in the toddler and preschool age-groups. (*) (IEC p. 1241)

35.

C. The most common type of burn injury suffered by children in the home is a scald injury, usually by pulling hot liquids off a table or stove. In cases of abuse, hot water immersion is the typical cause. (*) (IEC p. 1245)

36.

D. Prehospital fluid therapy for a child is accomplished with an isotonic solution, such as normal saline (0.9% sodium chloride) or lactated Ringer's, at 20 ml/kg initial bolus. (6-3.91) (IEC p. 1216)

37.

D. The initial dose of epinephrine for a child in asystolic cardiac arrest is 0.01 mg/kg of 1:10,000 IV/IO or 0.1 mg/kg of 1:1000 ET. (6-3.71) (IEC p. 1217)

38.

C. Prehospital management of a child with croup includes administering cool mist oxygen by face mask or blow-by, administering racemic epinephrine or albuterol via nebulizer if the attack is severe, and avoiding anything that will agitate the child, such as starting an IV. (6-3.28) (IEC p. 1222)

39.

B. Epiglottitis is caused by a bacterial infection—usually the Hemophilus influenza type B. With the advent of the *H. flu* vaccine, epiglottitis has become a rare pediatric disease. (6-3.33) (IEC p. 1222)

40.

D. If you suspect your pediatric patient may have croup (laryngotracheobronchitis) or epiglottitis, never put anything into his or her mouth. This may worsen the tissue swelling, cause further upper-airway obstruction, and even result in a complete obstruction and apnea. (6-3.28, 6-3.36) (IEC p. 1223)

Geriatrics

unit objectives

Questions in this unit relate to DOT objectives 6-4.1 to 6-4.21. The objectives are listed in the Appendix.

DIRECTIONS Each of the questions or incomplete statements below is followed by suggested answers or completions. Select the **one answer** that is best in each case.

1. Which of the following tends to complicate the assessment of the elderly?
   A. The elderly often suffer more than one disease at a time.
   B. The primary problem often is different from the chief complaint.
   C. The patient's perception of pain may be diminished or absent.
   D. all of the above

2. Assessing an elderly patient who presents with poor peripheral pulses, rales, and dependent edema may be difficult because
   A. his presentation is consistent with congestive heart failure.
   B. his signs and symptoms may be caused by the aging process.
   C. it is often difficult to distinguish acute from chronic problems.
   D. all of the above

3. Your patient who complains that the room is spinning and who is nauseated, pale, and sweating may be suffering from
   A. dementia.
   B. delirium.
   C. Alzheimer's.
   D. vertigo.

Match the following causes of syncope with their respective descriptions:

4. _____ vasodepressor
5. _____ orthostatic
6. _____ vasovagal
7. _____ cardiac
8. _____ TIA

   A. temporary stroke
   B. Stokes-Adams syndrome
   C. rising from a seated or supine position
   D. the common faint
   E. valsalva maneuver

9. Chronic global mental impairment is known as
   A. organic brain syndrome.
   B. senile dementia.
   C. senility.
   D. all of the above

10. Which of the following renders the elderly susceptible to making medication errors?
    A. forgetfulness
    B. limited income
    C. vision impairment
    D. all of the above

Scenario

Questions 11 and 12 refer to the following scenario:

Your patient is an 89-year-old female who presents with multiple bruises. She lives with her son, who says she is always falling down and is just generally clumsy. She appears somewhat undernourished and frightened. She cowers when you approach her and reluctantly allows you to inspect her bruises. Her son behaves very strangely toward you and your partner and nervously attempts to explain each bruise. She is incontinent of urine and appears not to have been washed in days. You suspect elderly abuse.

11. In which socioeconomic class is this problem most prevalent?

    A. lower

    B. middle class

    C. wealthy

    D. all classes

12. In this case, the EMT-Intermediate should do all of the following **except**

    A. obtain a complete patient and family history.

    B. report any suspicions to the ED staff.

    C. be honest with her son about your concerns.

    D. watch for inconsistencies in stories.

Scenario

Questions 13–15 refer to the following scenario:

Your patient is an 82-year-old woman who presents with some vague complaints about feeling weak and fatigued. She denies any chest pain. She has a long history of cardiac, respiratory, and diabetic problems. She takes a host of medications for each but cannot remember what she took today. In your exam, you notice her swollen ankles and weak peripheral pulses, and you auscultate some fine bibasilar rales. You suspect she is having a cardiac episode and begin appropriate prehospital management.

13. Which of the following is true regarding this elderly patient?

    A. Absence of chest pain does not rule out myocardial infarction.

    B. Her peripheral edema and rales may be normal findings.

    C. The first 2 hours after the onset of symptoms are critical.

    D. all of the above

14. Atypical presentations of myocardial infarction include

    A. dental pain.

    B. syncope.

    C. dyspnea.

    D. all of the above

15. All of the following statements are true regarding the management of the elderly cardiac patient **except**

    A. they are treated much the same as the younger patient.

    B. medication orders may be modified.

    C. oxygen administration must be carefully monitored.

    D. fluid administration may be decreased.

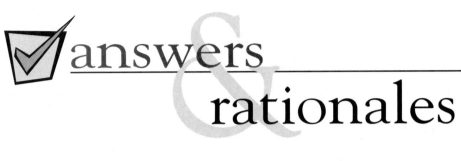

Following each rationale, you will find a reference to the corresponding objective in the DOT National Standard EMT-Intermediate curriculum. An asterisk denotes material that is supplemental to the DOT curriculum. Page numbers after a rationale indicate where the question topic may be discussed in the Brady text *Intermediate Emergency Care* (Bledsoe, Porter, Cherry).

1.

D. It is difficult to assess the elderly because they often suffer more than one disease at a time. Their primary problem is often different from the chief complaint, and their perception of pain may be diminished or absent. (6-4.8) (IEC p. 1264)

2.

D. Assessing elderly patients who present with poor peripheral pulses, rales, and edema may be difficult because their presentation is consistent with congestive heart failure, yet their signs and symptoms may be caused simply by the aging process. It is often difficult to distinguish the acute from the chronic problem. (6-4.8) (IEC p. 1264)

3.

D. Vertigo is a specific sensation of motion perceived by the patient as spinning or whirling. It is often accompanied by sweating, pallor, nausea, and vomiting. (6-4.9) (IEC p. 1286)

Matching (6-4.9) (IEC p. 1284)

4.	D	vasodepressor
5.	C	orthostatic
6.	E	vasovagal
7.	B	cardiac
8.	A	TIA

9.

D. Dementia, a chronic, global mental impairment, is often progressive or irreversible and usually is due to underlying neurological disease. This mental deterioration is often called organic brain syndrome, senile dementia, or senility. (6-4.14) (IEC p. 1287)

10.

D. Underdosing and overdosing of medication are very common in the elderly. This may be due to confusion, vision impairment, forgetfulness, or limited income. (6-4.11) (IEC p. 1265)

11.

D. Abuse of the elderly knows no socioeconomic bounds. It occurs in all classes of our society and is a major health and social problem. (6-4.9) (IEC p. 1302)

12.

C. In cases where you suspect geriatric abuse, you should obtain a complete patient and family history and watch for inconsistencies in the stories. You should report any suspicions to the ED staff and always avoid confrontations with the family. (*) (IEC p. 1303)

13.

D. In this case, the absence of chest pain does not rule out myocardial infarction because many elderly patients suffer silent myocardial infarctions. Her peripheral edema and rales may be normal findings of the aging process, and, as in all cardiac patients, the first 2 hours after the onset of symptoms are the most critical. (6-4.13) (IEC p. 1282)

14.

D. Atypical presentations of myocardial infarction include dental pain, syncope, dyspnea, confusion, neck pain, epigastric pain, and fatigue. (6-4.13) (IEC p. 1282)

15.

C. Managing the elderly cardiac patient is somewhat the same as managing the younger cardiac patient, with a few differences. Medication orders may be modified, and fluid administration may be decreased based on the presence of congestive heart failure, liver disease, and other metabolic problems. (6-4.13) (IEC p. 1283)

1

Assessment-Based Management

unit objectives

Questions in this unit relate to DOT objectives 7-1.1 to 7-1.21. The objectives are listed in the Appendix.

DIRECTIONS Each of the questions or incomplete statements below is followed by suggested answers or completions. Select the **one answer** that is best in each case.

1. Most of the time for a patient with a medical condition, you will formulate your field diagnosis based on the
   A. history.
   B. physical exam.
   C. vital signs.
   D. monitor strip.

2. Pattern recognition is based on experience and
   A. circumstances.
   B. knowledge.
   C. vital signs.
   D. protocols.

3. Which of the following statements is true regarding the use of protocols?
   A. Deviation from protocol is prohibited.
   B. Standing orders replace a paramedic's judgment.
   C. Exercising judgment is a dangerous proposition.
   D. Protocols are guidelines that require judicious application.

4. Which of the following circumstances can affect your on-scene decision-making capabilities?
   A. extreme environmental temperatures
   B. a loud, abusive patient
   C. gory injuries
   D. all of the above

5. In a two-paramedic ambulance crew, which of the following tasks is performed by the team leader?
   A. gathering scene information
   B. interrogating the patient
   C. starting the IV
   D. obtaining vital signs

6. Your patient presents with chest pain, normal mental status, and normal vital signs. The correct approach would be the _____ approach.
   A. contemplative
   B. resuscitative
   C. immediate evacuation
   D. none of the above

7. Which of the following patients requires a complete head-to-toe physical exam?
   A. patient with an isolated ankle sprain
   B. responsive patient with suspected AMI
   C. unresponsive stroke patient
   D. alert and oriented 14-year-old with moderate asthma attack

8. Your patient is unstable. You should perform an ongoing assessment every _____ minutes.
   A. 5
   B. 10
   C. 15
   D. 20

9. The "A" in SOAP stands for
   A. allergies.
   B. actions.
   C. acute.
   D. none of the above

10. An effective oral presentation should last no more than _____.
    A. 15 seconds.
    B. 1 minute.
    C. 2 minutes.
    D. 5 minutes.

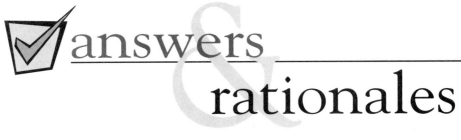

answers & rationales

Following each rationale, you will find a reference to the corresponding objective in the DOT National Standard EMT-Intermediate curriculum. An asterisk denotes material that is supplemental to the DOT curriculum. Page numbers after a rationale indicate where the question topic may be discussed in the Brady text *Intermediate Emergency Care* (Bledsoe, Porter, Cherry).

1.

A. Doctors will base 80% of their diagnosis on the history. Your ability to elicit a good history will determine your success in formulating an accurate field diagnosis. (7-1.1) (IEC p. 1310)

2.

B. Pattern recognition is based on your experience and knowledge base. The greater both are, the more likely you are to recognize patterns. This is why the perfect team is a seasoned paramedic (experienced, street savvy) and a new graduate (recent knowledge, enthusiasm). (7-1.1) (IEC p. 1311)

3.

D. Protocols and standing orders are guidelines only. You must add your clinical judgment when deciding to use or not use them. Of course, clinical judgment comes from experience. Experience comes from having had bad judgment. (7-1.1) (IEC p. 1311)

4.

D. A number of factors can affect your ability to make an on-scene decision. These include your personal attitude, your patient's attitude, distracting injuries, and environmental factors. Understanding this, try to maintain focus on the problem and disregard the distractions. (7-1.5) (IEC p. 1311)

5.

B. In a typical two-paramedic crew, the duties are sometimes divided into the team leader and patient care provider roles. The team leader obtains the history, performs the physical exam, presents the patient, and handles documentation. The patient care provider surveys the scene, obtains vital signs, and performs interventions. In a multiple-casualty incident, the team leader assumes EMS command, while his or her partner begins triage. (7-1.8) (IEC p. 1313)

6.

A. Use the contemplative approach when your patient does not require immediate intervention. In this case, a good history and physical exam are worth some added on-scene time because they will yield vital information. (7-1.11) (IEC p. 1317)

7.

C. A complete head-to-toe exam consists of a rapid trauma assessment for the trauma patient or a rapid medical assessment for the medical patient. These exams are performed on medical patients who are unresponsive and on trauma patients with significant mechanisms of injury or altered mental status. Responsive medical patients and patients with isolated injuries receive physical exams directed at the body systems involved. (7-1.17) (IEC p. 1317)

8.

A. The ongoing assessment must be performed on all patients to monitor for trends and changes in the patient's condition—every 5 minutes for an unstable patient, every 15 minutes for stable patients. The ongoing assessment includes reassessing the initial assessment and focused exam and reevaluating transport priorities and vital signs as well as the effectiveness of interventions and management plans. (7-1.11) (IEC p. 1318)

9.

D. SOAP is the universal format for presenting a patient to another health care professional. The mnemonic stands for **S**ubjective, **O**bjective, **A**ssessment, and **P**lan. You should always use SOAP or some variation of it when presenting your patient on the radio or in person at the ED. (7-1.12) (IEC p. 1319)

10.

B. An effective patient report, either on the radio or in person, should last no longer than 1 minute. Other health care providers, especially busy emergency department personnel, have little interest or time to listen to unimportant details. Use the SOAP format and get to the point quickly. (7-1.12) (IEC p. 1319)

Appendix: DOT Objectives

MODULE 1 PREPARATORY

UNIT 1-1 FOUNDATIONS OF THE EMT-INTERMEDIATE

Cognitive Objectives

At the completion of this unit, the EMT-Intermediate student will be able to:

1-1.1 Define the following terms:

    a. EMS Systems
    b. Certification
    c. Registration
    d. Profession
    e. Professionalism
    f. Health care professional
    g. Ethics
    h. Medical direction
    i. Protocols

1-1.2 Describe the attributes of an EMT-Intermediate as a health care professional.

1-1.3 Explain EMT-Intermediate licensure/certification, recertification, and reciprocity requirements in his or her state.

1-1.4 Describe the benefits of EMT-Intermediate continuing education.

1-1.5 List current state requirements for EMT-Intermediate education in his or her state.

1-1.6 Describe examples of professional behaviors in the following areas: integrity, empathy, self-motivation, appearance and personal hygiene, self-confidence, communications, time management, teamwork and diplomacy, respect, patient advocacy, and careful delivery of service.

1-1.7 Provide examples of activities that constitute appropriate professional behavior for an EMT-Intermediate.

1-1.8 Describe how professionalism applies to the EMT-Intermediate while on and off duty.

1-1.9 List and explain the primary and additional roles and responsibilities of the EMT-Intermediate.

1-1.10 Describe the importance and benefits of quality EMS research to the future of EMS.

1-1.11 Describe the role of the EMS physician in providing medical direction.

1-1.12 Describe the benefits of medical direction, both online and off-line.

1-1.13 Describe the relationship between a physician on the scene, the EMT-Intermediate on the scene, and the EMS physician providing medical direction.

1-1.14 Describe the components of continuous quality improvement.

1-1.14a Explain the components of wellness for the EMS provider.

1-1.15 Discuss the importance of universal precautions and body substance isolation practices and develop strategies to prevent the transmission of diseases.

1-1.16 Describe the steps to take for personal protection from airborne and blood-borne pathogens.

1-1.17 Explain what is meant by an exposure and describe principles for management.

1-1.18 Describe the incidence, morbidity, and mortality of preventable injury and illness.

1-1.19 Identify the human, environmental, and socioeconomic impact of preventable injury and illness.

1-1.20 Describe the feasibility of EMS involvement in illness and injury prevention.

1-1.21 Develop strategies for the implementation of EMS-related illness and injury prevention programs in the community.

1-1.22 Identify health hazards and potential crime areas within the community.

1-1.23 Identify local municipal and community resources available for physical and socioeconomic crises.

1-1.24 Identify the role of EMS in local municipal and community prevention programs.

1-1.25 Identify and explain the importance of laws pertinent to the EMT-Intermediate.

1-1.26 Identify and explain the importance of laws pertinent to the EMT-Intermediate.

1-1.27 Differentiate between licensure and certification as they apply to the EMT-Intermediate.

1-1.28 List the specific problems or conditions encountered while providing care that an EMT-Intermediate is required to report and identify in each instance to whom the report is to be made.

   a. Abandonment
   b. Advance directives
   c. Assault
   d. Battery
   e. Breach of duty
   f. Confidentiality
   g. Consent (expressed, implied, informed, involuntary)
   h. Do not resuscitate (DNR) orders
   i. Duty to act
   j. Emancipated minor
   k. False imprisonment
   l. Immunity
   m. Liability
   n. Libel
   o. Minor
   p. Negligence
   q. Proximate cause
   r. Scope of practice
   s. Slander
   t. Standard of care
   u. Tort

1-1.30 Differentiate between the scope of practice and the standard of care for EMT-Intermediate practice.

1-1.31 Discuss the concept of medical direction and its relationship to the standard of care of an EMT-Intermediate.

1-1.32 Review the four elements that must be present in order to prove negligence.

1-1.33 Given a scenario in which a patient is injured while an EMT-Intermediate is providing care, determine whether the four components of negligence are present.

1-1.34 Given a scenario, demonstrate patient care behaviors that would protect the EMT-Intermediate from claims of negligence.

1-1.35 Explain the concept of liability as it might apply to EMT-Intermediate practice, including physicians providing medical direction and EMT-Intermediate supervision of other care providers.

1-1.36 Review the legal concept of immunity, including Good Samaritan statutes and governmental immunity as it applies to the EMT-Intermediate.

1-1.37 Review the importance and necessity of patient confidentiality and the standards for maintaining patient confidentiality which apply to the EMT-Intermediate.

1-1.38 Review the steps to take if a patient refuses care.

1-1.39 Identify the legal issues involved in the decision not to transport a patient or to reduce the level of care being provided during transportation.

1-1.40 Review the conditions under which the use of force, including restraint, is acceptable.

1-1.41 Explain the purpose of advance directives relative to patient care and how the EMT-Intermediate should care for a patient who is covered by an advance directive.

1-1.42 Discuss the responsibilities of the EMT-Intermediate relative to resuscitation efforts for patients who are potential organ donors.

1-1.43 Review the importance of providing accurate documentation (oral and written) in substantiating an incident.

1-1.44 Review the characteristics of a patient care report required to make it an effective legal document.

1-1.45 Review the premise which should underlie the EMT-Intermediate's ethical decisions in out-of-hospital care.

1-1.46 Review the relationship between the law and ethics in EMS.

1-1.47 Identify the issues surrounding the use of advance directives in making an out-of-hospital resuscitation decision.

1-1.48 Describe the criteria necessary to honor an advance directive in your state.

Affective Objectives

At the completion of this unit, the EMT-Intermediate student will be able to:

1-1.49 Serve as a role model for others relative to professionalism in EMS.

1-1.50 Value the need to serve as the patient advocate, including of those with special needs, alternate lifestyles, and cultural diversity.

1-1.51 Defend the importance of continuing medical education and skills retention.

1-1.52 Advocate the need for supporting and participating in research efforts aimed at improving EMS systems.

1-1.53 Assess personal attitudes and demeanor that may distract from professionalism.

1-1.54 Advocate the need for injury prevention, including abusive situations.

1-1.55 Exhibit professional behaviors in the following areas: integrity, empathy, self-motivation, appearance and personal hygiene, self-confidence, communications, time management, teamwork and diplomacy, respect, patient advocacy, and careful delivery of service.

1-1.56 Advocate the benefits of working toward the goal of total personal wellness.

1-1.57 Serve as a role model for other EMS providers in regard to a total wellness program.

1-1.58 Value the need to assess his or her own lifestyle.

1-1.59 Challenge him- or herself to teach wellness concepts in his or her role as an EMT-Intermediate.

1-1.60 Defend the need to treat each patient as an individual, with respect and dignity.

1-1.61 Assess his or her own prejudices related to the various aspects of cultural diversity.

1-1.62 Improve personal physical well-being through achieving and maintaining proper body weight, regular exercise, and proper nutrition.

1-1.63 Defend the need to respect the emotional needs of dying patients and their families.

1-1.64 Advocate and practice the use of personal safety precautions in all scene situations.

1-1.65 Advocate and serve as a role model for other EMS providers relative to body substance isolation practices.

1-1.66 Value and defend tenets of prevention for patients and communities being served.

1-1.67 Value personal commitment to success of prevention programs.

1-1.68 Advocate the need to show respect for the rights and feelings of patients.

1-1.69 Assess his or her personal commitment to protecting patient confidentiality.

1-1.70 Defend personal beliefs about withholding or stopping patient care.

1-1.71 Defend the value of advance medical directives.

1-1.72 Reinforce the patient's autonomy in the decision-making process.

1-1.73 Given a scenario, defend an EMT-Intermediate's actions in a situation where a physician orders therapy the EMT-Intermediate feels to be detrimental to the patient's best interests.

Psychomotor Objectives

At the completion of this unit, the EMT-Intermediate student will be able to:

1-1.74 Demonstrate the proper procedures to take for personal protection from disease.

UNIT 1-2 OVERVIEW OF HUMAN SYSTEMS

Cognitive Objectives

At the completion of this unit, the EMT-Intermediate student will be able to:

1-2.1 Define anatomy, physiology, and pathophysiology.

1-2.2 Name the levels of organization of the body from simplest to most complex and explain each.

1-2.3 Define homeostasis.

1-2.4 State the anatomical terms for the parts of the body.

1-2.5 Identify terminology to describe the location of body parts with respect to one another.

1-2.6 Review the body cavities and the major organs within each.

1-2.7 Identify the anatomical planes.

1-2.8 Identify areas of the abdomen and underlying organs.

1-2.9 Define each of the cellular transport mechanisms and give an example of the role of each in the body: diffusion, osmosis, facilitated diffusion, active transport.

1-2.10 Define metabolism, anabolism, catabolism.

1-2.11 Describe how glucose is converted to energy during cellular respiration.

1-2.12 Describe the general characteristics of each of the four major categories of tissues.

1-2.13 Name the three major layers of the skin.

1-2.14 Describe the functions of the skeleton.

1-2.15 Explain how bones are classified.

1-2.16 Explain how joints are classified.

1-2.17 Describe the structure and function of muscles.

1-2.18 List the three types of muscles.

1-2.19 State the functions of the nervous system.

1-2.20 Name the divisions of the nervous system.

1-2.21 Explain the structure of neurons.

1-2.22 Describe the types of nerves.

1-2.23 Describe the role of polarization. depolarization, repolarization in nerve impulse transmission.

1-2.24 Identify the components of the central nervous system.

1-2.25 State the function of the meninges and cerebrospinal fluid.

1-2.26 Identify the divisions of the autonomic nervous system and define their functions.

1-2.27 Discuss the regulator processes of hormonal secretion.

1-2.28 State the functions of hormones.

1-2.29 State the function of the hormones of the pancreas.

1-2.30 State the functions of epinephrine and norepinephrine and explain their relationship to the sympathetic division of the autonomic nervous system.

1-2.31 Describe the characteristics of blood and its composition.

1-2.32 Explain the function of red blood cells, white blood cells, and platelets.

1-2.33 State the importance of blood clotting.

1-2.34 Describe the location of the heart.

1-2.35 Describe the function of the pericardium.

1-2.36 Identify the major vessels and chambers of the heart.

1-2.37 Identify the valves of the heart and explain their functions.

1-2.38 Describe coronary circulation and explain its purpose.

1-2.39 Describe the cardiac cycle.

1-2.40 Explain how heart sounds are created.

1-2.41 Name the parts of the cardiac conduction pathway.

1-2.42 Explain the relationship between stroke volume, heart rate, and cardiac output.

1-2.43 Explain how the nervous system regulates heart rate and force of contraction.

1-2.44 Describe the structure of arteries and veins and relate their structure to function.

1-2.45 Describe the structure of capillaries and explain the exchange processes that take place in capillaries.

1-2.46 Describe the pathway and purpose of pulmonary circulation.

1-2.47 Describe the pathway and purpose of systemic circulation.

1-2.48 Define blood pressure.

1-2.49 Explain the factors that maintain and regulate blood pressure.

1-2.50 Describe the functions of the lymphatic system.

1-2.51 Describe the immune response.

1-2.52 Describe the structure and functions of the components of the respiratory system.

1-2.53 Describe the structure and functions of the components of the respiratory system.

1-2.54 Describe normal inhalation and exhalation.

1-2.55 Differentiate between ventilation and respiration.

1-2.56 Explain the diffusion of gases across the alveolar-capillary junction.

1-2.57 Describe how oxygen and carbon dioxide are transported in the blood.

1-2.58 Explain the nervous and chemical mechanisms that regulate respiration.

1-2.59 Describe the functions of the digestive system and name its major divisions.

1-2.60 Describe the water compartments and the name for the fluid in each.

1-2.61 Explain how water moves between compartments.

1-2.62 Explain the regulation of the intake and output of water.

1-2.63 Describe the three buffer systems in body fluids.

1-2.64 Explain why the respiratory system has an effect on pH and describe respiratory compensating mechanisms.

1-2.65 Explain the renal mechanisms for pH regulation of extracellular fluid.

1-2.66 Describe the effects of acidosis and alkalosis.

Affective Objectives

At the completion of this unit, the EMT-Intermediate student will be able to:

1-2.67 Appreciate how anatomy and physiology are the foundation of medicine.

Psychomotor Objectives

None identified for this unit.

UNIT 1-3 EMERGENCY PHARMACOLOGY

Cognitive Objectives

At the completion of this unit, the EMT-Intermediate student will be able to:

1-3.1 Review the specific anatomy and physiology pertinent to pharmacology.

1-3.2 Discuss the standardization of drugs.

1-3.3 Differentiate among the chemical, generic (nonproprietary), and trade (proprietary) names of a drug.

1-3.4 List the four main sources of drug products.

1-3.5 Describe how drugs are classified.

1-3.6 List the authoritative sources for drug information.

1-3.7 Discuss special consideration in drug treatment with regard to pregnant, pediatric, and geriatric patients.

1-3.8 Discuss the EMT-Intermediate's responsibilities and scope of management pertinent to the administration of medications.

1-3.9 List and describe general properties of drugs.

1-3.10 List and describe liquid, solid, and gas drug forms.

1-3.11 List and differentiate routes of drug administration.

1-3.12 Differentiate between enteral and parenteral routes of drug administration.

1-3.13 Describe mechanisms of drug action.

1-3.14 List and differentiate the phases of drug activity, including the pharmaceutical, pharmacokinetic, and pharmacodynamic phases.

1-3.15 Describe pharmacokinetics, pharmacodynamics theories of drug action, drug-response relationship, factors altering drug responses, predictable drug responses, iatrogenic drug responses, and unpredictable adverse drug responses.

1-3.16 Discuss considerations for storing drugs.

1-3.17 List the components of a drug profile.

1-3.18 List and describe drugs which the EMT-Intermediate may administer in a pharmacological management plan according to local protocol.

1-3.19 Discuss procedures and measures to ensure security of controlled substances the EMT-Intermediate may administer.

Affective Objectives

At the completion of this unit, the EMT-Intermediate student will be able to:

1-3.20 Defend medication administration by an EMT-Intermediate to effect positive therapeutic affect.

Psychomotor Objectives

None identified for this unit.

UNIT 1-4 VENOUS ACCESS AND MEDICATION ADMINISTRATION

Cognitive Objectives

At the completion of this unit, the EMT-Intermediate student will be able to:

1-4.1 Review the specific anatomy and physiology pertinent to medication administration.

1-4.2 Review mathematical principles.

1-4.3 Review mathematical equivalents.

1-4.4 Differentiate temperature readings between the Centigrade and Fahrenheit scales.

1-4.5 Discuss formulas as a basis for performing drug calculations.

1-4.6 Calculate oral and parenteral drug dosages for all emergency medications administered to adults, infants, and children.

1-4.7 Calculate intravenous infusion rates for adults, infants, and children.

1-4.8 Discuss legal aspects affecting medication administration.

1-4.9 Discuss the "six rights" of drug administration and correlate these with the principles of medication administration.

1-4.10 Discuss medical asepsis and the differences between clean and sterile techniques.

1-4.11 Describe use of antiseptics and disinfectants.

1-4.12 Describe the use of universal precautions and body substance isolation (BSI) procedures when administering a medication.

1-4.13 Describe the indications, equipment needed, techniques utilized, precautions, and general principles of peripheral venous cannulation.

1-4.14 Describe the indications, equipment needed, techniques utilized, precautions, and general principles of intraosseous needle placement and infusion.

1-4.15 Describe the indications, equipment needed, techniques utilized, precautions, and general principles of administering medications by the inhalation route.

1-4.16 Differentiate among the different dosage forms for oral medications.

1-4.17 Describe the equipment needed and general principles of administering oral medications.

1-4.18 Describe the indications, equipment needed, techniques utilized, precautions, and general principles of rectal medication administration.

1-4.19 Differentiate among the different parenteral routes of medication administration.

1-4.20 Describe the equipment needed, techniques utilized, complications, and general principles for the preparation and administration of parenteral medications.

1-4.21 Differentiate among the different percutaneous routes of medication administration.

1-4.22 Describe the purpose, equipment needed, techniques utilized, complications, and general principles for obtaining a blood sample.

1-4.23 Describe disposal of contaminated items and sharps.

1-4.24 Synthesize a pharmacological management plan, including medication administration.

1-4.25 Integrate pathophysiological principles of medication administration with patient management.

Affective Objectives

At the completion of this unit, the EMT-Intermediate student will be able to:

1-4.26 Comply with EMT-Intermediate standards of medication administration.

1-4.27 Comply with universal precautions and body substance isolation (BSI).

1-4.28 Defend a pharmacologic management plan for medication administration.

1-4.29 Serve as a model for medical asepsis.

1-4.30 Serve as a model for advocacy while performing medication administration.

1-4.31 Serve as a model for disposing of contaminated items and sharps.

Psychomotor Objectives

At the completion of this unit, the
EMT-Intermediate student will be able to:

1-4.32 Use universal precautions and body substance isolation (BSI) procedures during medication administration.

1-4.33 Demonstrate cannulation of peripheral veins.

1-4.34 Demonstrate intraosseous needle placement and infusion.

1-4.35 Demonstrate clean technique during medication administration.

1-4.36 Demonstrate administration of medications by the inhalation route.

1-4.37 Demonstrate administration of oral medications.

1-4.38 Demonstrate rectal administration of medications.

1-4.39 Demonstrate preparation and administration of parenteral medications.

1-4.40 Demonstrate preparation and techniques for obtaining a blood sample.

1-4.41 Perfect disposal of contaminated items and sharps.

MODULE 2 AIRWAY

UNIT 2-1 AIRWAY MANAGEMENT AND VENTILATION

Cognitive Objectives

At the completion of this unit, the
EMT-Intermediate student will be able to:

2-1.1 Explain the primary objective of airway maintenance.

2-1.2 Identify commonly neglected prehospital skills related to airway.

2-1.3 Identify the anatomy and functions of the upper airway.

2-1.4 Describe the anatomy and functions of the lower airway.

2-1.5 Explain the differences between adult and pediatric airway anatomy.

2-1.6 Define normal tidal volumes for the adult, child, and infant.

2-1.7 Define atelectasis.

2-1.8 Define FiO_2.

2-1.9 Explain the relationship between pulmonary circulation and respiration.

2-1.10 List factors which cause decreased oxygen concentrations in the blood.

2-1.11 List the factors which increase and decrease carbon dioxide production in the body.

2-1.12 Describe the measurement of oxygen in the blood.

2-1.13 Describe the measurement of carbon dioxide in the blood.

2-1.14 List the concentration of gases which comprise atmospheric air.

2-1.15 List the factors which affect respiratory rate and depth.

2-1.16 Describe the voluntary and involuntary regulation of respiration.

2-1.17 Describe causes of upper airway obstruction.

2-1.18 Define normal respiratory rates for adult, child, and infant.

2-1.19 Describe causes of respiratory distress.

2-1.20 Define and differentiate between hypoxia and hypoxemia.

2-1.21 Define pulsus paradoxus.

2-1.22 Describe the modified forms of respiration.

2-1.23 Define gag reflex.

2-1.24 Explain safety considerations of oxygen storage and delivery.

2-1.25 Identify types of oxygen cylinders and pressure regulators (including a high-pressure regulator and a therapy regulator).

2-1.26 List the steps for delivering oxygen from a cylinder and regulator.

2-1.27 Describe the indications, contraindications, advantages, disadvantages, complications, liter flow range, and concentration of delivered oxygen for supplemental oxygen delivery devices.

2-1.28   Describe the use, advantages and disadvantages of an oxygen humidifier.

2-1.29   Define, identify, and describe a tracheostomy, stoma, and tracheostomy tube.

2-1.30   Explain the risk of infection to EMS providers associated with ventilation.

2-1.31   Describe the indications, contraindications, advantages, disadvantages, complications, and technique for ventilating a patient by:

   a.   Mouth-to-mouth
   b.   Mouth-to-nose
   c.   Mouth-to-mask
   d.   One-person bag-valve-mask
   e.   Two-person bag-valve-mask
   f.   Three-person bag-valve-mask
   g.   Flow-restricted, oxygen-powered ventilation device

2-1.32   Explain the advantage of the two person method when ventilating with the bag-valve-mask.

2-1.33   Describe indications, contraindications, advantages, disadvantages, complications, and technique for ventilating a patient with an automatic transport ventilator (ATV).

2-1.34   Describe the Sellick (cricoid pressure) maneuver.

2-1.35   Describe the use of cricoid pressure during intubation.

2-1.36   Compare the ventilation techniques used for an adult patient to those used for pediatric patients.

2-1.37   Define how to ventilate a patient with a stoma, including mouth-to-stoma and bag-valve-mask-to-stoma ventilation.

2-1.38   Define complete airway obstruction.

2-1.39   Define and explain the implications of partial airway obstruction with good and poor air exchange.

2-1.40   Describe complete airway obstruction maneuvers.

2-1.41   Describe laryngoscopy for the removal of a foreign body airway obstruction.

2-1.42   Identify types of suction catheters, including hard or rigid catheters and soft catheters.

2-1.43   Explain the purpose for suctioning the upper airway.

2-1.44   Identify types of suction equipment.

2-1.45   Describe the indications for suctioning the upper airway.

2-1.46   Identify the techniques of suctioning the upper airway.

2-1.47   Identify special considerations of suctioning the upper airway.

2-1.48   Describe the technique of tracheobronchial suctioning in the intubated patient.

2-1.49   Define gastric distention.

2-1.50   Describe the indications, contraindications, advantages, disadvantages, complications, equipment, and technique for inserting a nasogastric tube and orogastric tube.

2-1.51   Describe manual airway maneuvers.

2-1.52   Describe the use of an oral and nasal airway.

2-1.53   Describe the indications, contraindications, advantages, disadvantages, complications, and technique for inserting an oropharyngeal and nasopharyngeal airway.

2-1.54   Differentiate endotracheal intubation from other methods of advanced airway management.

2-1.55   Describe the indications, contraindications, advantages, disadvantages, and complications of endotracheal intubation.

2-1.56   Describe the visual landmarks for direct laryngoscopy.

2-1.57 Describe the methods of assessment for confirming correct placement of an endotracheal tube.

2-1.58 Describe methods for securing an endotracheal tube.

2-1.59 Describe the indications, contraindications, advantages, disadvantages, complications, equipment, and technique for extubation.

2-1.60 Describe methods of endotracheal intubation in the pediatric patient.

2-1.61 Describe the indications, contraindications, advantages, disadvantages, complications, equipment, and technique for using a dual lumen airway.

2-1.62 Define, identify, and describe a laryngectomy.

2-1.63 Describe the special considerations in airway management and ventilation for patients with facial injuries.

2-1.64 Describe the special considerations in airway management and ventilation for the pediatric patient.

Affective Objectives

At the completion of this unit, the EMT-Intermediate student will be able to:

2-1.65 Defend oxygenation and ventilation.

2-1.66 Defend the necessity of establishing and/or maintaining patency of a patient's airway.

2-1.67 Comply with standard precautions to defend against infectious and communicable diseases.

Psychomotor Objectives

At the completion of this unit, the EMT-Intermediate student will be able to:

2-1.68 Perform body substance isolation (BSI) procedures during basic airway management, advanced airway management, and ventilation.

2-1.69 Perform pulse oximetry.

2-1.70 Perform end-tidal CO_2 detection.

2-1.71 Perform oxygen delivery from a cylinder and regulator with an oxygen delivery device.

2-1.72 Deliver supplemental oxygen to a breathing patient using the following devices: nasal cannula, simple face mask, partial rebreather mask, nonrebreather mask, and Venturi mask.

2-1.73 Perform oxygen delivery with an oxygen humidifier.

2-1.74 Perform medication administration with an in-line small-volume nebulizer.

2-1.75 Demonstrate ventilating a patient by the following techniques:
   a. Mouth-to-mask ventilation
   b. One-person bag-valve-mask
   c. Two-person bag-valve-mask
   d. Three-person bag-valve-mask
   e. Flow-restricted, oxygen-powered ventilation device
   f. Automatic transport ventilator
   g. Mouth-to-stoma
   h. Bag-valve-mask-to-stoma ventilation

2-1.76 Perform the Sellick maneuver (cricoid pressure).

2-1.77 Ventilate a pediatric patient using the one- and two-person techniques.

2-1.78 Perform complete airway obstruction maneuvers, including:
   a. Heimlich maneuver
   b. Finger sweep
   c. Chest thrusts
   d. Removal with Magill forceps

2-1.79 Perform retrieval of foreign bodies from the upper airway.

2-1.80 Demonstrate suctioning the upper airway by selecting a suction device, catheter, and technique.

2-1.81 Perform tracheobronchial suctioning in the intubated patient by selecting a suction device, catheter, and technique.

2-1.82 Demonstrate insertion of a nasogastric tube.

2-1.83 Demonstrate insertion of an orogastric tube.

2-1.84 Perform gastric decompression by selecting a suction device, catheter, and technique.

2-1.85 Perform manual airway maneuvers, including:

   a.   Opening the mouth
   b.   Head tilt/chin lift maneuver
   c.   Jaw-thrust without head tilt maneuver
   d.   Modified jaw-thrust maneuver

2-1.86 Perform manual airway maneuvers for pediatric patients, including:

   a.   Opening the mouth
   b.   Head tilt/chin lift maneuver
   c.   Jaw-thrust without head tilt maneuver
   d.   Modified jaw-thrust maneuver

2-1.87 Demonstrate insertion of an oropharyngeal airway.

2-1.88 Demonstrate insertion of a nasopharyngeal airway.

2-1.89 Intubate the trachea by direct orotracheal intubation.

2-1.90 Perform assessment to confirm correct placement of the endotracheal tube.

2-1.91 Adequately secure an endotracheal tube.

2-1.92 Perform extubation.

2-1.93 Perform endotracheal intubation in the pediatric patient.

2-1.94 Insert a dual lumen airway.

2-1.95 Perform stoma suctioning.

2-1.96 Perform replacement of a tracheostomy tube through a stoma.

MODULE 3 PATIENT ASSESSMENT

UNIT 3-1 HISTORY TAKING

Cognitive Objectives

At the completion of this unit, the EMT-Intermediate student will be able to:

3-1.1 Describe the factors that influence the EMT-Intermediate's ability to collect medical history.

3-1.2 Describe the techniques of history taking.

3-1.3 Discuss the importance of using open- and closed-ended questions.

3-1.4 Describe the use of facilitation, reflection, clarification, empathetic responses, confrontation, and interpretation.

3-1.5 Differentiate between facilitation, reflection, clarification, empathetic responses, confrontation, and interpretation.

3-1.6 Describe the structure and purpose of a health history.

3-1.7 Describe how to obtain a health history.

3-1.8 List the components of a history of an adult patient.

3-1.9 List and describe strategies to overcome situations that represent special challenges in obtaining a medical history.

Affective Objectives

At the completion of this unit, the EMT-Intermediate student will be able to:

3-1.10 Demonstrate the importance of empathy when obtaining a health history.

3-1.11 Demonstrate the importance of confidentiality when obtaining a health history.

Psychomotor Objectives

None identified for this unit.

UNIT 3-2 TECHNIQUES OF PHYSICAL EXAMINATION

Cognitive Objectives

At the completion of this unit, the EMT-Intermediate student will be able to:

3-2.1 Define the terms inspection, palpation, percussion, auscultation.

3-2.2 Describe the techniques of inspection, palpation, percussion, and auscultation.

3-2.3 Review the procedure for taking and significance of vital signs (pulse, respiration, and blood pressure).

3-2.4 Describe the evaluation of mental status.

3-2.5 Evaluate the importance of a general survey.

3-2.6 Describe the examination of skin and nails.

3-2.7 Differentiate normal and abnormal findings of the assessment of the skin.

3-2.8 Distinguish the importance of abnormal findings of the assessment of the skin.

3-2.9 Describe the normal and abnormal assessment findings of the head (including the scalp, skull, face, and skin).

3-2.10 Describe the examination of the head (including the scalp, skull, face, and skin).

3-2.11 Describe the examination of the eyes.

3-2.12 Distinguish between normal and abnormal assessment findings of the eyes.

3-2.13 Describe the examination of the ears.

3-2.14 Differentiate normal and abnormal assessment findings of the ears.

3-2.15 Describe the examination of the nose.

3-2.16 Differentiate normal and abnormal assessment findings of the nose.

3-2.17 Describe the examination of the mouth and pharynx.

3-2.18 Differentiate normal and abnormal assessment findings of the mouth and pharynx.

3-2.19 Describe the examination of the neck and cervical spine.

3-2.20 Differentiate normal and abnormal assessment findings of the neck and cervical spine.

3-2.21 Describe the inspection, palpation, percussion, and auscultation of the chest.

3-2.22 Describe the examination of the thorax and ventilation.

3-2.23 Describe the examination of the anterior and posterior chest.

3-2.24 Differentiate the percussion sounds and their characteristics.

3-2.25 Differentiate the characteristics of breath sounds.

3-2.26 Differentiate normal and abnormal assessment findings of the chest examination.

3-2.27 Describe the examination of the arterial pulse, including rate, rhythm, and amplitude.

3-2.28 Differentiate normal and abnormal findings of arterial pulse.

3-2.29 Describe the assessment of jugular venous pressure and pulsations.

3-2.30 Differentiate normal and abnormal examination findings of jugular venous pressure and pulsations.

3-2.31 Describe the examination of the heart.

3-2.32 Differentiate normal and abnormal assessment findings of the heart.

3-2.33 Describe the auscultation of the heart.

3-2.34 Differentiate the characteristics of normal and abnormal findings associated with the auscultation of the heart.

3-2.35 Describe the examination of the abdomen.

3-2.36 Differentiate normal and abnormal assessment findings of the abdomen.

3-2.37 Describe the examination of the female external genitalia.

3-2.38 Differentiate normal and abnormal assessment findings of the genitalia.

3-2.39 Describe the examination of the male genitalia.

3-2.40 Differentiate normal and abnormal assessment findings of the male genitalia.

3-2.41 Describe the examination of the extremities.

3-2.42 Differentiate normal and abnormal assessment findings of the extremities.

3-2.43 Describe the examination of the peripheral vascular system.

3-2.44 Differentiate normal and abnormal assessment findings of the peripheral vascular system.

3-2.45 Describe the examination of the nervous system.

3-2.46 Differentiate normal and abnormal assessment findings of the nervous system.

3-2.47 Discuss the considerations of examination of an infant or child.

3-2.48 Describe the general guidelines of recording examination information.

Affective Objectives

At the completion of this unit, the EMT-Intermediate student will be able to:

3-2.49 Demonstrate a caring attitude when performing physical examination skills.

3-2.50 Discuss the importance of a professional appearance and demeanor when performing physical examination skills.

3-2.51 Appreciate the limitations of conducting a physical exam in the out-of-hospital environment.

Psychomotor Objectives

At the completion of this unit, the EMT-Intermediate student will be able to:

3-2.52 Demonstrate the examination of skin and nails.

3-2.53 Demonstrate the examination of the head and neck.

3-2.54 Demonstrate the examination of the eyes.

3-2.55 Demonstrate the examination of the ears.

3-2.56 Demonstrate the examination of the nose.

3-2.57 Demonstrate the examination of the mouth.

3-2.58 Demonstrate the examination of the neck.

3-2.59 Demonstrate the examination of the thorax and ventilation.

3-2.60 Demonstrate the examination of the anterior and posterior chest.

3-2.61 Demonstrate auscultation of the chest.

3-2.62 Demonstrate percussion of the chest.

3-2.63 Demonstrate the examination of the arterial pulse, including location, rate, rhythm, and amplitude.

3-2.64 Demonstrate the assessment of jugular venous pressure and pulsations.

3-2.65 Demonstrate the examination of the heart.

3-2.66 Demonstrate the examination of the abdomen.

3-2.67 Demonstrate auscultation of the abdomen.

3-2.68 Demonstrate the external visual examination of the female external genitalia.

3-2.69 Demonstrate the examination of the male genitalia.

3-2.70 Demonstrate the examination of the peripheral vascular system.

3-2.71 Demonstrate the examination of the extremities.

3-2.72 Demonstrate the examination of the nervous system.

UNIT 3-3 PATIENT ASSESSMENT

Cognitive Objectives

At the completion of this unit, the EMT-Intermediate student will be able to:

3-3.1 Recognize hazards/potential hazards.

3-3.2 Describe common hazards found at the scene of a trauma and a medical patient.

3-3.3 Determine hazards found at the scene of a medical or trauma patient.

3-3.4 Differentiate safe from unsafe scenes.

3-3.5 Describe methods of making an unsafe scene safe.

3-3.6 Discuss common mechanisms of injury/nature of illness.

3-3.7 Recognize the importance of determining the mechanism of injury.

3-3.8 Discuss the reason for identifying the total number of patients at the scene.

3-3.9 Organize the management of a scene following size-up.

3-3.10 Explain the reasons for identifying the need for additional help or assistance.

3-3.11 Summarize the reasons for forming a general impression of the patient.

3-3.12 Discuss methods of assessing mental status.

3-3.13 Categorize levels of consciousness.

3-3.14 Discuss methods of assessing the airway.

3-3.15 Describe why the cervical spine is immobilized during the assessment of the trauma patient.

3-3.16 Analyze a scene to determine if spinal precautions are required.

3-3.17 Describe methods used for assessing if a patient is breathing.

3-3.18 Differentiate between a patient with adequate and inadequate minute ventilation.

3-3.19 Discuss the need for assessing the patient for external bleeding.

3-3.20 Describe normal and abnormal findings when assessing skin color.

3-3.21 Describe normal and abnormal findings when assessing skin temperature.

3-3.22 Describe normal and abnormal findings when assessing skin condition.

3-3.23 Explain the reason for prioritizing a patient for care and transport.

3-3.24 Identify patients who require expeditious transport.

3-3.25 Describe orthostatic vital signs and evaluate their usefulness in assessing a patient in shock.

3-3.26 Apply the techniques of physical examination to the medical patient.

3-3.27 Differentiate between the assessment that is performed for a patient who has an altered mental status and other medical patients.

3-3.28 Discuss the reasons for reconsidering the mechanism of injury.

3-3.29 State the reasons for performing a rapid trauma assessment.

3-3.30 Recite examples and explain why patients should receive a rapid trauma assessment.

3-3.31 Apply the techniques of physical examination to the trauma patient.

3-3.32 Describe the areas included in the rapid trauma assessment and discuss what should be evaluated.

3-3.33 Differentiate cases when the rapid assessment may be altered in order to provide patient care.

3-3.34 Discuss the reason for performing a focused history and physical exam.

3-3.35 Describe when and why a detailed physical examination is necessary.

3-3.36 Discuss the components of the detailed physical exam in relation to the techniques of examination.

3-3.37 State the areas of the body that are evaluated during the detailed physical exam.

3-3.38 Explain what additional care should be provided while performing the detailed physical exam.

3-3.39 Distinguish between the detailed physical exam that is performed on a trauma patient and that of the medical patient.

3-3.40 Differentiate between patients requiring a detailed physical exam from those who do not.

3-3.41 Discuss the reasons for repeating the initial assessment as part of the ongoing assessment.

3-3.42 Describe the components of the ongoing assessment.

3-3.43 Describe the trending of assessment components.

3-3.44 Discuss medical identification devices/systems.

Affective Objectives

At the completion of this unit, the EMT-Intermediate student will be able to:

3-3.45 Explain the rationale for crew members to evaluate scene safety prior to entering.

3-3.46 Serve as a model for others explaining how patient situations affect your evaluation of mechanism of injury or illness.

3-3.47 Explain the importance of forming a general impression of the patient.

3-3.48 Explain the value of performing an initial assessment.

3-3.49 Demonstrate a caring attitude when performing an initial assessment.

3-3.50 Attend to the feelings that patients with medical conditions might be experiencing.

3-3.51 Value the need for maintaining a professional caring attitude when performing a focused history and physical examination.

3-3.52 Explain the rationale for the feelings that these patients might be experiencing.

3-3.53 Demonstrate a caring attitude when performing a detailed physical examination.

3-3.54 Explain the value of performing an ongoing assessment.

3-3.55 Recognize and respect the feelings that patients might experience during assessment.

3-3.56 Explain the value of trending assessment components to other health professionals who assume care of the patient.

Psychomotor Objectives

At the completion of this unit, the EMT-Intermediate student will be able to:

3-3.57 Demonstrate the techniques for assessing mental status.

3-3.58 Demonstrate the techniques for assessing the airway.

3-3.59 Demonstrate the techniques for determining if the patient is breathing.

3-3.60 Demonstrate the techniques for determining if the patient has a pulse.

3-3.61 Demonstrate the techniques for determining the patient for external bleeding.

3-3.62 Demonstrate the techniques for determining the patient's skin color, temperature, and condition.

3-3.63 Using the techniques of examination, demonstrate the assessment of a medical patient.

3-3.64 Demonstrate the techniques for assessing a patient who is responsive with no known history.

3-3.65 Demonstrate the techniques for assessing a patient who has an altered mental status.

3-3.66 Perform a rapid medical assessment.

3-3.67 Perform a focused history and physical exam of the medical patient.

3-3.68 Using the techniques of physical examination, demonstrate the assessment of a trauma patient.

3-3.69 Demonstrate the rapid trauma assessment used to assess a patient based on mechanism of injury.

3-3.70 Perform a focused history and physical exam on a non–critically injured patient.

3-3.71 Perform a focused history and physical exam on a patient with life-threatening injuries.

3-3.72 Perform a detailed physical examination.

3-3.73 Demonstrate the skills involved in performing the ongoing assessment.

UNIT 3-4 CLINICAL DECISION MAKING

Cognitive Objectives

At the completion of this unit, the EMT-Intermediate student will be able to:

3-4.1 Compare the factors influencing medical care in the out-of-hospital environment to other medical settings.

3-4.2 Differentiate between critical life-threatening, potentially life-threatening, and non–life-threatening patient presentations.

3-4.3 Evaluate the benefits and shortfalls of protocols, standing orders, and patient care algorithms.

3-4.4 Define the components, stages, and sequences of the critical thinking process for EMT-Intermediates.

3-4.5 Apply the fundamental elements of critical thinking for EMT-Intermediates.

3-4.6 Describe the effects of the "fight or flight" response and the positive and negative effects on an EMT-Intermediate's decision making.

3-4.7 Develop strategies for effective thinking under pressure.

3-4.8 Summarize the "six Rs" of putting it all together: Read the patient, Read the scene, React, Reevaluate, Revise the management plan, Review performance.

Affective Objectives

At the completion of this unit, the EMT-Intermediate student will be able to:

3-4.9 Defend the position that clinical decision making is the cornerstone of effective EMT-Intermediate practice.

3-4.10 Practice facilitating behaviors when thinking under pressure.

Psychomotor Objectives

None identified for this unit.

UNIT 3-5 COMMUNICATIONS

Cognitive Objectives

At the completion of this unit, the EMT-Intermediate student will be able to:

3-5.1 Identify the importance of communications when providing EMS.

3-5.2 Identify the role of verbal, written, and electronic communications in the provision of EMS.

3-5.3 Describe the phases of communications necessary to complete a typical EMS event.

3-5.4 Identify the importance of proper terminology when communicating during an EMS event.

3-5.5 Identify the importance of proper verbal communications during an EMS event.

3-5.6 List factors that impede effective verbal communications.

3-5.7 List factors which enhance verbal communications.

3-5.8 Identify the importance of proper written communications during an EMS event.

3-5.9 List factors which impede effective written communications.

3-5.10 List factors which enhance written communications.

3-5.11 Recognize the legal status of written communications related to an EMS event.

3-5.12 State the importance of data collection during an EMS event.

3-5.13 Identify technology used to collect and exchange patient and/or scene information electronically.

3-5.14 Recognize the legal status of patient medical information exchanged electronically.

3-5.15 Identify and differentiate among the following communications systems:
   a. Simplex
   b. Duplex
   c. Multiplex
   d. Trucked
   e. Digital communications
   f. Cellular telephone
   g. Facsimile
   h. Computer

3-5.16 Identify the components of the local dispatch communications system and describe their function and use.

3-5.17 Describe the functions and responsibilities of the Federal Communications Commission.

3-5.18 Describe how the emergency medical dispatcher functions as an integral part of the EMS team.

3-5.19 List appropriate information to be gathered by the emergency medical dispatcher.

3-5.20 Identify the role of Emergency Medical Dispatch in a typical EMS event.

3-5.21 Identify the importance of prearrival instructions in a typical EMS event.

3-5.22 Describe the procedure of verbal communication of patient information to the hospital.

3-5.23 Describe information that should be included in patient assessment information verbally reported to medical direction.

3-5.24 Diagram a basic model of communications.

3-5.25 Organize a list of patient assessment information in the correct order for electronic transmission to medical direction according to the format used locally.

Affective Objectives

At the completion of this unit, the EMT-Intermediate student will be able to:

3-5.26 Show appreciation for proper terminology when describing a patient or patient condition.

Psychomotor Objectives

At the completion of this unit, the EMT-Intermediate student will be able to:

3-5.27 Demonstrate the ability to use the local dispatch communications system.

3-5.28 Demonstrate the ability to use a radio.

3-5.29 Demonstrate the ability to use the biotelemetry equipment used locally.

UNIT 3-6 DOCUMENTATION

Cognitive Objectives

At the completion of this unit, the EMT-Intermediate student will be able to:

3-6.1 Identify the general principles regarding the importance of EMS documentation and ways in which documents are used.

3-6.2 Identify and use medical terminology correctly.

3-6.3 Recite appropriate and accurate medical abbreviations and acronyms.

3-6.4 Record all pertinent administrative information.

3-6.5 Explain the role of documentation in agency reimbursement.

3-6.6 Analyze the documentation for accuracy and completeness, including spelling.

3-6.7 Identify and eliminate extraneous or nonprofessional information.

3-6.8 Describe the differences between subjective and objective elements of documentation.

3-6.9 Evaluate a finished document for errors and omissions.

3-6.10 Evaluate a finished document for proper use and spelling of abbreviations and acronyms.

3-6.11 Evaluate the confidential nature of an EMS report.

3-6.12 Describe the potential consequences of illegible, incomplete, or inaccurate documentation.

3-6.13 Describe the special considerations concerning patient refusal of transport.

3-6.14 Record pertinent information using a consistent narrative format.

3-6.15 Explain how to properly record direct patient or bystander comments.

3-6.16 Describe the special considerations concerning mass casualty incident documentation.

3-6.17 Apply the principles of documentation to computer charting as access to this technology becomes available.

3-6.18 Identify and record the pertinent, reportable clinical data of each patient interaction.

3-6.19 Note and record "pertinent negative" clinical findings.

3-6.20 Correct errors and omissions using proper procedures as defined under local protocol.

3-6.21 Revise documents, when necessary, using locally approved procedures.

3-6.22 Assume responsibility for self-assessment of all documentation.

3-6.23 Demonstrate proper completion of an EMS event record used locally.

Affective Objectives

At the completion of this unit, the EMT-Intermediate student will be able to:

3-6.24 Advocate among peers the relevance and importance of properly completed documentation.

3-6.25 Resolve the common negative attitudes toward the task of documentation.

Psychomotor Objectives

None identified for this unit.

MODULE 4 TRAUMA

UNIT 4-1 TRAUMA SYSTEMS AND MECHANISM OF INJURY

Cognitive Objectives

At the completion of this unit, the EMT-Intermediate student will be able to:

4-1.1 List and describe the components of a comprehensive trauma system.

4-1.2 Describe the role of and differences between levels of trauma centers.

4-1.3 Describe the criteria for transport to a trauma center.

4-1.4 Describe the criteria and procedure for air medical transport.

4-1.5 Define energy and force as they relate to trauma.

4-1.6 Define laws of motion and energy and understand the role that increased speed has on injuries.

4-1.7 Describe each type of impact and its effect on unrestrained victims (e.g., frontal impacts, lateral impacts, rear impacts, rotational impacts, rollover).

4-1.8 Describe the pathophysiology of the head, spine, thorax, and abdomen that results from the above forces.

4-1.9 Describe the organ collisions that occur in blunt trauma and vehicular collisions.

4-1.10 Describe the effects that restraint systems (including seat belts, air bags, and child safety seats) have on the injury patterns found in motor vehicle crashes.

4-1.11 List specific injuries and their causes as related to interior and exterior vehicle damage.

4-1.12 Describe the kinematics of penetrating injuries.

4-1.13 List the motion and energy considerations of mechanisms other than motor vehicle crashes.

4-1.14 Define the role of kinematics as an additional tool for patient assessment.

Affective Objectives

None identified for this unit.

Psychomotor Objectives

None identified for this unit.

UNIT 4-2 HEMORRHAGE AND SHOCK

Cognitive Objectives

At the completion of this unit, the EMT-Intermediate student will be able to:

4-2.1 Describe the epidemiology, including the morbidity, mortality, and prevention strategies for shock and hemorrhage.

4-2.2 Discuss the various types and degrees of hemorrhage and shock.

4-2.3 Discuss the pathophysiology of hemorrhage and shock.

4-2.4 Discuss the assessment findings associated with hemorrhage and shock.

4-2.5 Identify the need for intervention and transport of the patient with hemorrhage or shock.

4-2.6 Discuss the treatment plan and management of hemorrhage and shock.

4-2.7 Discuss the management of external and internal hemorrhage.

4-2.8 Differentiate between controlled and uncontrolled hemorrhage.

4-2.9 Differentiate between the administration rate and amount of IV fluid in a patient with controlled versus uncontrolled hemorrhage.

4-2.10 Relate internal hemorrhage to the pathophysiology of compensated and decompensated hypovolemic shock.

4-2.11 Relate internal hemorrhage to the assessment findings of compensated and decompensated hypovolemic shock.

4-2.12 Describe the body's physiologic response to changes in perfusion.

4-2.13 Describe the effects of decreased perfusion at the capillary level.

4-2.14 Discuss the cellular ischemic phase related to hemorrhagic shock.

4-2.15 Discuss the capillary stagnation phase related to hypovolemic shock.

4-2.16 Discuss the capillary washout phase related to hypovolemic shock.

4-2.17 Discuss the assessment findings of hypovolemic shock.

4-2.18 Relate pulse pressure changes to perfusion status.

4-2.19 Define compensated and decompensated shock.

4-2.20 Discuss the pathophysiological changes associated with compensated shock.

4-2.21 Discuss the assessment findings associated with compensated shock.

4-2.22 Identify the need for intervention and transport of the patient with compensated shock.

4-2.23 Discuss the treatment plan and management of compensated shock.

4-2.24 Discuss the pathophysiological changes associated with decompensated shock.

4-2.25 Discuss the assessment findings associated with decompensated shock.

4-2.26 Identify the need for intervention and transport of the patient with decompensated shock.

4-2.27 Discuss the treatment plan and management of the patient with decompensated shock.

4-2.28 Differentiate between compensated and decompensated shock.

4-2.29 Relate external hemorrhage to the pathophysiology of compensated and decompensated hypovolemic shock.

4-2.30 Relate external hemorrhage to the assessment findings of compensated and decompensated hypovolemic shock.

4-2.31 Differentiate between the normotensive, hypotensive, and profoundly hypotensive patient.

4-2.32 Differentiate between the administration of fluid in the normotensive, hypotensive, and profoundly hypotensive patient.

4-2.33 Discuss the physiologic changes associated with the pneumatic antishock garment (PASG).

4-2.34 Discuss the indications and contraindications for the application and inflation of the PASG.

4-2.35 Apply epidemiology to develop prevention strategies for hemorrhage and shock.

4-2.36 Integrate the pathophysiological principles to the assessment of a patient with hemorrhage or shock.

4-2.37 Synthesize assessment findings and patient history information to form a field impression for the patient with hemorrhage or shock.

4-2.38 Develop, execute, and evaluate a treatment plan based on the field impression for the hemorrhage or shock patient.

4-2.39 Differentiate between the management of compensated and decompensated shock.

Affective Objectives

None identified for this unit.

Psychomotor Objectives

At the completion of this unit, the EMT-Intermediate student will be able to:

4-2.40 Demonstrate the assessment of a patient with signs and symptoms of hypovolemic shock.

4-2.41 Demonstrate the management of a patient with signs and symptoms of hypovolemic shock.

4-2.42 Demonstrate the assessment of a patient with signs and symptoms of compensated hypovolemic shock.

4-2.43 Demonstrate the management of a patient with signs and symptoms of compensated hypovolemic shock.

4-2.44 Demonstrate the assessment of a patient with signs and symptoms of decompensated hypovolemic shock.

4-2.45 Demonstrate the management of a patient with signs and symptoms of decompensated hypovolemic shock.

4-2.46 Demonstrate the assessment of a patient with signs and symptoms of external hemorrhage.

4-2.47 Demonstrate the management of a patient with signs and symptoms of external hemorrhage.

4-2.48 Demonstrate the assessment of a patient with signs and symptoms of internal hemorrhage.

4-2.49 Demonstrate the management of a patient with signs and symptoms of internal hemorrhage.

UNIT 4-3 BURNS

Cognitive Objectives

At the completion of this unit, the EMT-Intermediate student will be able to:

4-3.1 Describe the anatomy and physiology pertinent to burn injuries.

4-3.2 Describe the epidemiology, including incidence, morbidity/mortality, risk factors, and prevention strategies for the patient with a burn injury.

4-3.3 Describe the pathophysiologic complications and systemic complications of a burn injury.

4-3.4 Identify and describe types of burn injuries, including a thermal burn, an inhalation burn, a chemical burn, an electrical burn, and a radiation exposure.

4-3.5 Identify and describe the depth classifications of burn injuries, including a superficial burn, a partial thickness burn, a full-thickness burn, and other depth classifications described by local protocol.

4-3.6 Identify and describe methods for determining body surface area percentage of a burn injury, including the "rule of nines," the "rule of palms," and other methods described by local protocol.

4-3.7 Identify and describe the severity of a burn, including a minor burn, a moderate burn, a severe burn, and other severity classifications described by local protocol.

4-3.8 Differentiate criteria for determining the severity of a burn injury between a pediatric patient and an adult patient.

4-3.9 Describe special considerations for a pediatric patient with a burn injury.

4-3.10 Discuss considerations which impact management and prognosis of the burn injured patient.

4-3.11 Discuss mechanisms of burn injuries.

4-3.12 Discuss conditions associated with burn injuries, including trauma, blast injuries, airway compromise, respiratory compromise, and child abuse.

4-3.13 Describe the management of a burn injury, including airway and ventilation, circulation, pharmacologic, nonpharmacologic, transport considerations, psychological support/communication strategies, and other management described by local protocol.

4-3.14 Describe the epidemiology of a thermal burn injury.

4-3.15 Describe the specific anatomy and physiology pertinent to a thermal burn injury.

4-3.16 Describe the pathophysiology of a thermal burn injury.

4-3.17 Identify and describe the depth classifications of a thermal burn injury.

4-3.18 Identify and describe the severity of a thermal burn injury.

4-3.19 Describe considerations which impact management and prognosis of the patient with a thermal burn injury.

4-3.20 Discuss mechanisms of burn injury and conditions associated with a thermal burn injury.

4-3.21 Describe the management of a thermal burn injury, including airway and ventilation, circulation, pharmacologic, nonpharmacologic, transport considerations, and psychological support/communication strategies.

4-3.22 Describe the epidemiology of an inhalation burn injury.

4-3.23 Describe the specific anatomy and physiology pertinent to an inhalation burn injury.

4-3.24 Describe the pathophysiology of an inhalation burn injury,

4-3.25 Differentiate between supraglottic and infraglottic inhalation injuries.

4-3.26 Identify and describe the severity of an inhalation burn injury.

4-3.27 Describe considerations which impact management and prognosis of the patient with an inhalation burn injury.

4-3.28 Discuss mechanisms of burn injury and conditions associated with an inhalation burn injury.

4-3.29 Describe the management of an inhalation burn injury, including airway and ventilation, circulation, pharmacologic, nonpharmacologic, transport considerations, and psychological support/communication strategies.

4-3.30 Describe the epidemiology of a chemical burn injury and a chemical burn injury to the eye.

4-3.31 Describe the specific anatomy and physiology pertinent to a chemical burn injury and a chemical burn injury to the eye.

4-3.32 Describe the pathophysiology of a chemical burn injury, including types of chemicals and their burning processes and a chemical burn injury to the eye.

4-3.33 Identify and describe the depth classifications of a chemical burn injury.

4-3.34 Identify and describe the severity of a chemical burn injury.

4-3.35 Describe considerations which impact management and prognosis of the patient with a chemical burn injury and a chemical burn injury to the eye.

4-3.36 Discuss mechanisms of burn injury and conditions associated with a chemical burn injury.

4-3.37 Describe the management of a chemical burn injury to the eye, including airway and ventilation, circulation, pharmacologic, nonpharmacologic, transport considerations, and psychological support/communication strategies.

4-3.38 Describe the epidemiology of an electrical burn injury.

4-3.39 Describe the specific anatomy and physiology pertinent to an electrical burn injury.

4-3.40 Describe the pathophysiology of an electrical burn injury.

4-3.41 Identify and describe the depth classifications of an electrical burn injury.

4-3.42 Identify and describe the severity of an electrical burn injury.

4-3.43 Describe considerations which impact management and prognosis of the patient with an electrical burn injury.

4-3.44 Discuss mechanisms of burn injury and conditions associated with an electrical burn injury.

4-3.45 Describe the management of an electrical burn injury, including airway and ventilation, circulation, pharmacologic, nonpharmacologic, transport considerations, and psychological support/communication strategies.

4-3.46 Describe the epidemiology of a radiation exposure.

4-3.47 Describe the specific anatomy and physiology pertinent to a radiation exposure.

4-3.48 Describe the pathophysiology of a radiation exposure, including the types and characteristics of ionizing radiation.

4-3.49 Identify and describe the depth classifications of a radiation exposure.

4-3.50 Identify and describe the severity of a radiation exposure.

4-3.51 Describe considerations which impact management and prognosis of the patient with a radiation exposure.

4-3.52 Discuss mechanisms of burn injury associated with a radiation exposure.

4-3.53 Describe the management of a radiation exposure, including airway and ventilation, circulation, pharmacologic, nonpharmacologic, transport considerations, and psychological support/communication strategies.

4-3.54 Apply the information to formulate a field impression and implement the management plan for a thermal burn injury.

4-3.55 Apply the information to formulate a field impression and implement the management plan for an inhalation burn injury.

4-3.56 Apply the information to formulate a field impression and implement the management plan for a chemical burn injury.

4-3.57 Apply the information to formulate a field impression and implement the management plan for an electrical burn injury.

4-3.58 Apply the information to formulate a field impression and implement the management plan for a radiation exposure.

Affective Objectives

At the completion of this unit, the EMT-Intermediate student will be able to:

4-3.59 Value the changes of a patient's self-image associated with a burn injury.

4-3.60 Value the impact of managing a burn-injured patient.

4-3.61 Advocate empathy for a burn-injured patient.

4-3.62 Value and defend the sense of urgency in burn injuries.

Psychomotor Objectives

At the completion of this unit, the EMT-Intermediate student will be able to:

4-3.63 Take body substance isolation procedures during assessment and management of patients with a burn injury.

4-3.64 Perform assessment of a patient with a burn injury.

UNIT 4-4 THORACIC TRAUMA

Cognitive Objectives

At the completion of this unit, the EMT-Intermediate student will be able to:

4-4.1 Describe the incidence, morbidity, and mortality of thoracic injuries in the trauma patient.

4-4.2   Discuss the anatomy and physiology of the organs and structures related to thoracic injuries.

4-4.3   Predict thoracic injuries based on mechanism of injury.

4-4.4   Discuss the types of thoracic injuries.

4-4.5   Discuss the pathophysiology of thoracic injuries.

4-4.6   Discuss the assessment findings associated with thoracic injuries.

4-4.7   Discuss the management of thoracic injuries.

4-4.8   Identify the need for rapid intervention and transport of the patient with thoracic injuries.

4-4.9   Discuss the epidemiology and pathophysiology of specific chest wall injuries, including:

   a.   Rib fracture
   b.   Flail segment
   c.   Sternal fracture

4-4.10   Discuss the assessment findings associated with chest wall injuries.

4-4.11   Identify the need for rapid intervention and transport of the patient with chest wall injuries.

4-4.12   Discuss the management of chest wall injuries.

4-4.13   Discuss the pathophysiology of injury to the lung, including:

   a.   Simple pneumothorax
   b.   Open pneumothorax
   c.   Tension pneumothorax
   d.   Hemothorax
   e.   Hemopneumothorax
   f.   Pulmonary contusion

4-4.14   Discuss the assessment findings associated with lung injuries.

4-4.15   Discuss the management of lung injuries.

4-4.16   Identify the need for rapid intervention and transport of the patient with lung injuries.

4-4.17   Discuss the pathophysiology of myocardial injuries, including:

   a.   Pericardial tamponade
   b.   Myocardial contusion

4-4.18   Discuss the assessment findings associated with myocardial injuries.

4-4.19   Discuss the management of myocardial injuries.

4-4.20   Identify the need for rapid intervention and transport of the patient with myocardial injuries.

4-4.21   Discuss the pathophysiology of vascular injuries, including injuries to:

   a.   Aorta dissection/rupture
   b.   Vena cava
   c.   Pulmonary arteries/veins

4-4.22   Discuss the assessment findings associated with vascular injuries.

4-4.23   Discuss the management of vascular injuries.

4-4.24   Discuss the pathophysiology of diaphragmatic injuries.

4-4.25   Discuss the assessment findings associated with diaphragmatic injuries.

4-4.26   Discuss the management of diaphragmatic injuries.

4-4.27   Discuss the pathophysiology of esophageal injuries.

4-4.28   Discuss the assessment findings associated with esophageal injuries.

4-4.29   Discuss the management of esophageal injuries.

4-4.30   Discuss the pathophysiology of tracheobronchial injuries.

4-4.31   Discuss the assessment findings associated with tracheobronchial injuries.

4-4.32   Discuss the management of tracheobronchial injuries.

4-4.33   Discuss the pathophysiology of traumatic asphyxia.

4-4.34   Discuss the assessment findings associated with traumatic asphyxia.

4-4.35 Discuss the management of traumatic asphyxia.

4-4.36 Differentiate between thoracic injuries based on the assessment and history.

4-4.37 Formulate a field impression based on the assessment findings.

4-4.38 Develop a patient management plan based on the field impression.

Affective Objectives

At the completion of this unit, the EMT-Intermediate student will be able to:

4-4.39 Advocate the use of a thorough assessment to determine a differential diagnosis and treatment plan for thoracic trauma.

4-4.40 Advocate the use of a thorough scene survey to determine the forces involved in thoracic trauma.

4-4.41 Value the implications of failing to properly diagnose thoracic trauma.

4-4.42 Value the implications of failing to initiate timely interventions to patients with thoracic trauma.

Psychomotor Objectives

At the completion of this unit, the EMT-Intermediate student will be able to:

4-4.43 Demonstrate a clinical assessment for a patient with suspected thoracic trauma.

4-4.44 Demonstrate the following techniques of management for thoracic injuries.

   a. Needle decompression
   b. Fracture stabilization
   c. ECT monitoring
   d. Oxygenation and ventilation

UNIT 4-5 TRAUMA PRACTICAL LABORATORY

Cognitive Objectives

None identified for this unit.

Affective Objectives

None identified for this unit.

Psychomotor Objectives

At the completion of this unit, the EMT-Intermediate student will be able to:

4-5.1 Demonstrate the assessment of a patient with signs and symptoms of hypovolemic shock.

4-5.2 Demonstrate the management of a patient with signs and symptoms of hypovolemic shock.

4-5.3 Demonstrate the assessment of a patient with signs and symptoms of compensated shock.

4-5.4 Demonstrate the management of a patient with signs and symptoms of compensated shock.

4-5.5 Demonstrate the assessment of a patient with signs and symptoms of decompensated shock.

4-5.6 Demonstrate the management of a patient with signs and symptoms of decompensated shock.

4-5.7 Demonstrate the assessment of a patient with signs and symptoms of external hemorrhage.

4-5.8 Demonstrate the management of a patient with signs and symptoms of external hemorrhage.

4-5.9 Demonstrate the assessment of a patient with signs and symptoms of internal hemorrhage.

4-5.10 Demonstrate the management of a patient with signs and symptoms of internal hemorrhage.

4-5.11 Demonstrate a clinical assessment for a patient with suspected thoracic trauma.

4-5.12 Demonstrate the following techniques of management for thoracic injuries:

   a. Needle decompression
   b. Fracture stabilization
   c. ECG monitoring
   d. Oxygenation and ventilation

4-5.13 Demonstrate a clinical assessment to determine the proper treatment plan for a patient with a suspected musculoskeletal injury.

4-5.14 Demonstrate the proper use of fixation soft and traction splints for a patient with a suspected fracture.

4-5.15 Demonstrate the assessment and management of a patient with signs and symptoms of soft tissue injury, including:

   a. Contusion
   b. Hematoma
   c. Crushing
   d. Abrasion
   e. Laceration
   f. Avulsion
   g. Amputation
   h. Impaled object
   i. Penetration/puncture
   j. Blast

4-5.16 Demonstrate a clinical assessment to determine the proper management modality for a patient with a suspected traumatic spinal injury.

4-5.17 Demonstrate a clinical assessment to determine the proper management modality for a patient with suspected nontraumatic spinal injury.

4-5.18 Demonstrate immobilization of the urgent and nonurgent patient with assessment findings of spinal injury from the following presentations:

   a. Supine
   b. Prone
   c. Semiprone
   d. Sitting
   e. Standing

4-5.19 Demonstrate preferred methods for stabilization of a helmet from a potentially spine-injured patient.

4-5.20 Demonstrate helmet removal techniques.

4-5.21 Demonstrate alternative methods for stabilization of a helmet from a potentially spine-injured patient.

4-5.22 Demonstrate documentation of assessment before spinal immobilization.

4-5.23 Demonstrate documentation of assessment during spinal immobilization.

4-5.24 Demonstrate documentation of assessment after spinal immobilization.

MODULE 5 MEDICAL

UNIT 5-1 RESPIRATORY EMERGENCIES

Cognitive Objectives

At the completion of this unit, the EMT-Intermediate student will be able to:

5-1.1 Identify and describe the function of the structures located in the upper and lower airway.

5-1.2 Discuss the physiology of ventilation and respiration.

5-1.3 Identify common pathological events that affect the pulmonary system.

5-1.4 Discuss abnormal assessment findings associated with pulmonary diseases and conditions.

5-1.5 Compare various airway and ventilation techniques used in the management of pulmonary diseases.

5-1.6 Review the pharmacological preparations that EMT-Intermediates use for management of respiratory diseases and conditions.

5-1.7 Review the use of equipment used during the physical examination of patients with complaints associated with respiratory diseases and conditions.

5-1.8　Describe the epidemiology, pathophysiology, assessment findings, and management for the following respiratory diseases and conditions:

    a.　Bronchial asthma
    b.　Chronic bronchitis
    c.　Emphysema
    d.　Pneumonia
    e.　Pulmonary edema
    f.　Spontaneous pneumothorax
    g.　Hyperventilation syndrome
    h.　Pulmonary thromboembolism

Affective Objectives

At the completion of this unit, the EMT-Intermediate will be able to:

5-1.9　Recognize and value the assessment and treatment of patients with respiratory diseases.

5-1.10　Indicate appreciate for the critical nature of accurate field impressions of patients with respiratory diseases and conditions.

Psychomotor Objectives

At the completion of this unit, the EMT-Intermediate will be able to:

5-1.11　Demonstrate and record pertinent assessment findings associated with pulmonary diseases and conditions.

5-1.12　Review proper use of airway and ventilation devices.

5-1.13　Conduct a simulated history and patient assessment, record the findings, and report appropriate management of patients with pulmonary diseases and conditions.

UNIT 5-2 CARDIOVASCULAR EMERGENCIES

Cognitive Objectives

At the completion of this unit, the EMT-Intermediate student will be able to:

5-2.1　Describe the incidence, morbidity, and mortality of cardiovascular disease.

5-2.2　Review cardiovascular anatomy and physiology.

5-2.3　Discuss prevention strategies that may reduce morbidity and mortality of cardiovascular disease.

5-2.4　Identify the risk factors most predisposing to coronary artery disease.

5-2.5　Identify and describe the components of assessment as it relates to the patient with cardiovascular compromise.

5-2.6　Describe how ECG wave forms are produced.

5-2.7　Correlate the electrophysiological and hemodynamic events occurring throughout the entire cardiac cycle with the various ECG wave forms, segments, and intervals.

5-2.8　Identify how heart rates may be determined from ECG recordings.

5-2.9　List the limitations to the ECG.

5-2.10　Describe a systematic approach to the analysis and interpretation of cardiac arrhythmias.

5-2.11　Explain how to confirm asystole using more than one lead.

5-2.12　List the clinical indications for defibrillation.

5-2.13　Identify the specific mechanical, pharmacological, and electrical therapeutic interventions for patients with arrhythmias causing compromise.

5-2.14　List the clinical indications for an implanted defibrillation device.

5-2.15　Define angina pectoris and myocardial infarction.

5-2.16　List other clinical conditions that may mimic signs and symptoms of angina pectoris and myocardial infarction.

5-2.17　List the mechanisms by which an MI may be produced by traumatic and nontraumatic events.

5-2.18　List and describe the assessment parameters to be evaluated in a patient with chest pain.

5-2.19　Identify what is meant by the OPQRST of chest pain assessment.

5-2.20 List and describe the initial assessment parameters to be evaluated in a patient with chest pain that may be myocardial in origin.

5-2.21 Identify the anticipated clinical presentation of a patient with chest pain that may be angina pectoris or myocardial infarction.

5-2.22 Describe the pharmacological agents available to the EMT-Intermediate for use in the management of arrhythmias and cardiovascular emergencies.

5-2.23 Develop, execute, and evaluate a treatment plan based on the field impression for the patient with chest pain that may be indicative of angina or myocardial infarction.

5-2.24 Define the terms "congestive heart failure" and "pulmonary edema."

5-2.25 Define the cardiac and non-cardiac causes and terminology associated with pulmonary edema and pulmonary edema.

5-2.26 Describe the early and late signs and symptoms of pulmonary edema.

5-2.27 Explain the clinical significance of paroxysmal nocturnal dyspnea.

5-2.28 List and describe the pharmacological agents available to the EMT-Intermediate for use in the management of a patent with cardiac compromise.

5-2.29 Define the term "hypertensive emergency."

5-2.30 Describe the clinical features of the patient in a hypertensive emergency.

5-2.31 List the interventions prescribed for the patient with a hypertensive emergency.

5-2.32 Define the term "cardiogenic shock."

5-2.33 Identify the clinical criteria for cardiogenic shock.

5-2.34 Define the term "cardiac arrest."

5-2.35 Define the term "resuscitation."

5-2.36 Identify local protocol dictating circumstances and situations where resuscitation efforts would not be initiated.

5-2.37 Identify local protocol dictating circumstances and situations where resuscitation efforts would be discontinued.

5-2.38 Identify the critical actions necessary in caring for the patient in cardiac arrest.

5-2.39 Synthesize patient history, assessment findings to form a field impression for the patient with chest pain and cardiac arrhythmias that may be indicative of a cardiac emergency.

Affective Objectives

At the completion of this unit, the EMT-Intermediate will be able to:

5-2.40 Value the sense of urgency for initial assessment and intervention as it contributes to the treatment plan for the patient experiencing a cardiac emergency.

5-2.41 Defend patient situations where ECG rhythm analysis is indicated.

5-2.42 Value and defend the sense of urgency necessary to protect the window of opportunity for reperfusion in the patient with chest pain and arrhythmias that may be indicative of angina or myocardial infarction.

5-2.43 Value and defend the urgency in rapid determination and rapid intervention of patients in cardiac arrest.

Psychomotor Objectives

5-2.44 Demonstrate a working knowledge of various ECG lead systems.

5-2.45 Set up and apply a transcutaneous pacing system.

5-2.46 Given the model of a patient with signs and symptoms of pulmonary edema, position the patient to afford comfort and relief.

UNIT 5-3 DIABETIC EMERGENCIES

Cognitive Objectives

At the completion of this unit, the EMT-Intermediate student will be able to:

5-3.1   Describe the pathophysiology of diabetes mellitus.

5-3.2   Describe the effects of decreased levels of insulin on the body.

5-3.3   Correlate abnormal findings in assessment with clinical significance in the patient with a diabetic emergency.

5-3.4   Discuss the management of diabetic emergencies.

5-3.5   Describe the mechanism of ketone body formation and its relationship to ketoacidosis.

5-3.6   Describe the effects of decreased levels of insulin on the body.

5-3.7   Discuss the pathophysiology of hypoglycemia.

5-3.8   Recognize the signs and symptoms of the patient with hypoglycemia.

5-3.9   Describe the management of a hypoglycemic patient.

5-3.10 Integrate the pathophysiological principles and the assessment findings to formulate a field impression and implement a treatment plan for the patient with hypoglycemia.

5-3.11 Discuss the pathophysiology of hyperglycemia.

5-3.12 Recognize the signs and symptoms of the patient with hyperglycemia.

5-3.13 Describe the management of the hyperglycemic patient.

5-3.14 Differentiate between diabetic emergencies based on assessment and history.

5-3.15 Correlate abnormal findings in the assessment with clinical significance in the patient with a diabetic emergency.

5-3.16 Develop a patient management plan based on field impression in the patient with a diabetic emergency.

Affective Objectives

None identified for this unit.

Psychomotor Objectives

None identified for this unit.

UNIT 5-4 ALLERGIC REACTIONS

Cognitive Objectives

At the completion of this unit, the EMT-Intermediate student will be able to:

5-4.1   Define allergic reaction.

5-4.2   Define anaphylaxis.

5-4.3   Define allergens.

5-4.4   Describe the common methods of entry of substances into the body.

5-4.5   List common antigens most frequently associated with anaphylaxis.

5-4.6   Describe physical manifestations in anaphylaxis.

5-4.7   Recognize the signs and symptoms related to anaphylaxis.

5-4.8   Differentiate among the various treatment and pharmacological interventions used in the management of anaphylaxis.

5-4.9   Integrate the pathophysiological principles of the patient with anaphylaxis.

5-4.10 Correlate abnormal findings in assessment with the clinical significance in the patient with anaphylaxis.

5-4.11 Develop a treatment plan based on field impression in the patient with allergic reaction and anaphylaxis.

Affective Objectives

None identified for this unit.

Psychomotor Objectives

None identified for this unit.

UNIT 5-5 POISONING/OVERDOSE EMERGENCIES

Cognitive Objectives

At the completion of this unit, the EMT-Intermediate student will be able to:

5-5.1   Identify appropriate personal protective equipment and scene safety awareness concerns in dealing with toxicologic emergencies.

5-5.2   Identify the appropriate situations in which additional non-EMS resources need to be contacted.

5-5.3   Review the routes of entry of toxic substances into the body.

5-5.4   Discuss the role of the Poison Control Center in the United States.

5-5.5   List the toxic substances that are specific to your region.

5-5.6   Identify the need for rapid intervention and transport of the patient with a toxic substance emergency.

5-5.7   Review the management of toxic substances.

5-5.8   Differentiate among the various treatments and pharmacological interventions in the management of the most common poisonings by inhalation, ingestion, absorption, and injection.

5-5.9   Utilize assessment findings to formulate a field impression and implement a treatment plan for patients with the most common poisonings by inhalation, ingestion, absorption, and injection.

5-5.10   Review poisoning by overdose.

5-5.11   Review the signs and symptoms related to the most common poisonings by overdose.

5-5.12   Correlate the abnormal findings in assessment with the clinical significance in patients with the most common poisonings by overdose.

5-5.13   Differentiate among the various treatments and pharmacological interventions in the management of the most common poisonings by overdose.

5-5.14   Utilize assessment findings to formulate a field impression and implement a treatment plan for patients with the most common poisonings by overdose.

Affective Objectives

At the completion of this unit, the EMT-Intermediate student will be able to:

5-5.15   Appreciate the psychological needs for victims of drug abuse or overdose.

Psychomotor Objectives

None identified for this unit.

UNIT 5-6 NEUROLOGICAL EMERGENCIES

Cognitive Objectives

At the completion of this unit, the EMT-Intermediate student will be able to:

5-6.1   Discuss the general pathophysiology of nontraumatic neurologic emergencies.

5-6.2   Discuss the general assessment findings associated with nontraumatic neurologic emergencies.

5-6.3   Identify the need for rapid intervention and transport of the patient with nontraumatic emergencies.

5-6.4   Discuss the epidemiology, assessment findings, and management for stroke and intracranial hemorrhage.

5-6.5   Discuss the epidemiology, assessment findings, and management for transient ischemic attack.

5-6.6   Discuss the epidemiology, assessment findings, and management for epilepsy/seizure.

5-6.7   Discuss the epidemiology, assessment findings, and management for nonspecific coma or altered level of consciousness/syncope/weakness/headache.

5-6.8   Develop a patient management plan based on field impression in the patient with neurological emergencies.

Affective Objectives

At the completion of this unit, the EMT-Intermediate student will be able to:

5-6.9   Characterize the feelings of a patient who regains consciousness among strangers.

5-6.10   Formulate means of conveying empathy to patients whose ability to communicate is limited by their condition.

Psychomotor Objectives

At the completion of this unit, the EMT-Intermediate student will be able to:

5-6.11   Perform an appropriate assessment of a patient with a nontraumatic neurological emergency.

UNIT 5-7 NONTRAUMATIC ABDOMINAL EMERGENCIES

Cognitive Objectives

At the completion of this unit, the EMT-Intermediate student will be able to:

5-7.1   Discuss the pathophysiology of nontraumatic abdominal emergencies.

5-7.2   Discuss the signs and symptoms of nontraumatic acute abdominal pain.

5-7.3   Describe the technique for performing a comprehensive physical examination on a patient with nontraumatic abdominal pain.

5-7.4   Describe the management of the patient with nontraumatic abdominal pain.

Affective Objectives

None identified for this unit.

Psychomotor Objectives

None identified for this unit.

UNIT 5-8 ENVIRONMENTAL EMERGENCIES

Cognitive Objectives

At the completion of this unit, the EMT-Intermediate student will be able to:

5-8.1   Define the term "environmental emergency."

5-8.2   Identify risk factors most predisposing to environmental emergencies.

5-8.3   Identify environmental factors that may cause illness or exacerbate a preexisting illness.

5-8.4   Identify environmental factors that may complicate treatment or transport decisions.

5-8.5   List the principal types of environmental illnesses.

5-8.6   Identify normal, critically high, and critically low body temperatures.

5-8.7   Describe several methods of temperature monitoring.

5-8.8   Describe the body's compensatory process for overheating.

5-8.9   Describe the body's compensatory process for excess heat loss.

5-8.10   List the common forms of heat and cold disorders.

5-8.11   List the common predisposing factors associated with heat and cold disorders.

5-8.12   List the common preventative measures associated with heat and cold disorders.

5-8.13   Define heat illness.

5-8.14   Identify signs and symptoms of heat illness.

5-8.15   List the predisposing factors for heat illness.

5-8.16   List measures to prevent heat illness.

5-8.17   Relate symptomatic findings to the commonly used terms: heat cramps, heat exhaustion, and heat stroke.

5-8.18   Discuss how one may differentiate between fever and heat stroke.

5-8.19   Discuss the role of fluid therapy in the treatment of heat disorders.

5-8.20   Differentiate among the various treatments and interventions in the management of heat disorders.

5-8.21   Integrate the pathophysiological principles and the assessment findings to formulate a field impression and implement a treatment plan for the patient who has dehydration, heat exhaustion, or heat stroke.

5-8.22 Define hypothermia.

5-8.23 List predisposing factors for hypothermia.

5-8.24 List measures to prevent hypothermia.

5-8.25 Identify differences between mild and severe hypothermia.

5-8.26 Describe differences between chronic and acute hypothermia.

5-8.27 List signs and symptoms of hypothermia.

5-8.28 Correlate abnormal findings in assessment with their clinical significance in the patient with hypothermia.

5-8.29 Discuss the impact of severe hypothermia on standard BCLS and ACLS algorithms and transport considerations.

5-8.30 Integrate pathophysiological principles and the assessment findings to formulate a field impression and implement a treatment plan for the patient who has either mild or severe hypothermia.

5-8.31 Define near drowning.

5-8.32 List signs and symptoms of near drowning.

5-8.33 Discuss the complications and protective role of hypothermia in context of near drowning.

5-8.34 Correlate the abnormal findings in assessment with the clinical significance in the patient with near drowning.

5-8.35 Differentiate among the various treatments and interventions in the management of near drowning.

5-8.36 Integrate pathophysiological principles and the assessment findings to formulate a field impression and implement a treatment plan for the near-drowning patient.

5-8.37 Integrate pathophysiological principles of the patient affected by an environmental emergency.

5-8.38 Differentiate between environmental emergencies based on assessment findings.

5-8.39 Correlate abnormal findings in the assessment with the clinical significance in the patient affected by an environmental emergency.

5-8.40 Develop a patient management plan based on the field impression the patient affected by an environmental emergency.

Affective Objectives
None identified for this unit.

Psychomotor Objectives
None identified for this unit.

UNIT 5-9 BEHAVIORAL EMERGENCIES

Cognitive Objectives
At the completion of this unit, the EMT-Intermediate student will be able to:

5-9.1 Distinguish between normal and abnormal behavior.

5-9.2 Discuss the pathophysiology of behavioral emergencies.

5-9.3 Discuss appropriate measures to ensure the safety of the patient, EMT-Intermediate, and others.

5-9.4 Identify techniques for a physical assessment in a patient with behavioral problems.

5-9.5 Describe therapeutic interviewing techniques for gathering information from a patient with a behavioral emergency.

5-9.6 List factors that may indicate a patient is at increased risk for suicide.

5-9.7 Describe circumstances in which relatives, bystanders, and others should be removed from the scene.

5-9.8 Describe medical/legal considerations for managing a patient with a behavioral emergency.

5-9.9 List situations in which the EMT-Intermediate is expected to transport a patient against his or her will.

5-9.10   Describe methods of restraint that may be necessary in managing a patient with a behavioral emergency.

5-9.11   Formulate a field impression based on the assessment findings for patients with behavioral emergencies.

5-9.12   Develop a patient management plan based on the field impression for patients with behavioral emergencies.

Affective Objectives

At the completion of this unit, the EMT-Intermediate student will be able to:

5-9.13   Advocate for empathetic and respectful treatment for individuals experiencing behavioral emergencies.

Psychomotor Objectives

At the completion of this unit, the EMT-Intermediate student will be able to:

5-9.14   Demonstrate safe techniques for managing and restraining a violent patient.

UNIT 5-10 GYNECOLOGICAL EMERGENCIES

Cognitive Objectives

At the completion of this unit, the EMT-Intermediate student will be able to:

5-10.1   Review the anatomic structures and physiology of the female reproductive system.

5-10.2   Describe how to assess a patient with a gynecological complaint.

5-10.3   Explain how to recognize a gynecological emergency.

5-10.4   Describe the general care for any patient experiencing a gynecological emergency.

5-10.5   Describe the pathophysiology, assessment, and management of specific gynecological emergencies, including:

a.   Pelvic inflammatory disease
b.   Ruptured ovarian cyst
c.   Ectopic pregnancy
d.   Vaginal bleeding

5-10.6   Describe the general findings and management of the sexually assaulted patient.

Affective Objectives

At the completion of this unit, the EMT-Intermediate student will be able to:

5-10.7   Value the importance of maintaining a patient's modesty and privacy while still obtaining necessary information.

5-10.8   Defend the need to provide care for a patient of sexual assault while still preventing destruction of crime scene information.

5-10.9   Serve as a role model for other EMS providers when discussing or caring for patients with gynecological emergencies.

Psychomotor Objectives

At the completion of this unit, the EMT-Intermediate student will be able to:

5-10.10 Demonstrate how to assess a patient with a gynecological complaint.

5-10.11 Demonstrate how to provide care for a patient with:

a.   Excessive vaginal bleeding
b.   Abdominal pain
c.   Sexual assault

MODULE 6 SPECIAL CONSIDERATIONS

UNIT 6-1 OBSTETRICAL EMERGENCIES

Cognitive Objectives

At the completion of this unit, the EMT-Intermediate student will be able to:

6-1.1   Review the anatomic structures and physiology of the reproductive system.

6-1.2   Identify the normal events of pregnancy.

6-1.3   Describe how to assess an obstetrical patient.

6-1.4   Identify the stages of labor and the EMT-Intermediate's role in each stage.

6-1.5 Differentiate between normal and abnormal delivery.

6-1.6 Identify and describe complications associated with pregnancy and delivery.

6-1.7 Identify predelivery emergencies.

6-1.8 State indications of an imminent delivery.

6-1.9 Differentiate the management of a patient with predelivery emergencies from a normal delivery.

6-1.10 State the steps in the predelivery preparation of the mother.

6-1.11 State the steps to assist in the delivery of a newborn.

6-1.12 Describe how to care for the newborn.

6-1.13 Describe how and when to cut the umbilical cord.

6-1.14 Discuss the steps in the delivery of the placenta.

6-1.15 Describe the management of the mother postdelivery.

6-1.16 Describe the procedures for handling abnormal deliveries.

6-1.17 Describe the procedures of handling complications of pregnancy.

6-1.18 Describe the procedures for handling maternal complications of labor.

6-1.19 Describe special considerations when meconium is present in amniotic fluid or during delivery.

6-1.20 Describe special considerations of a premature baby.

Affective Objectives

At the completion of this unit, the EMT-Intermediate student will be able to:

6-1.21 Advocate the need for treating two patients (mother and baby).

6-1.22 Value the importance of maintaining a patient's modesty and privacy during assessment and management.

6-1.23 Serve as a role model for other EMS providers when discussing or performing the steps of childbirth.

6-1.24 Value the importance of body substance isolation.

Psychomotor Objectives

At the completion of this unit, the EMT-Intermediate student will be able to:

6-1.25 Demonstrate how to assess an obstetric patient.

6-1.26 Demonstrate how to provide care for a patient with:

    a. Excessive vaginal bleeding

    b. Abdominal pain

6-1.27 Demonstrate how to prepare the obstetric patient for delivery.

6-1.28 Demonstrate how to assist in normal cephalic delivery of the fetus.

6-1.29 Demonstrate how to deliver the placenta.

6-1.30 Demonstrate how to provide postdelivery care of the mother.

6-1.31 Demonstrate how to assist with abnormal deliveries.

6-1.32 Demonstrate how to care for the mother with delivery complications.

UNIT 6-2 NEONATAL RESUSCITATION

Cognitive Objectives

At the completion of this unit, the EMT-Intermediate student will be able to:

6-2.1 Define the term newborn.

6-2.2 Define the term neonate.

6-2.3 Identify important antepartum factors that can affect childbirth.

6-2.4 Identify important intrapartum factors that can term the newborn high risk.

6-2.5 Identify the primary signs utilized for evaluating a newborn during resuscitation.

6-2.6 Formulate an appropriate treatment plan for providing initial care to a newborn.

6-2.7 Identify the appropriate use of the APGAR score in caring for a newborn.

6-2.8 Calculate the APGAR score given various newborn situations.

6-2.9 Determine when ventilatory assistance is appropriate for a newborn.

6-2.10 Prepare appropriate ventilation equipment, adjuncts, and technique for a newborn.

6-2.11 Determine when chest compressions are appropriate for a newborn.

6-2.12 Discuss appropriate chest compression techniques for a newborn.

6-2.13 Reassess a patient following chest compressions and ventilations.

6-2.14 Determine when blow-by oxygen delivery is appropriate for a newborn.

6-2.15 Discuss appropriate blow-by oxygen delivery devices and technique for the newborn.

6-2.16 Assess patient improvement due to assisted ventilations.

6-2.17 Discuss the initial steps in resuscitation of a newborn.

6-2.18 Assess patient improvement due to blow-by oxygen delivery.

6-2.19 Discuss appropriate transport guidelines for a newborn.

6-2.20 Describe the epidemiology, including the incidence, morbidity/mortality, and risk factors for meconium aspiration in the neonate.

6-2.21 Discuss the pathophysiology of meconium aspiration in the neonate.

6-2.22 Discuss the assessment findings associated with meconium aspiration in the neonate.

6-2.23 Discuss the management/treatment plan for meconium aspiration in the neonate.

6-2.24 Describe the epidemiology, including the incidence, morbidity/mortality, and risk factors for bradycardia in the neonate.

6-2.25 Discuss the pathophysiology of bradycardia in the neonate.

6-2.26 Discuss the assessment findings associated with bradycardia in the neonate.

6-2.27 Discuss the management/treatment plan for bradycardia in the neonate.

6-2.28 Describe the epidemiology, including the incidence, morbidity/mortality, and risk factors for respiratory distress/cyanosis in the neonate.

6-2.29 Discuss the pathophysiology of respiratory distress/cyanosis in the neonate.

6-2.30 Discuss the assessment findings associated with respiratory distress/cyanosis in the neonate.

6-2.31 Discuss the management/treatment plan for respiratory distress/cyanosis in the neonate.

6-2.32 Describe the epidemiology, including the incidence, morbidity/mortality, and risk factors for hypothermia in the neonate.

6-2.33 Discuss the pathophysiology of hypothermia in the neonate.

6-2.34 Discuss the assessment findings associated with hypothermia in the neonate.

6-2.35 Discuss the management/treatment plan for hypothermia in the neonate.

6-2.36 Describe the epidemiology, including the incidence, morbidity/mortality, and risk factors for cardiac arrest in the neonate.

6-2.37 Discuss the pathophysiology of cardiac arrest in the neonate.

6-2.38 Discuss the assessment findings associated with cardiac arrest in the neonate.

6-2.39 Discuss the management/treatment plan for cardiac arrest in the neonate.

Affective Objectives

At the completion of this unit, the EMT-Intermediate student will be able to:

6-2.40 Demonstrate and advocate appropriate interaction with a newborn/neonate that conveys respect for their position in life.

6-2.41 Recognize the emotional impact of newborn/neonate injuries/illnesses on parents/guardians.

6-2.42　Recognize and appreciate the physical and emotional difficulties associated with separation of the parent/guardian and a newborn/neonate.

6-2.43　Listen to the concerns expressed by parents/guardians.

6-2.44　Attend to the need for reassurance, empathy, and compassion for the parent/guardian.

Psychomotor Objectives

At the completion of this unit, the EMT-Intermediate student will be able to:

6-2.45　Demonstrate preparation of a newborn resuscitation area.

6-2.46　Demonstrate appropriate assessment technique for examining a newborn.

6-2.47　Demonstrate appropriate assisted ventilations for a newborn.

6-2.48　Demonstrate appropriate insertion of an orogastric tube.

6-2.49　Demonstrate appropriate chest compression and ventilation technique for a newborn.

6-2.50　Demonstrate the initial steps in resuscitation of a newborn.

6-2.51　Demonstrate blow-by oxygen delivery for a newborn.

UNIT 6-3 PEDIATRICS

Cognitive Objectives

At the completion of this unit, the EMT-Intermediate student will be able to:

6-3.1　Identify methods/mechanisms that prevent injuries to infants and children.

6-3.2　Identify the growth and developmental characteristics of infants and children.

6-3.3　Identify anatomy and physiology characteristics of infants and children.

6-3.4a　Describe techniques for successful interaction with families of acutely ill or injured infants and children.

6-3.4b　Identify the common responses of families to acute illness and injury of an infant or child.

6-3.5　Describe techniques for successful interaction with families of acutely ill or injured infants and children.

6-3.6　Outline differences in adult and childhood anatomy and physiology.

6-3.7　Discuss pediatric patient assessment.

6-3.8　Identify "normal" age-group–related vital signs.

6-3.9　Discuss the appropriate equipment utilized to obtain pediatric vital signs.

6-3.10　Determine appropriate airway adjuncts for infants and children.

6-3.11　Discuss complications of improper utilization of airway adjuncts with infants and children.

6-3.12　Discuss appropriate ventilation devices for infants and children.

6-3.13　Discuss complications of improper utilization of ventilation devices with infants and children.

6-3.14　Discuss appropriate endotracheal intubation equipment for infants and children.

6-3.15　Identify complications of improper endotracheal intubation procedures in infants and children.

6-3.16　Define respiratory distress.

6-3.17　Define respiratory failure.

6-3.18　Define respiratory arrest.

6-3.19　Describe the epidemiology, including the incidence morbidity/mortality, risk factors, and prevention strategies for respiratory distress/failure in infants and children.

6-3.20　Discuss the pathophysiology of respiratory distress/failure in infants and children.

6-3.21　Discuss the assessment findings associated with respiratory distress/failure in infants and children.

6-3.22　Discuss the management/treatment plan for respiratory distress/failure in infants and children.

6-3.23　List the indications for gastric decompression for infants and children.

6-3.24 Differentiate between upper- and lower-airway obstruction.

6-3.25 Describe the epidemiology, including the incidence, morbidity/mortality, risk factors, and prevention strategies for croup in infants and children.

6-3.26 Discuss the pathophysiology of croup in infants and children.

6-3.27 Discuss the assessment findings associated with croup in infants and children.

6-3.28 Discuss the management/treatment plan for croup in infants and children.

6-3.29 Describe the epidemiology, including the incidence, morbidity/mortality, risk factors, and prevention strategies for foreign body aspiration in infants and children.

6-3.30 Discuss the pathophysiology of foreign body aspiration in infants and children.

6-3.31 Discuss the assessment findings associated with foreign body aspiration in infants and children.

6-3.32 Discuss the management/treatment plan for foreign body aspiration in infants and children.

6-3.33 Describe the epidemiology, including the incidence, morbidity/mortality, risk factors, and prevention strategies for epiglottitis in infants and children.

6-3.34 Discuss the pathophysiology of epiglottitis in infants and children.

6-3.35 Discuss the assessment findings associated with epiglottitis in infants and children.

6-3.36 Discuss the management/treatment plan for epiglottitis in infants and children.

6-3.37 Describe the epidemiology, including the incidence, morbidity/mortality, risk factors, and prevention strategies for asthma/bronchiolitis in infants and children.

6-3.38 Discuss the pathophysiology of asthma/bronchiolitis in infants and children.

6-3.39 Discuss the assessment findings associated with asthma/bronchiolitis in infants and children.

6-3.40 Discuss the management/treatment plan for asthma/bronchiolitis in infants and children.

6-3.41 Describe the epidemiology, including the incidence, morbidity/mortality, risk factors, and prevention strategies for pneumonia in infants and children.

6-3.42 Discuss the pathophysiology of pneumonia in infants and children.

6-3.43 Discuss the assessment findings associated with pneumonia in infants and children.

6-3.44 Discuss the management/treatment plan for pneumonia in infants and children.

6-3.45 Describe the epidemiology, including the incidence, morbidity/mortality, risk factors, and prevention strategies for foreign body lower-airway obstruction in infants and children.

6-3.46 Discuss the pathophysiology of foreign body lower-airway obstruction in infants and children.

6-3.47 Discuss the assessment findings associated with foreign body lower-airway obstruction in infants and children.

6-3.48 Discuss the management/treatment plan for foreign body lower-airway obstruction in infants and children.

6-3.49 Discuss the common causes of shock in infants and children.

6-3.50 Evaluate the severity of shock in infants and children.

6-3.51 Describe the epidemiology, including the incidence, morbidity/mortality, risks factors, and prevention strategies for shock in infants and children.

6-3.52 Discuss the pathophysiology of shock in infants and children.

6-3.53 Discuss the assessment findings associated with shock in infants and children.

6-3.54   Discuss the management/treatment plan for shock in infants and children.

6-3.55   Identify the major classifications of pediatric cardiac rhythms.

6-3.56   Describe the epidemiology, including the incidence, morbidity/mortality, risks factors, and prevention strategies for cardiac dysrhythmias in infants and children.

6-3.57   Discuss the pathophysiology of cardiac dysrhythmias in infants and children.

6-3.58   Discuss the assessment findings associated with cardiac dysrhythmias in infants and children.

6-3.59   Discuss the management/treatment plan for cardiac dysrhythmias in infants and children.

6-3.60   Describe the epidemiology, including the incidence, morbidity/mortality, risk factors, and prevention strategies for tachydysrhythmias in infants and children.

6-3.61   Discuss the pathophysiology of tachydysrhythmias in infants and children.

6-3.62   Discuss the assessment findings associated with tachydysrhythmias in infants and children.

6-3.63   Discuss the management/treatment plan for tachydysrhythmias in infants and children.

6-3.64   Describe the epidemiology, including the incidence, morbidity/mortality, risk factors, and prevention strategies for bradydysrhythmias in infants and children.

6-3.65   Discuss the pathophysiology of bradydysrhythmias in infants and children.

6-3.66   Discuss the assessment findings associated with bradydysrhythmias in infants and children.

6-3.67   Discuss the management/treatment plan for bradydysrhythmias in infants and children.

6-3.68   Discuss the primary etiologies of cardiopulmonary arrest in infants and children.

6-3.69   Discuss basic cardiac life support (CPR) guidelines for infants and children.

6-3.70   Identify appropriate parameters for performing infant and child CPR.

6-3.71   Integrate advanced life support skills with basic cardiac life support for infants and children.

6-3.72   Describe the epidemiology, including the incidence, morbidity/mortality, risk factors, and prevention strategies for seizures in infants and children.

6-3.73   Discuss the pathophysiology of seizures in infants and children.

6-3.74   Discuss the assessment findings associated with seizures in infants and children.

6-3.75   Discuss the management/treatment plan for seizures in infants and children.

6-3.76   Describe the epidemiology, including the incidence, morbidity/mortality, risk factors, and prevention strategies for hypoglycemia in infants and children.

6-3.77   Discuss the pathophysiology of hypoglycemia in infants and children.

6-3.78   Discuss the assessment findings associated with hypoglycemia in infants and children.

6-3.79   Discuss the management/treatment plan for hypoglycemia in infants and children.

6-3.80   Describe the epidemiology, including the incidence, morbidity/mortality, risk factors, and prevention strategies for hyperglycemia in infants and children.

6-3.81   Discuss the pathophysiology of hyperglycemia in infants and children.

6-3.82   Discuss the assessment findings associated with hyperglycemia in infants and children.

6-3.83 Discuss the management/treatment plan for hyperglycemia in infants and children.

6-3.84 Discuss age-appropriate vascular access sites for infants and children.

6-3.85 Discuss the appropriate equipment for vascular access in infants and children.

6-3.86 Identify complications of vascular access for infants and children.

6-3.87 Identify common lethal mechanisms of injury in infants and children.

6-3.88 Discuss anatomical features of children that predispose or protect them from certain injuries.

6-3.89 Describe aspects of infant and children airway management that are affected by potential cervical spine injury.

6-3.90 Identify infant and child trauma patients who require spinal immobilization.

6-3.91 Discuss fluid management and shock treatment for infant and child trauma patients.

6-3.92 Discuss the pathophysiology of trauma in infants and children.

6-3.93 Discuss the assessment findings associated with trauma in infants and children.

6-3.94 Discuss the management/treatment plan for trauma in infants and children.

6-3.95 Discuss the assessment findings and management considerations for pediatric trauma patients with the following specific injuries: head/neck injuries, chest injuries, abdominal injuries, extremities injuries, and burns.

6-3.96 Define child abuse.

6-3.97 Define child neglect.

6-3.98 Describe the epidemiology, including the incidence, morbidity/mortality, risk factors, and prevention strategies for abuse and neglect in infants and children.

6-3.99 Discuss the assessment findings associated with abuse and neglect in infants and children.

6-3.100 Discuss the management/treatment plan for abuse and neglect in infants and children.

6-3.101 Define sudden infant death syndrome (SIDS).

6-3.102 Discuss the parent/caregiver responses to the death of an infant or child.

6-3.103 Describe the epidemiology, including the incidence, morbidity/mortality, risk factors, and prevention strategies for SIDS infants.

6-3.104 Discuss the pathophysiology of SIDS in infants.

6-3.105 Discuss the assessment findings associated with SIDS infants.

6-3.106 Discuss the management/treatment plan for SIDS in infants.

Affective Objectives

At the completion of this unit, the EMT-Intermediate student will be able to:

6-3.107 Demonstrate and advocate appropriate interactions with the infant/child that conveys an understanding of their developmental stage.

6-3.108 Recognize the emotional dependence of the infant/child to their parent/guardian.

6-3.109 Recognize the emotional impact of the infant/child injuries and illnesses on the parent/guardian.

6-3.110 Recognize and appreciate the physical and emotional difficulties associated with separation of the parent/guardian of a special needs child.

6-3.111 Demonstrate the ability to provide reassurance, empathy, and compassion for the parent/guardian.

Psychomotor Objectives

At the completion of this unit, the EMT-Intermediate student will be able to:

6-3.112 Demonstrate the appropriate approach for treating infants and children.

6-3.113 Demonstrate appropriate intervention techniques with families of acutely ill or injured infants and children.

6-3.114 Demonstrate an appropriate assessment for different developmental age-groups.

6-3.115 Demonstrate appropriate technique for measuring pediatric vital signs.

6-3.116 Demonstrate the use of a length-based resuscitation device for determining equipment sizes, drug doses, and other pertinent information for a pediatric patient.

6-3.117 Demonstrate the techniques/procedures for treating infants and children with respiratory distress.

6-3.118 Demonstrate proper technique for administering blow-by oxygen to infants and children.

6-3.119 Demonstrate the proper utilization of a pediatric nonrebreather oxygen mask.

6-3.120 Demonstrate appropriate use of airway adjuncts with infants and children.

6-3.121 Demonstrate appropriate use of ventilation devices for infants and children.

6-3.122 Demonstrate endotracheal intubation procedures in infants and children.

6-3.123 Demonstrate appropriate treatment/management of intubation complications for infants and children.

6-3.124 Demonstrate proper placement of a gastric tube in infants and children.

6-3.125 Demonstrate appropriate technique for insertion of peripheral intravenous catheters for infants and children.

6-3.126 Demonstrate appropriate technique for administration of intramuscular, subcutaneous, rectal, endotracheal, and oral medication for infants and children.

6-3.127 Demonstrate appropriate technique for insertion of an intraosseous line for infants and children.

6-3.128 Demonstrate age-appropriate interventions for infants and children with an obstructed airway.

6-3.129 Demonstrate appropriate airway control maneuvers for infant and child trauma patients.

6-3.130 Demonstrate appropriate treatment of infants and children requiring advanced airway and breathing control.

6-3.131 Demonstrate appropriate immobilization techniques for infant and child trauma patients.

6-3.132 Demonstrate treatment of infants and children with head injuries.

6-3.133 Demonstrate appropriate treatment of infants and children with chest injuries.

6-3.134 Demonstrate appropriate treatment of infants and children with abdominal injuries.

6-3.135 Demonstrate appropriate treatment of infants and children with extremity injuries.

6-3.136 Demonstrate appropriate treatment of infants and children with burns.

6-3.137 Demonstrate appropriate parent/caregiver interviewing techniques for infant and child death situations.

6-3.138 Demonstrate proper infant CPR.

6-3.139 Demonstrate proper child CPR.

6-3.140 Demonstrate proper techniques for performing infant and child defibrillation.

UNIT 6-4 GERIATRICS

Cognitive Objectives

At the completion of this unit, the EMT-Intermediate student will be able to:

6-4.1 Describe dependent and independent living environments.

6-4.2 Identify local resources available to assist the elderly and discuss strategies to refer at-risk patients to appropriate community services.

6-4.3 Discuss expected physiological changes associated with aging.

6-4.4 Describe common psychological reactions associated with aging.

6-4.5 Discuss problems with mobility in the elderly.

6-4.6 Discuss problems with continence and elimination.

6-4.7 Describe communication strategies used to provide psychological support.

6-4.8 Discuss factors that may complicate the assessment of the elderly patient.

6-4.9 Discuss common complaints, injuries, and illnesses of elderly patients.

6-4.10 Discuss pathophysiology changes associated with the elderly in regard to drug distribution, metabolism, and elimination.

6-4.11 Discuss the impact of polypharmacy, dosing errors, medication noncompliance, and drug sensitivity on patient assessment and management.

6-4.12 Discuss various body system changes associated with age.

6-4.13 Discuss the assessment and management of the elderly patient with complaints related to the following body systems:

- Respiratory
- Cardiovascular
- Nervous
- Endocrine
- Gastrointestinal

6-4.14 Describe the assessment of nervous system diseases in the elderly, including cerebral vascular disease, delirium, dementia, Alzheimer's disease, and Parkinson's disease.

6-4.15 Discuss the assessment of an elderly patient with gastrointestinal problems, including GI hemorrhage and bowel obstruction.

6-4.16 Discuss the normal and abnormal changes with age related to toxicology.

6-4.17 Discuss the assessment of the elderly patient with complaints related to toxicology.

6-4.18 Describe the assessment and management of the elderly patient with toxicological problems.

6-4.19 Discuss the assessment and management of the patient with environmental considerations.

6-4.20 Discuss the normal and abnormal changes of the musculoskeletal system with age.

6-4.21 Discuss the assessment and management of the elderly patient with complaints associated with trauma.

Affective Objectives

At the completion of this unit, the EMT-Intermediate student will be able to:

6-4.22 Demonstrate and advocate appropriate interactions with the elderly that convey respect for their position.

6-4.23 Recognize and appreciate the many impediments to physical and emotional well-being in the elderly.

Psychomotor Objectives

At the completion of this unit, the EMT-Intermediate student will be able to:

6-4.24 Demonstrate the ability to assess a geriatric patient.

6-4.25 Demonstrate the ability to apply assessment findings to the management plan for a geriatric patient.

MODULE 7 ASSESSMENT-BASED MANAGEMENT

UNIT 7-1 FOUNDATIONS OF THE EMT-INTERMEDIATE

Cognitive Objectives

At the completion of this unit, the EMT-Intermediate student will be able to:

7-1.1 Explain how effective assessment is critical to clinical decision making.

7-1.2   Explain how the EMT-Intermediate's attitude affects assessment and decision making

7-1.3   Explain how uncooperative patients affect assessment and decision making.

7-1.4   Explain strategies to prevent labeling and tunnel vision.

7-1.5   Develop strategies to decrease environmental distractions.

7-1.6   Describe how manpower considerations and staffing configurations affect assessment and decision making.

7-1.7   Synthesize concepts of scene management and choreography to simulated emergency calls.

7-1.8   Explain the roles of the team leader and the patient care person.

7-1.9   List and explain the rationale for carrying the essential patient care items.

7-1.10   When given a simulated call, list the appropriate equipment to be taken to the patient.

7-1.11   Explain the general approach to the emergency patient.

7-1.12   Describe how to effectively communicate patient information face to face, over the telephone, by radio, and in writing.

7-1.13   Explain the general approach, patient assessment, and management priorities for patients who complain of chest pain.

7-1.14   Explain the general approach, patient assessment, and management priorities for medical and traumatic cardiac arrest patients.

7-1.15   Explain the general approach, patient assessment, and management priorities for patients who complain of acute abdominal pain.

7-1.16   Explain the general approach, patient assessment, and management priorities

for patients who complain of GI bleeding.

7-1.17   Explain the general approach, patient assessment, and management priorities for altered mental status patients.

7-1.18   Explain the general approach, patient assessment, and management priorities for patients who complain of dyspnea.

7-1.19   Explain the general approach, patient assessment, and management priorities for trauma or multitrauma patients.

7-1.20   Explain the general approach, patient assessment, and management priorities for a patient who is having an allergic reaction.

7-1.21   Explain the general approach, patient assessment, and management priorities for pediatric patients.

Affective Objectives

At the completion of this unit, the EMT-Intermediate student will be able to:

7-1.22   Appreciate the use of scenarios to develop high-level clinical decision-making skills.

7-1.23   Advocate and practice the process of complete patient assessment on all patients.

7-1.24   Value the importance of presenting the patient accurately and clearly.

Psychomotor Objectives

At the completion of this unit, the EMT-Intermediate student will be able to:

7-1.25   While serving as team leader, choreograph the EMS response team, perform a patient assessment, provide local/regionally appropriate treatment, and present cases verbally and in writing given a moulaged and programmed simulated patient.

7-1.26   While serving as team leader, assess a programmed patient or mannequin; make decisions relative to interventions and transportation; provide the interventions, patient packaging, and transportation; work as a team; and practice various roles for the following common emergencies:

a. Chest pain
b. Cardiac arrest
   - Traumatic arrest
   - Medical arrest
c. Acute abdominal pain
d. GI bleeding
   - Lower GI bleeding
   - Upper GI bleeding
e. Altered mental status
f. Dyspnea
g. Syncope
h. Trauma
   - Isolated extremity fracture (tibia/fibula or radius/ulna)
   - Femur fracture
   - Spine injury (no neurologic deficit, with neurologic deficit)
   - Multiple trauma—blunt
   - Penetrating trauma
   - Impaled object
   - Elderly fall
   - Athletic injury
   - Head injury (concussion, subdural/epidural)
i. Allergic reactions/bites, envenomation
   - Local allergic reaction
   - Systemic allergic reaction
j. Pediatric
   - Respiratory distress
   - Fever
   - Seizures

Index